Personal Information

This handbook becomes a personal notebook and record of positioning and technique notes. Therefore it is a very valuable and personal document. **Please return to:**

Jim Linderman
____
Name

AF713619

____
Home Address

_______________________ _______________________
Day phone Evening phone

____
Institution

Ordering Information:

Additional copies of this handbook are available from your book distributor, or you may order directly from:

Bontrager Publishing Inc.

6851 West Emile Zola Avenue

Peoria, Arizona 85381

1-800-889-XRAY (9729)

In Arizona, call 602-878-5207

FAX 1-602-486-4584

About the Author

Kenneth L. Bontrager, M.A., R.T. (R) received his training in radiologic technology at St. Luke's Hospital in Denver, Colorado. He received a B.A. degree from the University of Colorado, an M.A. in Education and Instructional Media from the University of Northern Colorado, and an M.A. degree in education from Denver Seminary.

Mr. Bontrager has served as a staff and emergency call technologist, as a chief technologist and technical director of a hospital-based radiologic technology program, and as director and instructor of a college-based associate degree program.

He began his writing and publishing career in 1972 when he founded Multi-Media Publishing, Inc. , Denver, CO. which produced and published programmed self-instructional media and educational textbooks in radiologic technology and other allied health fields. Bontrager's most successful and most widely used educational media in radiologic technology are his textbook and workbooks shown below, and an AV series on the same subject. These works are published and distributed by Mosby-Year Book, Inc. to whom he sold Multi-Media Publishing in 1985.

Mr. Bontrager now resides in Peoria, Arizona where he once again continues writing and producing instructional media for radiologic technology.

Additional books by author: Available from Mosby-Year Book, Inc., St. Louis, MO.

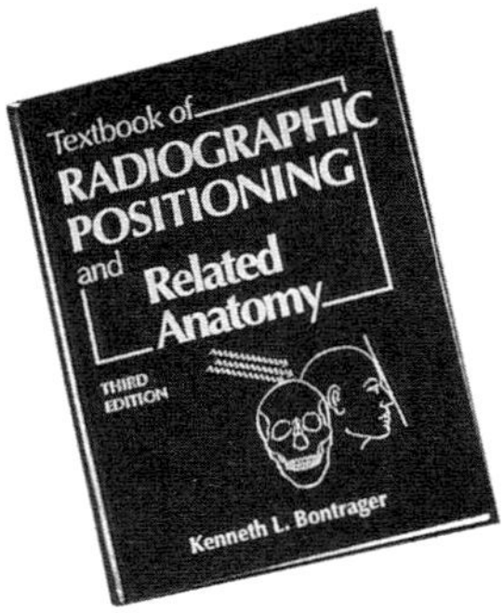

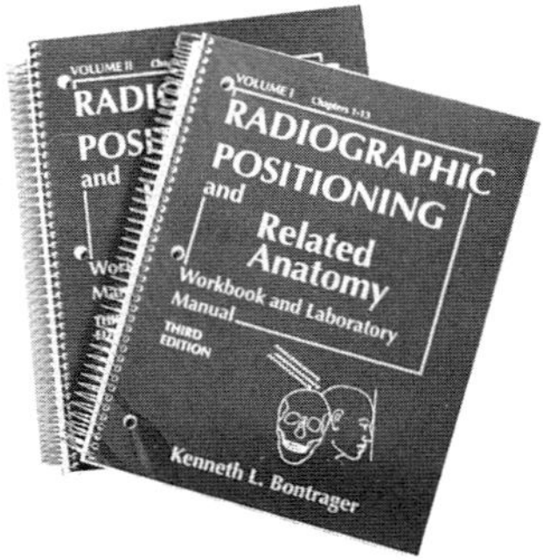

Bontrager's

Pocket Handbook

Radiographic Positioning
and Techniques

Second Edition

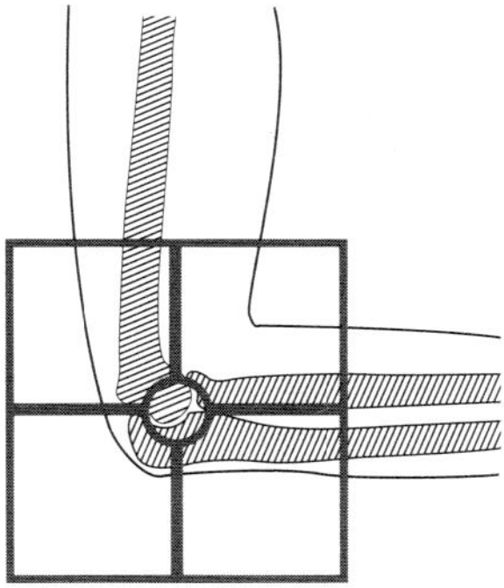

Kenneth L. Bontrager
M.A., R.T. (R)

Second Edition

210 projections demonstrated
305 illustrations
13 charts

BPI
BONTRAGER PUBLISHING INC.

6851 West Emile Zola Avenue
Peoria, AZ 85381

1-800-889-XRAY (9729)

Published and Distributed by:

BONTRAGER PUBLISHING INC.

Publisher:	Kenneth L. Bontrager
Designer:	Neil Bontrager
Compositors:	Mary Lou Bontrager Troy Bontrager Kim Wagler Bontrager
Illustrators:	Sally Schmitt and Deborah Raven
Cover Design:	Aart-Werk Graphic Design Inc.
Photography:	Kenneth L. Bontrager
Computer Graphics:	Neil Bontrager, James and Diana Sanderson
Facilities for Photography:	St. Joseph's Hospital and Medical Center, Phoenix, AZ Phoenix Baptist Hospital and Medical Center, Phoenix, AZ

Second Edition

Printed in the United States of America
First edition copyrighted in 1994

Bontrager Publishing Inc.
6851 West Emile Zola Avenue, Peoria, Arizona 85381

ISBN 0-9641723-1-3
Library of Congress Catalog Card Number 94-94590

95 96 97 98 MP/RG 9 8 7 6 5 4 3 2

Preface

This pocket handbook was developed in response to requests by students and technologists for a thorough and practical pocket guide covering the applied aspect of both positioning and techniques (exposure factors). They asked for a durable and long-lasting pocket-sized handbook that included a review of all the common procedures but would still be small enough to carry with them in clinical situations. They wanted sufficient space for writing in personal notes and techniques that they found worked for them with specific equipment, or in certain rooms or departments.

Some radiographic procedures are also done so infrequently that the students and/or technologists need to refer to notes and brief positioning descriptions and photographs to refresh their memories of CR locations, degrees of obliquity or specific CR angles. A quick review of this information prior to beginning the procedure can provide the assurance that the exam is being done correctly.

Another useful feature of this handbook is the ability to check or mark those projections as listed on the contents page at the beginning of each chapter that are routine for the department in which they are working. This is especially helpful for students or newly hired technologists that are not yet fully familiar with departmental routines or protocol.

Becoming familiar with new equipment in different rooms is easier if personal notes including proven techniques for these rooms can be written in this handbook and can be quickly referred to when needed.

Second Edition: Thirty additional projections have been added as well as new chapters 12 and 13 which include current information on principles and applied aspects of computed radiography.

Patient dosages are now included with each projection for the technique factors provided. This will remind the radiographer of potential radiation hazzards and encourages the use of optimum protection practices to keep radiation exposure to patients as low as possible.

Acknowledgments

As with any project of this type, there are many persons who contributed in significant ways, beginning with my wife, Mary Lou who, as with all my writing projects, is my best typist, spell proofer and overall contributor and supporter. I am also thankful to our son Troy for taking time between his semesters of graduate school and many Saturdays to use his expert computer and typing skills in entering much of this information. I also thank our son and partner in this project Neil, for his graphic layout and design skills which were severely tested in his attempts to contain on each page in a legible manner all of the information I felt needed to be included. Thanks, Neil, for your patience and persistence.

I am also very grateful to the administration and staff at St. Joseph's Hospital and Medical Center and Phoenix Baptist Hospital and Medical Center, Phoenix, Arizona for the use of their facilities, and to Karen Brown, R.T., Dell Hershberger, R.T. and Jim Sanderson, B.S., R.T. for their expert assistance during the photography sessions with the models and for their help in providing suggested exposure factors for each projection.

I also thank the models David Babington, Amy Trevett , Elaine Modena and my little friends, Tanya Fry and Joey Swartzendruber for agreeing to model for the positioning pages.

I am grateful and indebted to the following persons who reviewed and made valuable suggestions for the format and contents of this handbook: Eugene Frank, M.A., R.T. (R) FASRT, David Hall, M.A., R.T. (R), Kathy Martensen, B.S., R.T. (R), and Fred Price, M.S., R.T. (R) FASRT. Also thanks to Jim Sanderson, B.S., R.T. for his contributions to the CR chapter and to Richard Geise, Ph.D. for patient dose calculations.

Finally I am most indebted to my former students, fellow technologists and those many educator colleagues throughout the U.S. and Canada who challenged and inspired me early in my career, and throughout the years have advised, supported and encouraged me. I thank all of you and hope this pocket handbook becomes a valuable aid in improving and maintaining that high level of radiological services for which we all strive.

KLB

Contents

Contents

Explanations for Use

This handbook is intended as a quick reference and review and assumes that each user has successfully completed courses in positioning and in principles of exposure and techniques including radiation protection practices.

Radiation protection: Certain radiation protection practices and shielding descriptions are included with each projection and **it is the responsibility of the user to ensure that maximum shielding is used wherever possible.**

Patient doses: Patient doses are provided for each projection according to the technique factors listed for the "model" patient. (See Appendix E for more details.)

Estimated technique factors: Each projection includes suggested technique factors for the model "patient" which **should be used only as a starting reference for determining specific techniques** for the screen-film speed being used and the equipment as calibrated in each department. The techniques provided are for 3∅ generators with Kodak lanex™ regular screens (400 speed) or lanex extremity (100 speed), both with TMG film. Other brands of intensifying screens and film combinations may be considerably slower or faster even though rated at the same speed. Each user must determine this difference and adjust all techniques accordingly. Proven techniques can then be written in (in pencil) for small, medium and large patients.

AEC cells: Suggested specific ionization chamber cells locations are shown in black in the small upper left box drawing on projections where AEC can be used successfully.

Chapter title pages: The list of projections on each chapter title page is provided for ease in locating specific projections and also as a reference for marking the basic department routines for each examination. A small check ☑ can be placed in the box by each projection that is part of the preferred departmental routine. (Suggest these boxes be marked in pencil.)

Blank pages are provided to write in descriptions and techniques for any specialized projections and procedures not included.

Positioning Pages

Each positioning page has a format similar to this sample page.

- Suggested location of patient ID info.. For table exams this represents the top of film, which is to your left as you face patient.
- Recommended AEC cell (darkened R and L cells indicated on this PA chest example).
- Collimation field size with CR location in center.
- Cassette size recommended for average adult, placed lengthwise (L.W.) or crosswise (C.W.) in reference to the patient.
- Grid or TT (table top) screen.
- Patient position description.
- CR location and CR angle.
- Calculated patient doses based on suggested techniques and estimated field sizes.
- Suggested SID range.
- Suggested kVp range. (Pencil in kVp range for your department.)
- **Estimated** technique factors for the model "patient" on this page using Kodak lanex regular (400) and extremity screens (100) and TMG film.
- To be filled in (in pencil) as determined best for specific rooms or equipment for small (S), medium (M) or large (L) patients.
- InSight™: This additional space is provided for techniques for special screen-films such as Kodak's Insight™ thoracic imaging system which requires a technique adjustment.
- Page number in textbook.

PA Chest

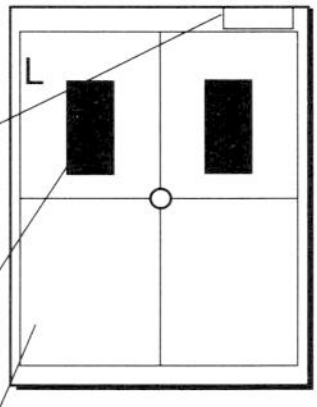

- 14 x 17" L.W. or C.W. (35 x 43 cm)
- Grid

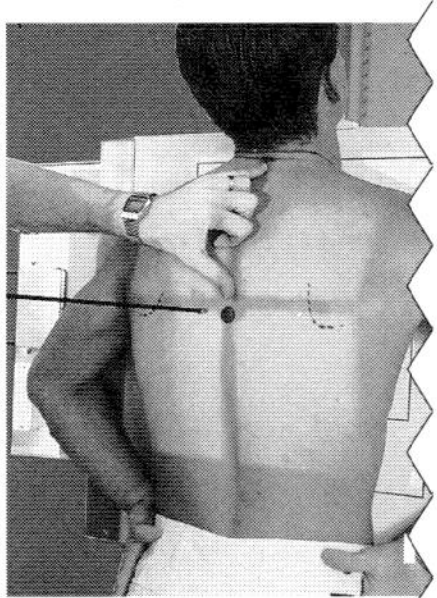

PA chest (≈8" below
(average female 7")

Position

- Erect, chin raised, hands on hips with palms out, shoulders forward.
- Center CR to T7 region (film should automatically be centered to CR).
- Center thorax bilaterally to film borders with equal margins on both sides, ensure there is **no rotation** of thorax.

Central Ray: CR ⊥ to T7 or 7–8" or 18–20 cm below vertebra prominens (is also near level of inferior angle of scapula).

SID: 72–120" (183–305 cm)

Collimation: Upper border to vertebra prominens; sides to lateral skin borders.

Respiration: Expose at end of 2nd deep inspiration.

Technique: kVp (110–125) ____ mrad | S 10 | ML 3

	cm	kVp	mA	Time	mAs	SID	I
Model	21	125			1.5	72"	
Room							
S							
M							
L							
InSight							

Bontrager Textbook, 3rd ed., p. 66

36

Explanations for Use

Symbols and Abbreviations

The following symbols and abbreviations are used throughout this handbook:

Symbols

<	Less than
>	Greater than
⊥	Perpendicular to
≈	Approximately
±	Plus or minus
x	Multiplied by
"	Inches
cm	Centimeter
°	Degrees of angle
1ø	Single phase
3ø	Three phase

Abbreviations

General Positioning/Anatomy Terms

ASIS	Anterior Superior Iliac Spine (pelvis landmark)
MCP	Mid-Coronal Plane (plane dividing the body into anterior and posterior halves)
MSP	Mid-Sagittal Plane (plane dividing the body into equal right and left halves)
Ext.	External
Int.	Internal
Obli.	Oblique
Lat.	Lateral
R & L	Right and Left
C	Specific Cervical vertebrae
T	Specific Thoracic vertebrae
L	Specific Lumbar vertebrae
S	Specific Sacral segment
LS	Lumbo-Sacral vertebrae
SI Joints	Sacroiliac Joints
AC Joints	Acromioclavicular Joints

Technical Factors

AEC	Automatic Exposure Controls
CR	Central Ray and/or Computed Radiography
DF	Digital Fluoroscopy
OID	Object Image receptor Distance
SID	Source Image receptor Distance
C.W.	Crosswise (cassette orientation)
L.W.	Lengthwise (cassette orientation)
RS	Relative Speed (intensifying screens)
RE	Rare Earth (intensifying screens)
TT	Table Top (non-Bucky)
F.S.	Focal Spot (large or small)

Terms related to Joints of Limbs (Extremities)

CM	Carpo-Metacarpal
MP	Metacarpo-Phalangeal
IP	Inter-Phalangeal
DIP	Distal Inter-Phalangeal
PIP	Proximal Inter-Phalangeal

Terms Related to Cranium

AML	Acanthio-Meatal Line
EAM	External Acoustic Meatus
GAL	Glabello-Alveolar Line
IOML	Infra-Orbital Meatal Line
IPL	Inter-Pupillary Line
LML	Lips-Meatal Line (modified Waters)
MML	Mento-Meatal Line (Waters)
OML	Orbito-Meatal Line

Terms Related to Mammography

CC	Cranio-Caudal projection
MLO	Medio-Lateral projection
XLCC	Exaggerated-Lateral-Cranio-Caudal projection

Glossary of Positioning Terms
(Named Positions)

Certain positions have been named after the person first describing them in a published form. Sometimes physicians will use these names to request a specific position and the radiographer needs to know to which position or projection they are referring. Following are some of these "named" terms listed alphabetically by body parts.

Method	Description	References
	Chest and Bony Thorax	
Lindblom	Chest, AP lordotic	[2] Bontrager Hndbk. p. 41 [3] Bontrager Textbk. p. 72 [1] Merrill's Atlas p. 1-468
	Lower Limb and Pelvis	
Beclere	**Intercondylar fossa,** AP, axial, curved cassette	[3] Bontrager Textbk. p. 208 [1] Merrill's Atlas p. 1-228
Camp-Coventry	**Intercondylar fossa,** prone, axial	[2] Bontrager Hndbk. p. 124 [3] Bontrager Textbk. p. 207 [1] Merrill's Atlas p. 1-252
Chassard-Lapine	**Pelvic area** and **rectosigmoid colon**, axial projection	[3] Bontrager Textbk. p. 481 [1] Merrill's Atlas p. 1-280 and 2-147
Cleaves	**Hips**, bilateral "frog-leg"	[2] Bontrager Hndbk. p. 142 [3] Bontrager Textbk p. 235 [1] Merrill's Atlas p. 1-284
Clements-Nakayama	**Lateral hip,** modified axiolateral projection, patient supine	[3] Bontrager Textbk. p. 233 [1] Merrill's Atlas p. 1-292
Hickey (also see Lauenstein)	**Lateral hip,** (unilateral "frog-leg") leg abducted, CR 20–25° cephalad	[2] Bontrager Hndbk. p.142 [3] Bontrager Textbk. p. 231 [1] Merrill's Atlas p.1-288

Glossary

Method	Description	References
Lower limb continued		
Holly (and Lewis)	**Foot**, tangential for sesamoids, AP (and PA)	[2] Bontrager Hndbk. p.106 [3] Bontrager Textbk. p. 190 [1] Merrill's Atlas p. 1-194
Holmblad	**Intercondylar fossa,** erect or kneeing, tunnel view	[2] Bontrager Hndbk. p. 124 [3] Bontrager Textbk p. 207 [1] Merrill's Atlas p. 1-250
Hughston	**Patella,** tangential prone, axial	[2] Bontrager Hndbk p. 128 [3] Bontrager Textbk. p. 212 [1] Merrill's Atlas p. 1-261
Kite	**Pediatric feet**, AP and lateral for club feet	[2] Bontrager Hndbk. p.134 [1] Merrill's Atlas p. 1-212
Lauenstein (also see Hickey)	**Lateral hip** (unilateral "frog-leg") leg abducted, CR ⊥	[2] Bontrager Hndbk. p. 142 [3] Bontrager Textbk. p. 231 [1] Merrill's Atlas p. 1-288
Lorenz(Danelius-Miller modification)	**Trauma hip** (cross-table lateral)	[2] Bontrager Handbk. p.144 [3] Bontrager Textbk. p. 232 [1] Merrill's Atlas p. 1-290
Merchant	**Patellofemoral joint** and **patella**, tangential	[2] Bontrager Hndbk. p. 127 [3] Bontrager Textbk. p. 211 [1] Merrill's Atlas p. 1-262
Settegast	**Patellofemoral joint** and **patella**, tangential	[2] Bontrager Hndbk. p. 128 [3] Bontrager Textbk. p. 212 [1] Merrill's Atlas p. 1-264
Taylor	**Pelvis** (pubic area) AP, CR 20-45° cephalad	[2] Bontrager Hndbk. p. 146 [3] Bontrager Textbk. p. 236 [1] Merrill's Atlas p. 1-305
Teufel (also Judet)	**Pelvis** (acetabulum) 35-40° anterior oblique, CR 12° cephalad or ⊥	[3] Bontrager Textbk. p. 236 [1] Merrill's Atlas p. 1-302 [4] Long/Rafert p. 308

Method	Description	References
	Upper Limb and Shoulder	
Coyle	**Lateral elbow,** trauma views, CR 45° toward and away from shoulder	[2] Bontrager Hndbk. p. 79 [3] Bontrager Textbk. p. 139 [4] Long/Rafert p. 134
Fisk	**Intertubercular** (bicipi-tal) **groove**, tangential	[2] Bontrager Hndbk. p. 91 [1] Merrill's Atlas p. 1-148 [4] Long/Rafert p. 180
Garth	**Apical oblique shoulder** 45° obli., CR 45° caudad	[2] Bontrager Hndbk. p. 95 [3] Bontrager Textbk. p. 162 [4] Long/Rafert p. 182
Gaynor-Hart	**Carpal canal**, tangential view	[2] Bontrager Hndbk. p. 73 [3] Bontrager Textbk. p. 127 [1] Merrill's Atlas p. 1-94
Grashey	**Shoulder** for glenoid cavity, 35-45° post. obli. and **Foot**, PA oblique	[2] Bontrager Hndbk. p. 90 [3] Bontrager Textbk. p. 158 [1] Merrill's Atlas p. 1-144 [1] Merrill's Atlas p. 1-202
Lawrence	**Shoulder** and **proximal humerus,** transthoracic lateral	[2] Bontrager Hndbk. p. 94 [3] Bontrager Textbk. p. 157 [1] Merrill's Atlas p. 1-130
Neer	**Lateral scapula** for supraspinatus outlet, scapular "Y" view	[2] Bontrager Hndbk. p. 92 [1] Merrill's Atlas p. 1-146 [4] Long/Rafert p. 194
Stecher (modified)	**Wrist**, scaphoid view, with angled support	[2] Bontrager Hndbk. p. 71 [1] Merrill's Atlas p. 1-91 [4] Long/Rafert p. 94
Stryker	**Shoulder** "notch" projection	[1] Merrill's Atlas p. 1-147 [4] Long/Raefert p. 190
West Point (and Clements mod.)	**Shoulder**, prone or lateral recumbent, inferosuperior	[1] Merrill's Atlas p. 1-134 [1] Merrill's Atlas p. 1-136 [4] Long/Rafert p. 204

Glossary

Method	Description	References
	Vertebral Column	
Ferguson	**Spine**, scoliosis series, AP or PA, erect with elevation support	[2] Bontrager Hndbk. p. 170 [3] Bontrager Textbk. p. 268 [1] Merrill's Atlas p. 1-394
Fuchs (Reverse Judd)	**C1-2 (Dens)** through foramen magnum, chin elevated, AP (supine)	[2] Bontrager Hndbk. p. 155 [1] Merrill's Atlas p.1-328 [4] Long/Rafert p. 252
Grandy	**Lateral C. spine,** erect, shoulders down	[2] Bontrager Hndbk. p. 158 [3] Bontrager Textbk. p. 289 [1] Merrill's Atlas p. 1-336
Judd (see Fuchs)	**C1-2 (Dens)** through foramen magnum, chin elevated, PA (prone)	[2] Bontrager Hndbk. p. 155 [1] Merrill's Atlas p. 1-330
Ottonello	**C1-2**, "Wagging Jaw" or "chewing" view	[3] Bontrager Textbk. p. 293 [1] Merrill's Atlas p. 1-344
Pawlow or Twining	**C7-T1**, "Swimmers" view, erect or recumbent	[2] Bontrager Hndbk. p. 159 [3] Bontrager Textbk. p. 291 [1] Merrill's Atlas p. 1-352
	Skull	
Arcelin (Reverse Stenvers)	**Temporal bone**, AP, 45° oblique, CR 10° cephalad	[2] Bontrager Hndbk. p. 209 [1] Merrill's Atlas p. 2-410
Caldwell	**Skull & Facial bones**, PA, CR 15° caudad	[2] Bontrager Hndbk. p. 183 [3] Bontrager Textbk. p. 331 [1] Merrill's Atlas p. 2-242
Haas	**Cranium**, PA axial, CR 25° cephalad	[2] Bontrager Hndbk. p. 181 [3] Bontrager Textbk. p. 339 [1] Merrill's Atlas p. 2-251
Law	**Skull (mastoids or TMJ)** 15° rotation from lateral, CR 15° caudad	[2] Bontrager Hndbk. p. 207 [3] Bontrager Textbk. p. 405 [1] Merrill's Atlas p. 2-398

Method	Description	References
Skull continued		
Mayer and Owen modification	**Mastoids**, AP, 45° rotation, CR 45° caudad	[2] Bontrager Hndbk. p. 211 [3] Bontrager Textbk. p.408 [1] Merrill's Atlas p. 2-412
Rhese	**Optic foramen**, PA, 53° rotation, CR ⊥	[2] Bontrager Hndbk. p. 191 [3] Bontrager Textbk. p. 374 [1] Merrill's Atlas p. 2-272
Schuller (Henchen) (Lysholm)	**Mastoids**, CR 15–30° caudad, no rotation	[2] Bontrager Hndbk. p. 202 [3] Bontrager Textbk. p.384 [1] Merrill's Atlas p. 2-404
Stenvers	**Mastoids**, PA, 45° rotation, CR 12° cephalad, no rotation	[2] Bontrager Hndbk. p. 208 [3] Bontrager Textbk. p. 406 [1] Merrill's Atlas p. 2-408
Towne	**Skull**, AP axial, CR 30° caudad	[2]Bontrager Hndbk. p. 181 [3] Bontrager Textbk. p. 328 [1] Merrill's Atlas p. 2-246
Waters	**Facial bones** and **Sinuses**	[2] Bontrager Hndbk. pp. 188 and 205 [3] Bontrager Textbk. pp. 359, 402 [1] Merrill's Atlas pp. 2-304 and 382
Other:		

[1] Ballinger, PW *Merrill's Atlas of Radiographic Positions and Radiologic Procedures*, 8th ed., Vol I and II, St. Louis: Mosby-Year Book Inc., 1995

[2] Bontrager, KL *Pocket Handbook; Radiographic Positioning and Techniques*, 2nd ed. Peoria, AZ, Bontrager Publishing, Inc., 1995

[3] Bontrager, KL *Textbook of Radiographic Positioning and Related Anatomy*, 3rd ed. St. Louis: Mosby-Year Book Inc., 1993

[4] Long, BW, Rafert, JA *Orthopaedic Radiography,* Philadelphia: WB Saunders, 1995

Chapter 1

Exposure Factor Considerations and Conversions

Exposure – Density Correction Rule

Calculating Exposure

Formula: (milliamps) x (seconds) = (milliampere-seconds)

mA x T = mAs

See **Appendix A** at end of book for mAs chart. This chart includes time in both fractions and decimals.

Total exposure is measured in **mAs**, therefore exposure technique can be changed by changing **mA** or **T**. As a combination of both mA and T, **mAs is the primary controlling factor for density.**

Density Change Rules[1]

In practice there is a tendency to undercorrect for density changes on repeats. This may be due to experience with 2 kVp interval changes in certain technique charts and from this may come the wrong assumption that even 2 kVp changes make a visible difference on radiographs.

A general rule states that it requires a minimum **30% change in exposure** to make a change on the radiograph that is discernible to the human eye.

A 50% change in exposure is required if only a slight density correction is desired.

A 100% change in exposure (doubling or cutting in half) is generally required to correct a radiograph requiring a repeat.

kVp – Density Factors

Kilovoltage (kVp) is **a secondary controlling factor for density**.

<u>**15% Rule**</u>**:** This rule indicates **a 15% change in kVp is equivalent to a 100% change in mAs.** Thus a 15% change in kVp will approximately double or cut in half the density of a radiograph.[2,3]

Fifteen Percent kVp Change:
- Lower kVp (60–70) requires **9–10 kVp** change
- Medium kVp (80–90) requires **12–14 kVp** change
- High kVp (100+) requires **15–18 kVp** change

Example 1. A chest radiograph taken at **10 mAs**, **110 kVp** is underexposed and requires a repeat. Which exposure factors should be changed and how much on this repeat?

Answer: With kVp already at 110, the mAs should probably be increased by at least 50% to **15 mAs** if only a slight correction is needed, or by 100% to **20 mAs** if a major correction is needed.

Example 2. An ankle taken at **10 mAs** and **52 kVp** was underpenetrated due to excessive swelling. A repeat was required with an increase in kVp. How much would the kVp need to be increased to correct the underexposure?

Answer: Increase kVp 15% to double the density (100% change). 52 x .15 = 7.8 (8)
New kVp = 52 + 8 = <u>**60**</u>

Exposure – Distance Conversions

The exposure or radiographic density **is directly proportional to the square of the distance from the source.** This is based on the inverse square law which states that the intensity of the x-ray beam is inversely proportional to the square of the distance from the source. Therefore at two times the distance, the intensity of the x-ray beam is only one-fourth. The exposure (mAs) would then need to be increased by a factor of four times to maintain the radiographic density.

Formula: $$\frac{{}_{0}\text{mAs}}{{}_{N}\text{mAs}} = \frac{{}_{0}D^2}{{}_{N}D^2}$$

See **Appendix B: Exposure–Distance Conversion Chart** to determine exposure factors when SID is to be changed.

Common Examples for Changing of SID

Traditionally a common SID has been 40 inches (102 cm). However, increasing the SID not only improves image quality due to less magnification and distortion, but also reduces patient dose. Studies have shown that increasing the SID from 40 to 48" reduces patient exposure by 11 to 12%.[4]

Standard SID: Some departments have changed their standard SID to 48" and others have changed to only 44" due to the difficulty of shorter technologists being able to reach the x-ray tube at 48". (Grid limitations also need to be determined due to focal ranges of under-table grids to prevent grid cutoff on the edges of larger-size films at increased SID.)

Routine Chest SID: In some departments chest radiographs are routinely taken at 120" (300 cm) rather than 72" (180 cm). Grids are available which can be used at these longer distances.

Portables: Portable procedures frequently require a change in SID and therefore a change in mAs.

Rather than using the formula to calculate new mAs each time the SID is changed, the Exposure Distance Conversion Chart in Appendix B can be used more quickly.

Density–Collimation Field Size Conversions

Accurate collimation of the primary x-ray beam to the area of interest reduces the area and volume of tissue irradiated. This not only reduces patient dose but also improves image quality by reducing the amount of undesirable scatter radiation reaching the film. Therefore reducing the collimation field size reduces the amount of scatter reaching the film, resulting in less film density. This requires an adjustment in mAs or kVp to maintain adequate film density when the collimation field size is significantly reduced.

Both the **tissue density** and the **part thickness** affect these factors, but for general purposes the following conversion factors can be used as **a suggested starting guide** for exposure adjustments. (Each technologist should determine what works best for the equipment, procedures and techniques they are using.)

Exposure Conversion Factors

Exposure field size change	Increase in mAs required	Multiplication factors
14 x 17" (35 x 43 cm) → 10 x 12" (20 x 24 cm)	25–35% ________	1.25–1.35 x ________x
14 x 17" (34 x 43 cm) → 8 x 10" (20 x 24 cm)	50–75% ________	1.5–1.75 x ________x
14 x 17" (34 x 43 cm) → 4 x 4" (10 x 10 cm)	100–150% ________	2.0–2.5 x ________x

Example: Calculate the new mAs range required for an abdomen when the collimation field size is decreased from 14 x 17" to 8 x 10". Original mAs = 65 @ 80 kVp.

Solution: Increase mAs 50–75%.
New mAs = (50%) 1.5 x 65 = 97.5
(75%) 1.75 x 65 = 113.75
Answer: **new mAs = <u>98–114</u>**

Increase in CR angle causes a decrease in density

As the angle of the central ray (CR) is increased from directly perpendicular or right angle to the film and body part, the density on the radiograph will be decreased unless the exposure is adjusted accordingly.

The two reasons for this decrease in radiographic density are (A) the increase in SID which occurs as the CR angle is increased, and (B) the increase in part thickness as the CR angle increases.

A. SID increases as CR angle increases (if x-ray tube is not lowered)

As the CR angle is changed from directly vertical or perpendicular to the film, to some angle of less than 90°, **the distance (SID) increases** by the amounts shown on the following chart. Therefore the height of the x-ray tube must be lowered by these amounts to maintain a constant SID. (The tape on the x-ray tube should be used if available to maintain a constant SID.)

CR Angle	Increase in SID if tube height is not changed	
0°	0	SID 40" (102 cm)
10°	+.5" (1 cm)	40.5" (103 cm)
20°	+1.75" (4 cm)	41.75" (106 cm)
30°	+4" (10 cm)	44" (112 cm)
40°	+8" (20 cm)	48" (122 cm)
45°	+11" (28 cm)	51" (130 cm)

Example: How much would the x-ray tube need to be lowered on an AP axial of the sacro-iliac joints where the CR angle is angled 40° cephalad?

Answer: Lower tube 8" (20 cm) to maintain a constant SID.

B. Part thickness increases as CR angle increases

The thickness of the body part penetrated by the central ray increases as the degree of angle from perpendicular increases. Therefore **in addition to lowering the x-ray tube to maintain a constant SID, the mAs or kVp must be increased as the CR angle is increased to compensate for increased body part thickness.** The following chart indicates the **approximate** percent of increase, and the mAs increase multiplier, or the increase in kVp required to maintain adequate density as the CR angle is increased. (These conversions are suggested as a starting guide only and each technologist should determine what works best for their situations when AEC is not used.)

CR Angle change from 90°	Exposure increase required	mAs multiplier or	kVp increase (75–80 kVp range)
0°	0	0	0
10°	0	0	0
20°	*15–20%	*0 (unobservable)	*0 (unobservable)
30°	30–50%	1.3 to 1.5x	+4–5 kVp
40°	60–75%	1.6 to 1.75x	+7–8 kVp
45°	80–150%	1.8 to 2.5x	+9–14 kVp

*The exposure–density change rule states that at least a **30% change in exposure** is required to make a **visible density change** on the radiograph.

Example: Using the above table, what mAs or kVp would be required on an AP semi-axial of the sacroiliac joints taken at a 40° cephalic angle if the following AP pelvis technique is known? (Tube height is lowered 8" to maintain a 40" SID.)

AP Pelvis: 300 mA, .2 sec (60 mAs) 75 kVp

Answer: New mAs = **96 – 105** (60 x 1.6 = 96 or 60 x 1.75 = 105)
60-75% increase

or

New kVp **82 – 83** (75 + 7 = 82, or 75 + 8 = 83)
7-8 kVp increase

Cast Conversion Rule

A cast applied to upper or lower limbs (extremities) requires an increase in exposure. One suggested method for determining exposure compensation is to measure for the increased thickness of the part including the cast and adjust the exposure factors accordingly.[5]

The above method can be used in general, but in addition to the added thickness of the cast, the different densities of cast materials also affect the required exposure adjustments. Therefore the following general cast conversion guide which makes allowances for the wetness and the type of cast material is suggested.[6]

Cast size and type	Exposure adjustment
Fiberglass cast	+3 to 4 kVp or 1.3–1.4 x mAs (+30-40%)
Small to average size dry plaster cast	+5 to 7 kVp or 1.6–1.7 x mAs (+60-70%)
Large dry cast or average wet plaster cast	+8 to 10 kVp or 2 x mAs (+100%)
Large wet plaster cast	+10 kVp and (+300%) 2 x mAs

Single-phase (1ø) <—> Three-phase (3ø) Conversions

There are three basic types of high-voltage x-ray generators in x-ray machines currently in use. These are:

– **Single-phase (1ø):** Generally are lower power generators (full-wave rectification most common)

– **Three-phase (3ø):** Generally are higher power generators (12 pulse most common)

– **High-frequency:** Similar to 3-phase except more efficient due to near monoenergetic wave form. Used primarily for newer type mammography or mobile (portable) machines, but may become more common for higher power machines in the future.[7]

Exposure factors differ markedly between (1ø) and (3ø) and each technologist should know which type of equipment they are using and how to convert techniques from one type to another. Three phase generators require less exposure (mAs) than single phase. For conversion purposes, the 3-phase and high-frequency are grouped together since they are somewhat similar in output.

Conversion Table [8,9]

(Approximate exposure [mAs] conversion factors)

kVp range	Multiplication Factors 3ø to 1ø	Multiplication Factors 1ø to 3ø
70-80	1.4x	x .7 (70%)
85-95	2x	x .5 (50%)
110-120	5x	x .2 (20%)

Example: Convert 3ø exposure factors of 90 kVp, 10 mAs, to 1ø exposure factors

Answer: mAs conversion factor at 90 kVp range is 2x
10 x 2 = **<u>20 mAs</u>**

Intensifying Screens and Screen Speed – Exposure Conversions

Intensifying screens are generally identified in groups according to their speed or intensification factor. Technologists should know relative speeds of screens in use and be able to convert exposure factors when needed.

The higher the speed factor, the faster the screen with more light emitted when struck by x-rays resulting in greater film density. Therefore less exposure (mAs) is required with faster screens. Par or medium speed screens are assigned a relative speed (RS) factor of 100 and a density factor of 1 and are used as the standard for comparing other screen speeds.

Screen–Speed Factor Table[10,11,12]

Type	Relative speed (RS)	Density Conversion factor - (mAs)
Ultra detail (ultra slow extremity)	25	4x
Fine detail (extremity)	50 (20–80)	2x
Par or medium	100	1x
*High speed (RE)	200–400	.5–.25x
*Ultra high (RE)	500–1,200	.2–.08x

*Rare earth (RE) screens (speed factors vary depending on screen manufacturers and the specific phosphors used, specific screen-film combinations, temperature and other factors). RS speeds of 800–1,200 in general may cause some loss of image quality.[11]

Formula: $\frac{{}_{0}RS}{{}_{N}RS} = \frac{{}_{N}mAs}{{}_{0}mAs}$ mAs is inversely proportional to the RS (relative speed) of screens

Example: Original technique for ankle using extremity (fine detail) screens with a speed of 50 RS was 60 kVp, 16 mAs. Motion was a problem so high speed screens with 400 RS were to be used to reduce exposure time. What should be the new mAs?
Answer: 16 mAs x .13 = **2 mAs.**

See **Appendix C: Screen-Speed Conversion Chart** for correction conversion factor (.13).

Asymmetric Emulsion Film-Screen Imaging System for Thoracic and Pediatric Imaging

Conventional Film-Screen Systems

Conventional film-screen systems as commonly used in general radiography consist of two intensifying screens of equal thickness and equal emulsions. Conventional films also consist of identical emulsion on both sides of the film, which with the cross-over effect from the screens **equalizes the exposure on both emulsion sides of the film**.

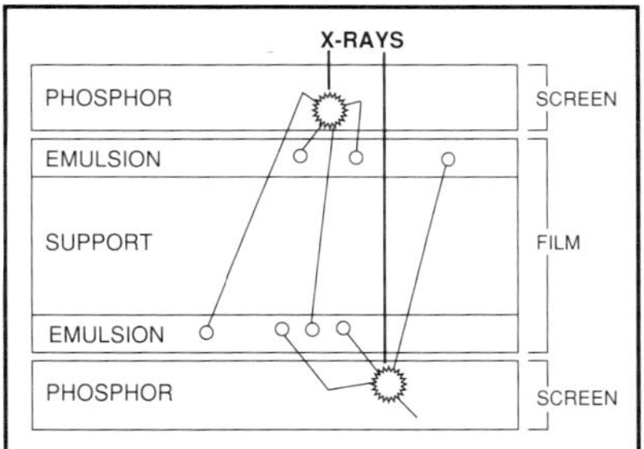

Courtesy of Eastman Kodak, Rochester, N.Y.

Conventional Screen-Film System

New Asymmetric Screen-Film System

A new type of asymmetric screen and film combination has been developed and is now being used in thoracic and pediatric imaging systems (Kodak In-Sight™ Imaging System, introduced in 1990).

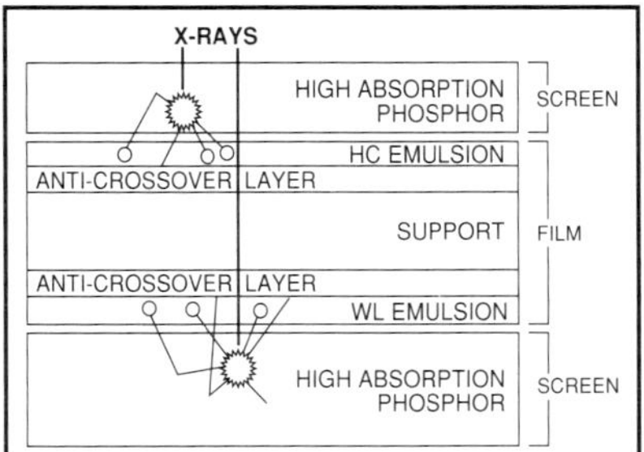

Courtesy of Eastman Kodak, Rochester, N.Y.

Asymmetric Screen-Film System
(with cross-over barriers)

In chest radiography there is a need to visualize details behind the high density mediastinum or behind ribs without losing or "burning out" the detail in the less dense air-filled lung regions.

As the term **asymmetric** implies, this film has **a different emulsion on each side of the film**. The **front side emulsion** is a relatively slow, fine grain, high-contrast and high resolution emulsion needed to record fine lung detail. The **back side emulsion** is a faster, lower-contrast emulsion recording even very low densities in the area behind the mediastinum receiving low x-ray exposure.

In addition to the asymetric film emulsion, a second important and necessary feature of this film is **the cross-over barrier** under each emulsion preventing significant cross-over of exposure such as occurs with conventional films.

The third feature of this system is the difference in front and back screens. The **front screen** of this system is a slower, high-resolution screen providing excellent visualization of fine lung structures and edges of larger structures. The **back screen** is a thicker, faster and lower resolution screen providing a lower contrast image behind the mediastinum where detail may not have been recorded at all with conventional screen-film combinations.

Two Images Superimposed on One Film: The final image from this system is therefore actually made up of two separate images which when combined provide an enhanced and higher resolution chest image at overall lower densities.[13] Low contrast structures such as behind the mediastinum and under ribs can be visualized more readily without "burning out" the fine detail structures in the lung fields.

Loading Film into Cassette: The asymmetric screen-film system requires special attention to the way the film is loaded into the cassette to ensure that the correct film emulsion is matched with the correct screen. To assist with this, each film with the Kodak Insight system has a notch which must be placed in the cassette where the word "NOTCH" appears (see illustration).

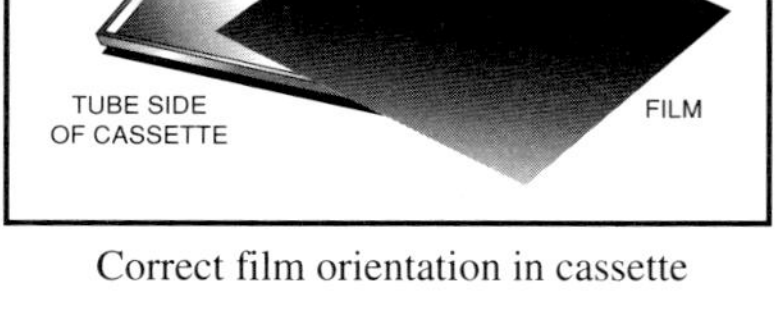

Correct film orientation in cassette

When a PA chest is viewed on the viewbox in the normal viewing position with the patient's right to the viewer's left, the notch should always appear on the upper right or lower left corner.

Note: If the film were loaded and exposed backwards, the image would be visibly darker and appear more "grainy", and on the viewbox the notch would be incorrectly placed to the upper left or lower right for a PA chest.

Uses of this System: Due to its unusually wide exposure latitude and high resolution, this system can also be used for pediatric procedures and for adult trauma ribs, cervical or thoracic spine, shoulder, foot or other exams requiring wide exposure latitude.

This also provides for a good **portable chest imaging system** when used in cassettes with the **special built-in InSight flexible grid**. Due to its dual receptor technology, the InSight film-screen-grid system provides a wider gray scale and a **greater exposure latitude,** which reduce the number of repeats on portables due to under or over exposure.[14] (Allows up to 50-75% overexposure and 50% underexposure, while conventional film-screen systems allow only ~20% over and under exposure.)[15]

Exposure Factors: Due to the wider range of visible contrast at lower densities, studies have also shown that this asymmetric screen-film system **reduces the required exposure about 40%** from that of a similar speed conventional screen-film system.[16] A common kVp range is 100-115 for this new system rather than the higher 110-125 kVp range common for conventional chest systems. With the portable InSight screen-film system with the built-in flexible grid, a common kVp range is 80-95.

Screen-Film Speeds: The Kodak InSight system has various speed screens and films available as follows:[17]

- *InSight Pediatric Ultra-Detail Screen & IP Film - 100 speed
- *InSight Pediatric Detail Screens and IP Film - 250 speed
- *InSight Pediatric Detail Screens and IT Film - 330 speed
- InSight Standard Screen and IT Film - 250 speed
- InSight HC (higher contrast) Screen and IT Film - 350 speed
- InSight VHC (very high contrast) Screen and IT Film - 400 sp
- InSight VHC Screen and IT Film and Flexible Grid - 250 speed (with grid included)

*Pediatric screens are mounted in special cassettes with low absorption carbon-fiber fronts for use with lower kVp. (**IP** = InSight Pediatric film; **IT** = InSight Thoracic asymmetric film.)

General Grid Use Rule

Grids improve image quality on radiographs by removing unwanted scatter radiation. A general rule states that grids should be used **for body parts measuring 10 cm or more and where 60–70 or greater kVp is used.**[18,19] Some prefer that grids be used for parts measuring 13 cm or greater with 70 or greater kVp.[20]

Grid Ratio

The effectiveness of grids in absorbing unwanted scatter radiation is primarily determined by their ratio, which is the height of the lead strips compared to the space between them.

Grid Frequency

The effectiveness of a grid is also determined by the grid frequency, which is defined as the **number of lead strips per inch**. The most commonly used grids have a frequency of 85-103 lines/inch (33-41 lines/cm).[21]

Types of Grids

Linear focused grids are the most common wherein the lead strips are tilted and focused to allow x-rays at certain distances (SID) to pass through unobstructed. Thus focused grids have certain focal ranges called the **grid radius** wherein grid cutoff does not occur.

Common portable grids in use today are 6:1 ratio with a medium focal range of 34–44"(86–112 cm), or a long focal range of 48–72"(122–183 cm). Common table Bucky grids are 12:1 ratio with a medium focal range of 34–44" (86–112 cm).

Linear parallel grids wherein the lead strips are parallel to each other and not tilted or focused were used as portable grids in the past but generally are not in common use today.

Cross-hatch grids have focused lead strips in two directions and in general are twice as effective in absorbing scatter. Centering and focal range however, are much more critical with cross-hatch guides which makes them impractical for portable use.

Grids and Angling of the CR

Linear grids allow angling of the CR **if the CR angle is along the length of the lead strips**, which most commonly run parallel to the longest dimension of the grids (except for decubitus type grids wherein the lead strips run along the shorter dimension). The **CR also must be near the centerline** of the focused linear grid. Only a **very limited angle of ~3° off center crosswise** to the lead strips is possible without grid cutoff .

InSight™ Flexible Grid [22]

This is a portable cassette-mounted grid which provides scatter absorption equivalent to a conventional 4:1 or 5:1 linear grid. This special purpose grid is unique in its construction of a series of eight stacked and precisely aligned sheets of lead foil with very small circular openings (14,400 holes per square inch).

As a portable or non-Bucky grid, it has certain distinct advantages over conventional linear grids. Due to its construction it is flexible and lightweight with **a wide focal range**. It does **not require that the CR be centered** to the centerline of the grid. It also tolerates up to **10° off center CR angles in all directions** without grid cutoff, which is important for non-Bucky or portable use.

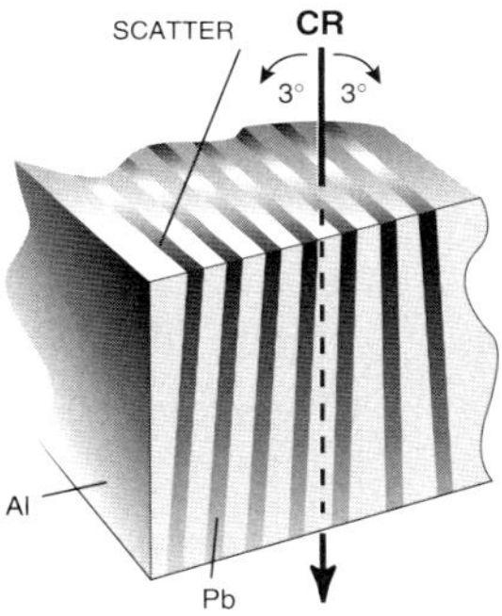

Courtesy of Eastman Kodak, Rochester

Conventional Linear Grid
- Lead strips absorb scatter in two directions only.
- Allows unlimited CR angle along length of lead strips but only ~3° off center crosswise.
- Limited focal range of ±4" from focal point. (Medium focal range grid.)

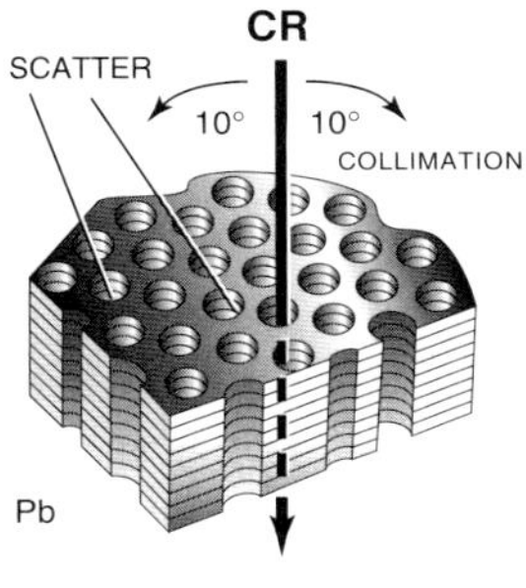

Courtesy of Eastman Kodak, Rochester

InSight™ Flexible Grid
- Collimation design absorbs scatter in all directions.
- Allows 10° angle of CR off center in all directions.
- Focal range of 20 inches (50 cm) to infinity.

Air-Gap Technique

The air-gap technique, which places the patient 4–6 inches (10–15 cm) from the film, can be used as an alternative to the use of a grid. This air-gap space allows for fewer scattered x-rays reaching the film thereby reducing unwanted exposure from scatter rays, similar to the effect of grids. In general an air-gap technique is approximately equivalent in effect to that of a 7:1 ratio grid.[23] (Generally when an air-gap is used the SID is increased to prevent increased penumbra and magnification.)

Grid Conversion Factors

Converting exposure factors from a non-grid to a grid, and from one grid ratio to another requires certain conversion factors which are multiples of a non-grid technique that is used as a standard.

Grid Use Guidelines and Approximate Conversion Factors [24,25]

Recommended kVp Ranges	Grid Ratios	Exposure Conversion Factors		
		60-75 kVp	75-95 kVp	95-125 kVp
up to 60 kVp	Non grid	1	1	1
25–30 kVp (mammogram)	4:1 or 5:1 Linear	–	–	–
up to 80-95 kVp	InSight flexible grid	2	2.5	–
up to 80 kVp	5:1 or 6:1 Linear	3	–	–
up to 100 kVp	8:1 Linear	3.5	4	–
up to 120 kVp	12:1 Linear 6:1 Crosshatch	4	5	6
over 100 kVp	16:1 Linear 8:1 Crosshatch	5	6	7

Example: Original technique for a non-grid leg to include the knee was 6 mAs, 64 kVp. If a 5:1 portable grid was to be used, what should be the new mAs if other factors remain unchanged?
Answer: Increase exposure by a factor of 3x.

New mAs: 6 x 3 = **<u>18 mAs</u>**

See **Appendix D: Grid Ratio Conversion Chart** for easy-to-use conversion factors.

Anode Heel Effect Rule

The anode heel effect alters the intensity of the x-ray beam along the long axis of the x-ray tube between the cathode and anode ends. **The intensity is always greater at the cathode end.** Studies have shown the intensity at the cathode end is from 30 to 50% greater than at the anode end using a 14 x 17" (35 x 43 cm) film at 40" SID.[26]

The heel effect is more evident with a fractional focal spot x-ray tube with an anode angle of 12° or less. Therefore an anode target angle of no steeper than 12° should be used with 14 x 17" (35 x 43 cm) film at 40" (102 cm) SID.[27] With a dual focal spot tube the heel effect is greatest with the large focal spot. The anode-heel effect can best be utilized for body parts with significant difference in thickness from one end of a 14 x 17" film to the other. When it is practical to do so, **the thickest part of the patient should be placed at the cathode end of the x-ray table.** (Cathode and anode parts of the x-ray tube are usually marked on the tube housing.)

Body parts and projections wherein the anode-heel effect can be used are as follows: (Listed in suggested order of the greatest to the least importance for utilizing the anode-heel effect.)

Projection	Anode End	Cathode End
1. Thoracic spine		
- lateral	Feet	Head
- AP	Head	Feet
2. Lumbar spine		
- lateral	Head	Feet
3. Femur - AP and lateral	Foot	Pelvis
4. Humerus - AP and lateral	Elbow	Shoulder
5. Leg (tibia-fibula)		
- AP and lateral	Foot	Knee
6. Forearm - AP and lateral	Wrist	Elbow

AEC Guidelines (Automatic Exposure Control)

AEC systems are commonly used on modern x-ray equipment to terminate the exposure time when a preset quantity of radiation has passed through the patient and reached strategically located ionization chamber cells. Kilovoltage (kVp) and mA settings are selected manually. **Only the exposure time is controlled by the AEC**.

Ionization Chamber Cell Selections

Most AEC systems have three ionization chamber cells located in **central** and in **right** and **left** slightly higher locations. The specific cell or combination of cells must be selected at the control panel. Some x-ray machines permit only one cell to be selected but most allow the selection of any combination of cells.

If more than one cell is selected, the AEC system averages the readings to more accurately reflect the desired overall density for that radiograph.[28] This averaging is desirable for some body parts such as the abdomen or pelvis. However for other parts such as the chest or spine this can result in false readings. On chests for example, the right and left cells measure under the air-filled lungs which provides for accurate lung technique. An activated center cell over the heart and mediastinum may result in overexposed lung fields and thus generally should not be used for PA chest radiographs.

The spine requires only the center cell to provide sufficient exposure for correctly visualizing the vertebral regions only.

The technologist must know what cell or combination of cells to select for each body part being radiographed when using the AEC system. This pocket handbook provides suggestions for which cell to use throughout the positioning chapters.

Adjustable Density Settings

AEC systems have adjustable density settings on the control panel. This includes an "0" neutral setting and multiples of plus (+) and minus (-) density settings. The neutral setting can generally be used for all types and sizes of patients. The plus (+) or minus (-) density settings can be used to compensate for changes in film or screen types, or for calibration or other temporary solutions to density contrast problems.[29]

Since AEC systems control only the exposure time (or the mAs), the kVp must be set manually and can be increased for larger or more muscular type patients when increased penetration is required. Likewise the kVp can be decreased for older or thin hyposthenic type patients without changing AEC controls or settings.

AEC controls should not be used for body parts that are too small to completely cover the selected ionization chamber cell. Examples of this are parts of the upper or lower limbs, or parts of the skull and/or facial bones such as sinuses, TMJ's, mastoids, mandibles, optic foramina, nasal bones or sinuses.[30]

Accurate Positioning

The use of AEC systems **require very precise and accurate positioning.** If the center cell is selected, **the correct central ray location is essential** for correctly exposed radiographs. AEC systems do not forgive inaccurate CR locations or incorrectly positioned parts in the same way that manually set technique factors do.

Accurate Collimation

Accurate collimation is also essential for consistent optimal density radiographs with AEC systems. Overly large collimation fields for example will result in increased scatter rays which also reach the ionization cells causing premature termination of the exposure creating underexposed radiographs.

Marker Placement and Correct Placement of Radiographs for Viewing

Markers and Placement

Each radiograph must have **a minimum of two types of identification markers**. First is a **right** or **left marker** which must be on every radiograph to indicate the patient's right or left side, or to indicate which limb is being radiographed.

The second marker which must be on every radiograph is the **patient identification** including at least the **name, date** and **case number** and the **name of the institution**. For legal purposes most institutions require a radiograph to be repeated if it does not have at least these two markers.

Other markers which may also be used are **radiographer's initials**, **body position** if not recumbent, and **time markers** if a timed sequence of radiographs are being taken.

ID Blocker Location

Each cassette has one screen cut out or a lead blocker at one corner on which the patient information is photographically flashed from the back of the cassette before processing. This ID blocker should be placed so as to be least likely to cover up essential anatomy. For most brands of cassettes the only possible two locations for this marker on vertical or lengthwise placed cassettes are **the upper right** corner, or the **lower left corner** as shown on these photographs.

If the cassettes are placed crosswise, the two possible locations are upper left or lower right.

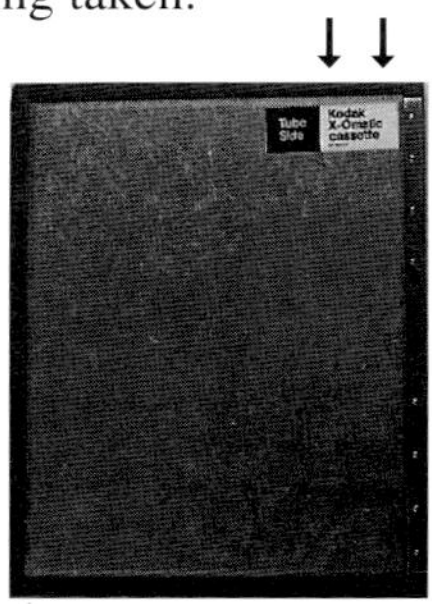

Upper right corner

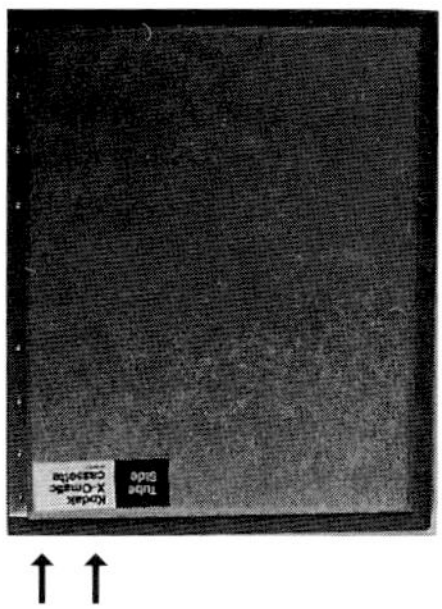

Lower left corner

First General Rule: The first general rule for placement of radiographs for viewing is to **place the radiograph in the anatomical position, so the patient is facing the viewer.** (The viewer should be able to "shake hands" with the patient.) **This always places the patient's right to the viewer's left**.

AP Projection: By knowing that for most cassettes the only patient ID blocker positions on a lengthwise cassette are to the upper right or lower left, one can determine if the radiograph is a PA or an AP projection. For an **AP projection** the ID blocker would have to be to the **upper right or lower left**, if the radiograph is placed on the view box so the patient's right is to the viewer's left.[31]

PA Projection: For a PA projection one would need to turn the radiograph over so the patient's right is again to the viewer's left (to be able to shake hands). Now the ID marker will have to be to the **upper left** or **lower right** indicating this was a PA projection.

Determining Patient's Right or Left Side: If one forgot to use a right or left marker when taking the radiograph,but knew which brand of cassette was used and which projection was taken (an AP or a PA), one could determine which is the patient's right and left side. However this should **not** be an acceptable reason for not using right and left markers.

Second General Rule: The second general rule for placing radiographs for viewing is that radiographs including the digits of the upper and lower limbs are placed on the view box with the **digits up** (opposite of anatomical position). Thus radiographs of the hands and wrist and of the feet are generally placed with the digits up rather than down.[32]

Radiographs of the forearm to include the elbow are generally placed with digits down as in the anatomical position. The same is true of the leg and/or ankle which are also generally placed in the anatomical position, digits down.

Personal Notes on Exposure Factors and/or Special Conversion Techniques:

Chapter 2

Chest and Bony Thorax

Adult Chest

Pediatric Chest

Bony Thorax

Other

Chest – Positioning Considerations and Radiation Protection

Collimation

Restricting the primary beam coverage is a very effective way to reduce patient exposure in chest radiography. This requires accurate and correct location of the central ray (CR).

Correct CR Location

Correct CR location to the mid chest (T7) allows for accurate collimation and protection to the upper radiosensitive region of the neck area. It also prevents exposure to the dense abdominal area below the diaphragm which produces scatter and secondary radiation to the radiosensitive reproductive organs.

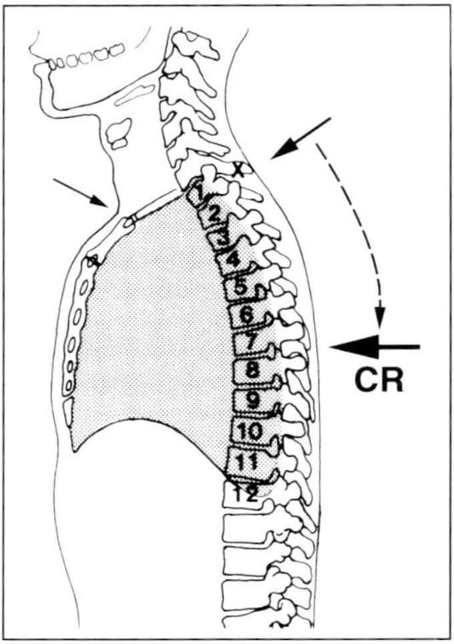

Correct CR location

T7 can be located posteriorly in reference to the long spinous process of C7, the **vertebra prominens**.[1] (This also generally corresponds to approximately the inferior angle of the scapula on most patients.) Anteriorly the mid chest (T7) is located by the **jugular notch**.[2]

Gonadal Shielding

Shielding should be used on patients of reproductive age and younger.

Backscatter Protection

Shields placed between the patient and the chest board and wall can also be used to prevent scatter and secondary radiation from these structures reaching the patient's gonadal regions.

Exposure and Patient Dose

Calculated patient doses in mrads, based on the suggested "model" exposure factors, are listed on each positioning page as skin (S), midline (ML) and gonadal (G) dose for male and female.

Bony Thorax – Positioning Considerations

Sternum

The routine for a sternum generally includes a lateral and an oblique wherein the sternum is shifted to the left of the spine and superimposed over the homogeneous heart shadow. A 15-20° RAO achieves this best. A breathing technique is generally used to blur out the lung markings and the ribs overlying the sternum.

Ribs

Each person should determine the preferred routine for their department.

Two-Film Routine: One suggested two-film routine is an **AP or PA** with the area of injury closest to the film (above or below diaphragm), and an **oblique** wherein the spine is shifted away from the side of the injury. Therefore the oblique for this routine on an injury to the left anterior ribs would be an RAO shifting the spine away from the area of injury. The oblique for an injury to the right posterior ribs would be an RPO wherein the spine is again rotated away from the area of injury.

Four-Film Routine: Another four-film routine required in some departments for all rib trauma is: **AP above diaphragm**, **AP below diaphragm**, **RPO** and **LPO** of entire thorax.

Above and Below Diaphragm: The location of the injury site in relationship to the diaphragm is important for all routines. Those injuries above the diaphragm require less exposure (nearer to a chest technique), and those below the diaphragm require an exposure nearer to that of an abdomen technique.

Screens, Films, Grids and Suggested Techniques

The positioning pages of this chapter include suggested starting techniques for chests and ribs for both conventional screen-film-grid systems and for the newer asymmetric emulsion (InSight™) system. These newer asymmetric emulsion films and intensifying screens (described in chapter one) are used primarily for thoracic imaging and for pediatrics.

PA Chest

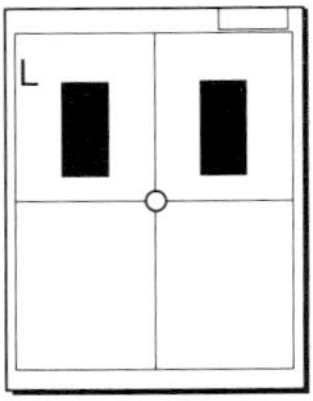

- 14 x 17" L.W. or C.W. (35 x 43 cm)
- Grid

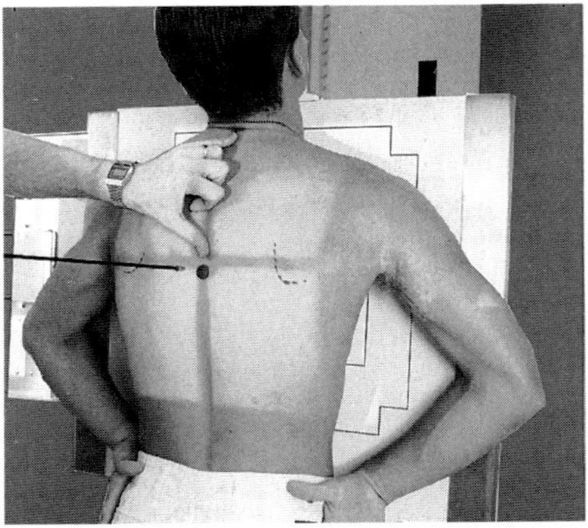

PA chest (≈8" below vertebra prominens) (average female 7")

Position

- Erect, chin raised, hands on hips with palms out, shoulders forward.
- Center CR to T7 region (film should automatically be centered to CR).
- Center thorax bilaterally to film borders with equal margins on both sides, ensure there is **no rotation** of thorax.

Central Ray: CR ⊥ to T7 or 7–8" or 18–20 cm below vertebra prominens (is also near level of inferior angle of scapula).

SID: 72–120" (183–305 cm)

Collimation: Upper border to vertebra prominens; sides to lateral skin borders.

Respiration: Expose at end of 2nd deep inspiration.

Technique: kVp (110–125) _____

mrad		
	S 10	G<0.01 M
	ML 3	0.1 F

	cm	kVp	mA	Time	mAs	SID	Film–Screen	Grid	F.S.
Model Room	21	125			1.5	72"	Kodak 400	12:1	L
S									
M									
L									
InSight									

Bontrager Textbook, 3rd ed., p. 66

Lateral Chest

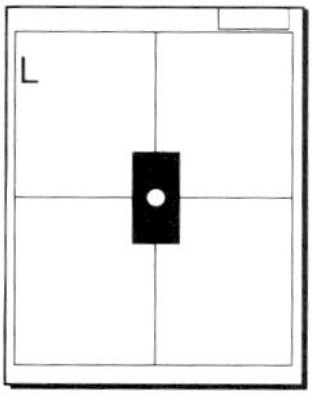

- 14 x 17" L.W. (35 x 43 cm)
- Grid

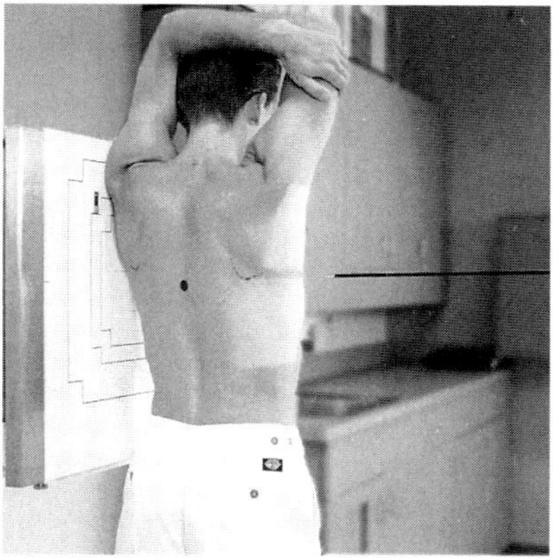

Left lateral chest

Position

- Erect, left side against film (unless right lateral indicated).
- Arms raised, crossed above head, chin up.
- **True lateral**, as viewed from x-ray tube (requires slight anterior rotation of side away from film to superimpose post. ribs).[2]
- Thorax centered to CR, and to film anteriorly and posteriorly.

Central Ray: CR ⊥, to mid thorax at level of T7.

SID: 72–120" (183–305 cm)

Collimation: Upper border to level of vertebra prominens, sides to anterior and posterior skin margins.

Respiration: Expose at end of 2nd full inspiration.

Technique: kVp (110–125) _____

mrad		
	S 73	G<0.01 M
	ML 19	0.2 F

	cm	kVp	mA	Time	mAs	SID	Film–Screen	Grid	F.S.
Model Room	38	125			8	72"	Kodak 400	12:1	L
S									
M									
L									
InSight									

Bontrager Textbook, 3rd ed., p. 68

Lateral Chest (Wheelchair or Stretcher)

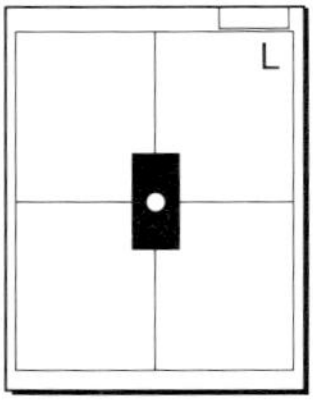

- 14 x 17" L.W. (35 x 43 cm)
- Grid

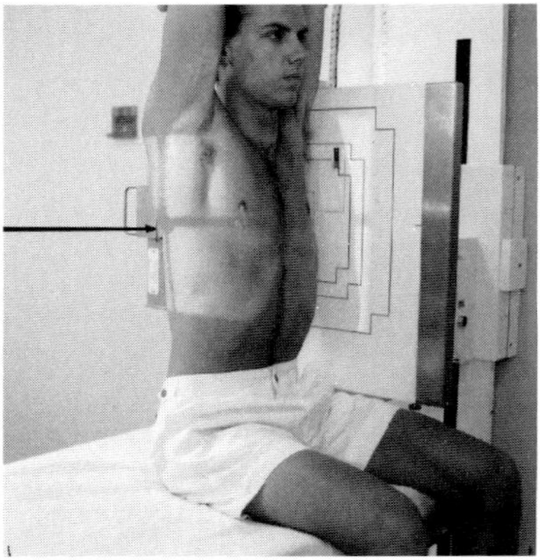

Left lateral on stretcher

Position

- Erect, on stretcher or in wheelchair.
- Arms raised, crossed above head, or hold on to support bar.
- Center thorax to CR, and to film anteriorly and posteriorly.
- Ensure no rotation as viewed from x-ray tube, keep chin up.

Central Ray

- CR ⊥, to mid thorax at level of T7.

SID: 72–120" (183–305 cm)

Collimation: Upper border to level of vertebra prominens, sides to anterior and posterior skin margins.

Respiration: Expose at end of 2nd full inspiration.

Technique: kVp (110–125) _____

mrad

S 73	G<0.01 M
ML 19	0.2 F

	cm	kVp	mA	Time	mAs	SID	Film–Screen	Grid	F.S.
Model Room	38	125			8	72"	Kodak 400	12:1	L
S									
M									
L									
InSight									

Bontrager Textbook, 3rd ed., p. 69

AP Chest (also portable)

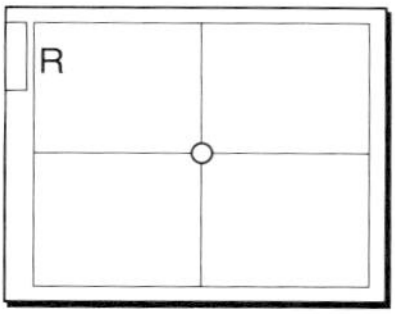

- 14 x 17" C.W. (35 x 43 cm)
- TT (Grids or screens)

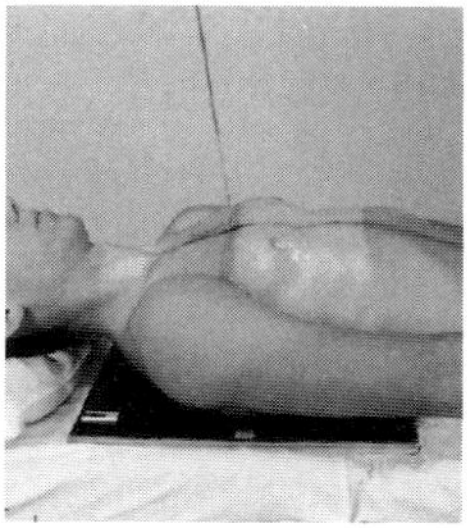

AP supine

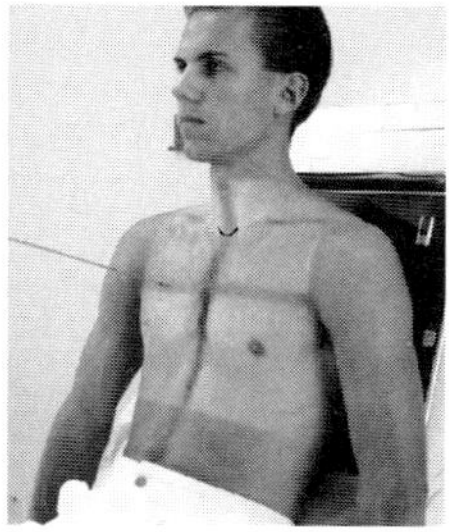

AP semi-erect

Position

- Supine, or if possible raise head end of stretcher or bed.
- Center film and T7 region to CR (upper cassette border should be ≈1.5–2" [4–5 cm] above shoulders).
- Patient to be centered to film with equal margins on both sides.
- Roll shoulders forward if possible, keep chin up.

Central Ray: CR ⊥ to sternum (3-5° caudal angle prevents clavicles from obscuring apices).[3]

- CR centered to mid sternum (T7) (3-4" below jugular notch).

SID: 40–72" (102–180 cm), (greatest SID possible).

Collimation: On four sides to lung fields.

Respiration: Expose at end of 2nd full inspiration.

Technique: kVp with grid (100–120)_____ with screen (80-90) _____

mrad

S	10	G<0.01 M
ML	3	0.1 F

	cm	kVp	mA	Time	mAs	SID	Film–Screen	Grid	F.S.
Model Room	21	110			2	72"	Kodak 400	6:1	L
S									
M									
L									
InSight									

Lateral Decubitus Chest – AP

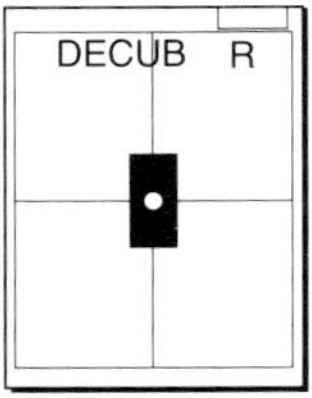

- 14 x 17" C.W. with respect to patient (35 x 43 cm)
- Grid

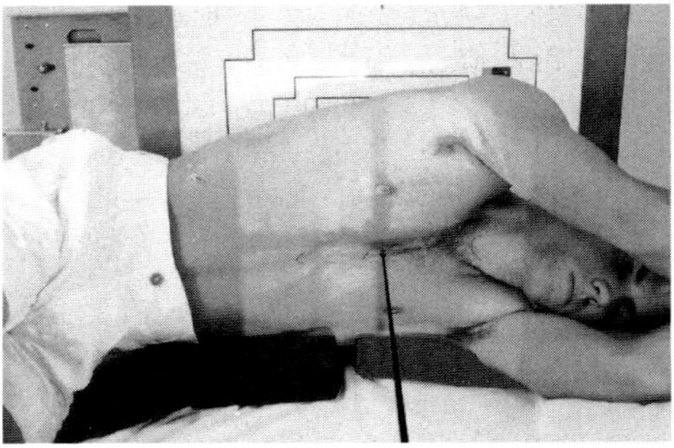

Left lateral decubitus chest (AP)

Position

- Patient on side (R or L, see Note) with pad under patient.
- Ensure that stretcher does not move (lock wheels).
- Raise both arms above head, chin up.
- True AP, no rotation, patient centered to CR at level of T7.
- Film centered to CR, ensure entire thorax is included on film.

Central Ray: CR horizontal, to T7 and center of film.

SID: 72–120" (183–305 cm) with chest film holder;
40–48" (102–122 cm) with erect table and Bucky.

Collimation: On four sides to lung fields.

Respiration: End of 2nd full inspiration.

Note: For possible fluid (pleural effusion), suspected side down; possible air (pneumothorax), suspected side up.

Technique: kVp (110–125) _____

mrad

S	22	G<0.01 M
ML	7	.0.2 F

	cm	kVp	mA	Time	mAs	SID	Film–Screen	Grid	F.S.
Model	21	125			3	72"	Kodak 400	12:1	L
Room									
S									
M									
L									
InSight									

Bontrager Textbook, 3rd ed., p. 71

AP Lordotic Chest

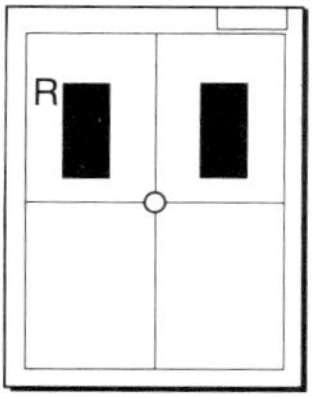

- 14 x 17" L.W. (35 x 43 cm)
- Grid

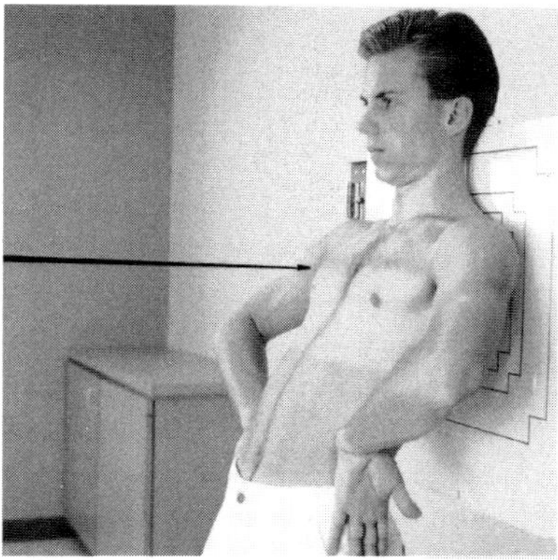

AP lordotic
(Best demonstrates apices of lungs)

Position

- Patient stands ≈1 ft. (30 cm) away from film, leans back against chest board.
- Hands on hips, palms out, shoulders rolled forward.
- Center mid sternum and film to CR, top of cassette should be 3–4" (8–10 cm) above shoulders.

Central Ray: CR ⊥ to film, 4–5" below jugular notch.

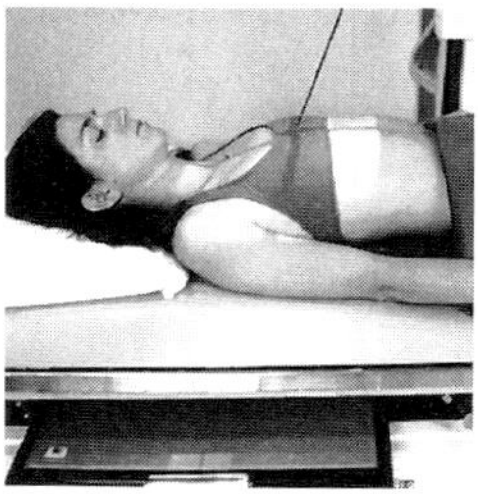

AP supine

SID: 72–120" (183–305 cm)

Collimation: On four sides to lung fields.

Respiration: End of 2nd full inspiration.

Exception: With patient supine, angle CR 15-20° cephalad.

Technique: kVp (110-125) _____

mrad

S 23	G<0.01 M
ML 7	.0.2 F

	cm	kVp	mA	Time	mAs	SID	Film–Screen	Grid	F.S.
Model Room	21	125			3	72"	Kodak 400	12:1	L
S									
M									
L									
InSight									

Anterior Oblique Chest
(RAO and/or LAO)

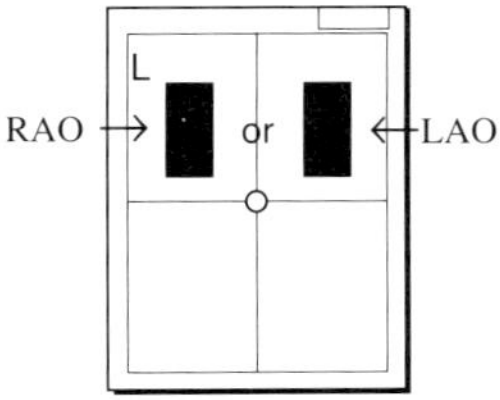

- 14 x 17" L.W. (35 x 43 cm)
- Grid

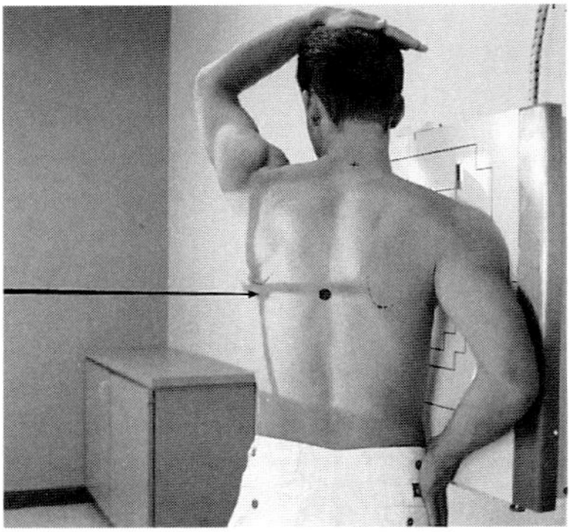
45° RAO

Position
- Erect, rotated 45°, right shoulder against film holder (RAO). (Certain heart studies require LAO, 60° rotation from PA.)
- Arm away from film up resting on head or on film holder.
- Arm nearest film down on hip, keep chin up.
- Center thorax laterally to film margins; vertically to CR at T7.

Central Ray
- CR ⊥, to level of T7.

SID: 72–120" (183–305 cm)

Collimation: On four sides to lung fields.

Respiration: End of 2nd full inspiration.

Technique: kVp (110-125) _____

mrad

S 25	G<0.01 M
ML 7	0.2 F

	cm	kVp	mA	Time	mAs	SID	Film–Screen	Grid	F.S.
Model Room	22	125			3	72"	Kodak 400	12:1	L
S									
M									
L									
InSight									

Bontrager Textbook, 3rd ed., p. 73

AP and Lateral Upper Airway
(Trachea and Larynx)

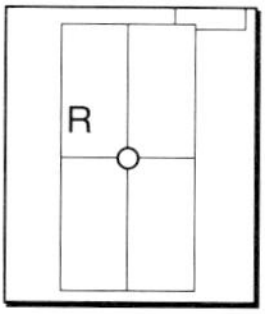

- 10 x 12" L.W. (24 x 30 cm) or 11 x 14"
- Grid

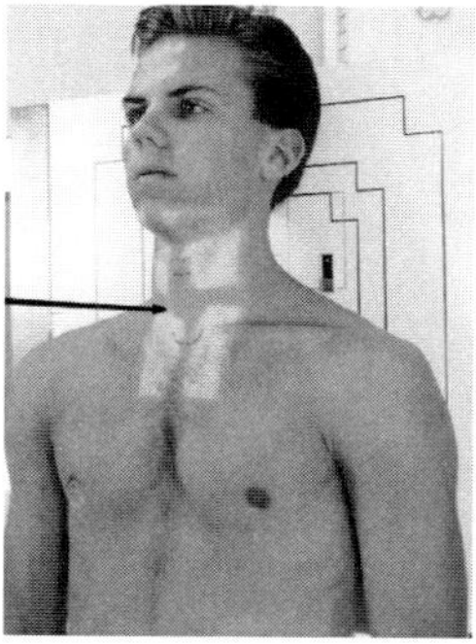
AP

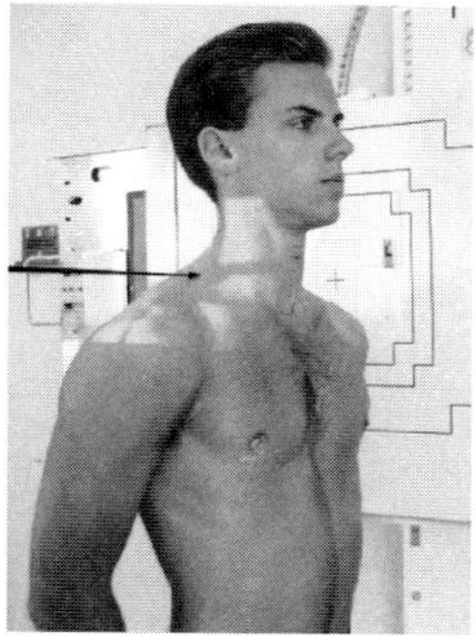
Lateral

Position
- Erect, seated or standing, center upper airway to CR.
- Arms down, chin raised slightly.
  Lateral: Depress shoulders and pull shoulders back.
- Center of cassette to level of CR.

Central Ray: CR ⊥, to midpoint between lower margin of thyroid cartilage and jugular notch (C 6-7); or ≈2" (5 cm) lower if trachea is of primary interest.

SID: 72–120" (183–305 cm)

Collimation: To area of interest.

Respiration: Expose during slow gentle inspiration.

Technique: kVp (80±5) _____

mrad, two projections		
	S 64	Thyroid 50
	ML 22	

	cm	kVp	mA	Time	mAs	SID	Film–Screen	Grid	F.S.
Model	15	80			10	72"	Kodak 400	12:1	S
Room									
S									
M									
L									
InSight									

AP Pediatric Chest

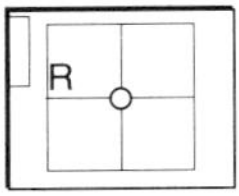

- 8 x 10" or 10 x 12" C.W. (20 x 24 cm or 24 x 30 cm)
- TT (Screens, non-grid)

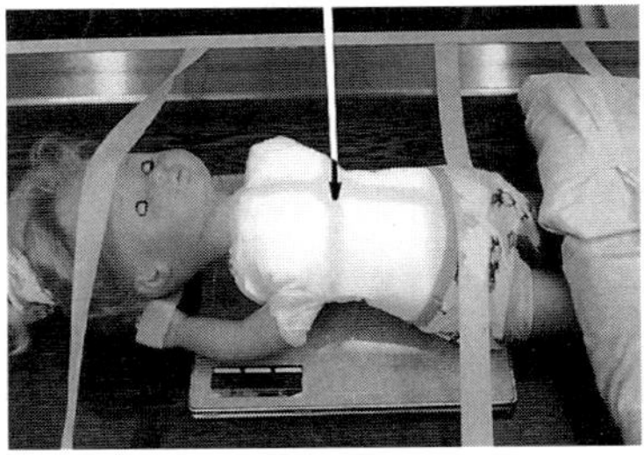

Immobilization with tape and sandbags

Position

- Supine, arms and legs extended, tape and sandbags or other immobilization of arms and legs.
- No rotation of thorax, gonadal shield over pelvic area.
- Film and thorax centered to CR.

Central Ray

- CR ⊥, to mid lung fields, mammillary (nipple) line.

SID: 40–48" (102–122 cm)

Collimation: To area of lungs.

Respiration: Full inspiration; if crying, time the exposure at full inhalation.

Note: If parental assistance is necessary, have parent hold arms overhead and head tilted back with one hand, and other hand holding down legs (provide with lead apron and gloves).

Technique: kVp (70±5) _____

mrad		
S 6	G NDC M	
ML 3	0.1 F	

	cm	kVp	mA	Time	mAs	SID	Film–Screen	Grid	F.S.
Model	1 yr	70			1.5	48"	Kodak 400	–	S
Room									
S									
M									
L									
8-Lb. Newborn, InSight		56			1.25	48"	Kodak Ped. IP 300	–	S

Bontrager Textbook, 3rd ed., p. 554

Erect PA Pediatric Chest
(with Pigg-O-Stat)

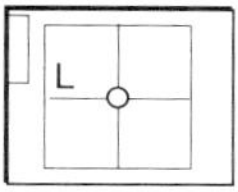

- 8 x 10" or 10 x 12" C.W. (20 x 24 cm or 24 x 30 cm)
- Screens (non-grid)

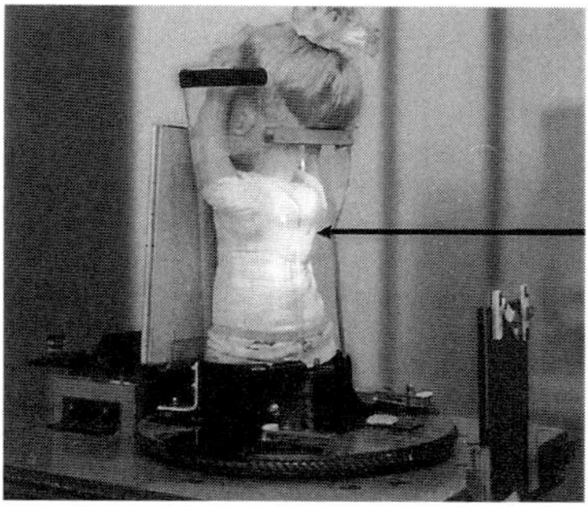

PA chest (Pigg-O-Stat, for 6 mo.-3 yrs.)

Position

- Patient on seat, legs through openings.
- Adjust height of seat to place shoulders ≈1" (2.5 cm) below upper margin of cassette.
- Raise arms and gently but firmly place side body clamps to hold raised arms and head in place.
- Set upper border of lead shield with R and L markers 1–2" (2.5–5 cm) above level of iliac crest.

Central Ray

- CR ⊥, to mid lung fields, mammillary (nipple) line.

SID: 72–120" (183–305 cm)

Collimation: On four sides to lung field borders.

Respiration: Full inspiration; if crying, expose at full inhalation.

Technique: kVp (70±5) _____ mrad

S 5	G NDC M
ML 3	0.01 F

	cm	kVp	mA	Time	mAs	SID	Film–Screen	Grid	F.S.
Model Room	≈1 yr	70			3	72"	Kodak 400	–	S
S									
M									
L									
InSight									

Lateral Pediatric Chest

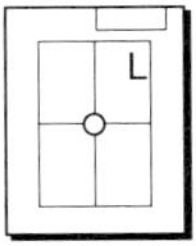

- 8 x 10" or 10 x 12" L.W. (20 x 24 cm or 24 x 30 cm)
- TT (Screens, non-grid)

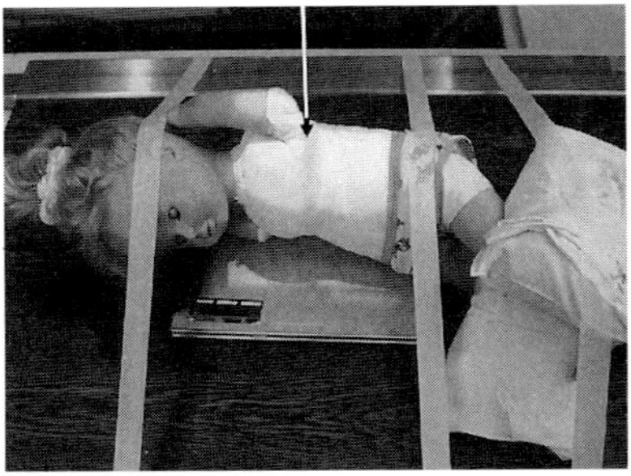

Lateral chest (with tape and sandbags)

Position

- Lying on side, arms up with head between arms.
- Support arms with tape and sandbags, ensure a true lateral.
- Flex legs; secure with tape and sandbags or with retention band across legs and hips. Lead Shield over pelvic region.

Central Ray

- CR ⊥, to mid lung fields, level of mammillary line.

SID: 40–48" (102–122 cm)

Collimation: On four sides to area of lung field.

Respiration: Full inspiration; if crying, time exposure at full inhalation.

Note: If parental assistance is necessary, have parent hold arms overhead and head tilted back with one hand, and other hand holding down legs (provide with lead apron and gloves).

Technique: kVp (75±5) _____

mrad

S 15	G NDC M
ML 7	0.2 F

	cm	kVp	mA	Time	mAs	SID	Film–Screen	Grid	F.S.
Model Room	≈1 yr	75			3	48"	Kodak 400	–	S
S									
M									
L									
8-Lb. Newborn, InSight									

Bontrager Textbook, 3rd ed., p. 556

Erect Lateral Pediatric Chest
(with Pigg-O-Stat)

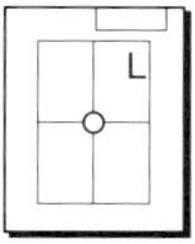

- 8 x 10" or 10 x 12" L.W. (20 x 24 cm or 24 x 30 cm)
- Screens (non-grid)

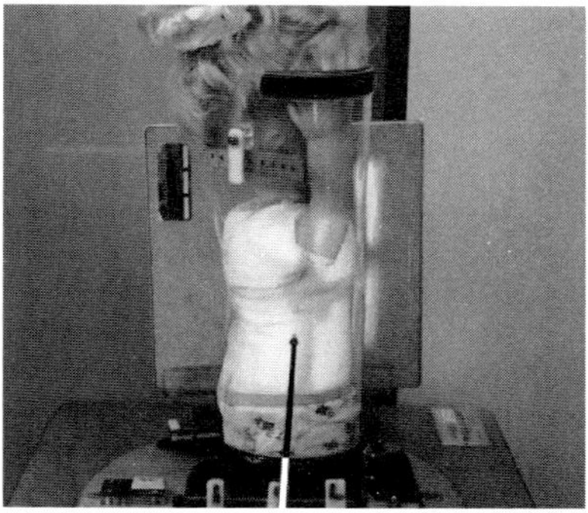
Lateral chest (Pigg-O-Stat, for 6 mo.-3yrs.)

Position

- With patient remaining in same position as for PA chest, change cassette and rotate entire seat and body clamps 90° into a left lateral position. Lead shield just above iliac crest.
- Change lead marker to indicate left lateral.

Central Ray

- CR ⊥, to mid lung fields, mammillary (nipple) line.

SID: 72–120" (183–305 cm)

Collimation: On four sides to lung field borders.

Respiration: Full inspiration; if crying, time exposure at full inhalation.

Technique: kVp (75±5) _____ mrad

S 11	G NDC M
ML 6	0.1 F

	cm	kVp	mA	Time	mAs	SID	Film–Screen	Grid	F.S.
Model Room	≈1 yr	80			5	72"	Kodak 400	–	S
S									
M									
L									
InSight									

Bontrager Textbook, 3rd ed., p. 557

Oblique Sternum

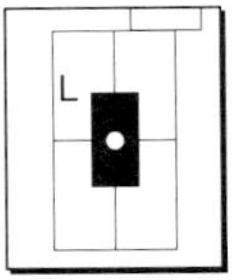

- 10 x 12" L.W. (24 x 30 cm)
- Grid
- 3–4 sec with breathing technique

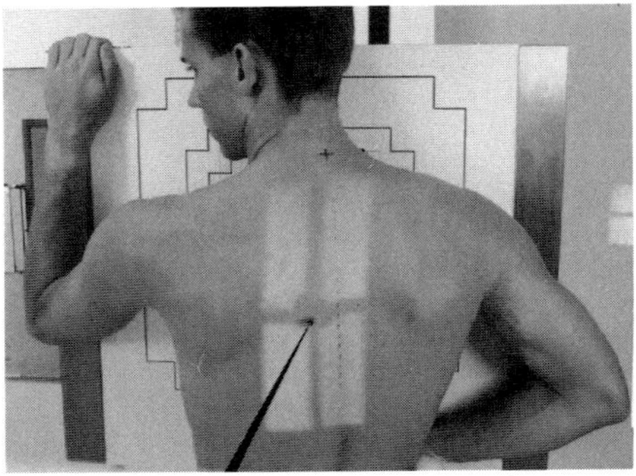

Erect 15–20° RAO sternum

Position

- Erect (preferred) or semiprone, turned 15–20° with right side down. (A thin-chested person requires more obliquity than a thick-chested patient.)
- Center sternum to CR at midline of table or cassette holder.

Central Ray

- CR ⊥, to mid sternum (midway between jugular notch and xiphoid tip).

SID: 40–48" (102–122 cm)

Collimation: Long narrow collimation field, to area of sternum.

Respiration: Gentle even breathing during exposure.

Technique: kVp (65±5) ______

mrad

S 254	G<0.01 M
ML 43	0.4 F

	cm	kVp	mA	Time	mAs	SID	Film–Screen	Grid	F.S.
Model	20	65			45	44"	Kodak 400	12:1	S
Room									
S									
M									
L									
InSight									

Bontrager Textbook, 3rd ed., p. 306

Lateral Sternum

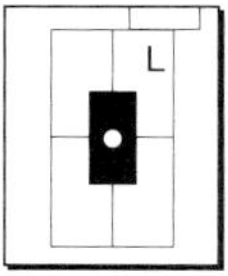

- 10 x 12" L.W. (24 x 30 cm)
- Grid
- Place lead blocker anterior to sternum.

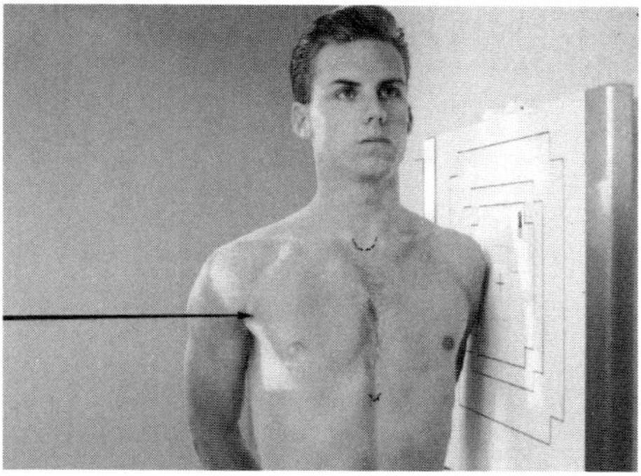

Lateral, erect sternum

Position

- Erect (seated or standing), or recumbent lying on side with vertical CR; or supine with cross table CR for severe trauma.
- Draw shoulders and arms back.
- Align sternum to CR at midline of cassette holder.
- Top of cassette 1 1/2" (4 cm) superior to level of jugular notch.

Central Ray

- CR ⊥, to mid sternum.

SID: 40–48" (102–122 cm)

Collimation: Collimate on four sides to area of sternum.

Respiration: Expose upon full inspiration.

Technique: kVp (75±5) _____

mrad

S 625	G<0.01 M
ML 141	0.5 F

	cm	kVp	mA	Time	mAs	SID	Film–Screen	Grid	F.S.
Model Room	29	80			40	44"	Kodak 400	12:1	S
S									
M									
L									
InSight									

Sternoclavicular Joints
PA and Anterior Obliques

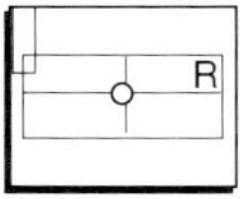

- 8 x 10 C.W. (20 x 24 cm)
- Grid

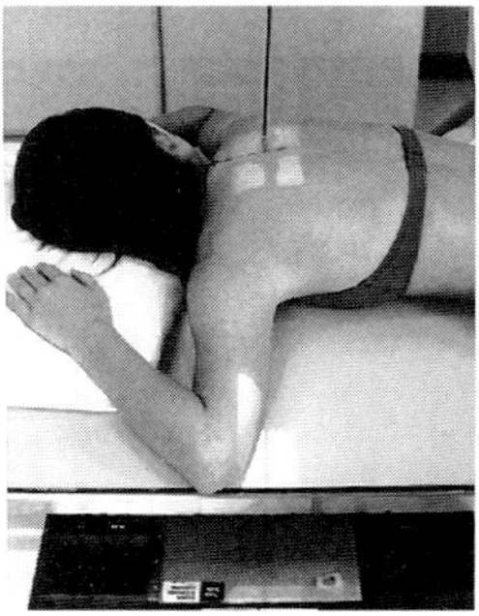

Bilateral PA

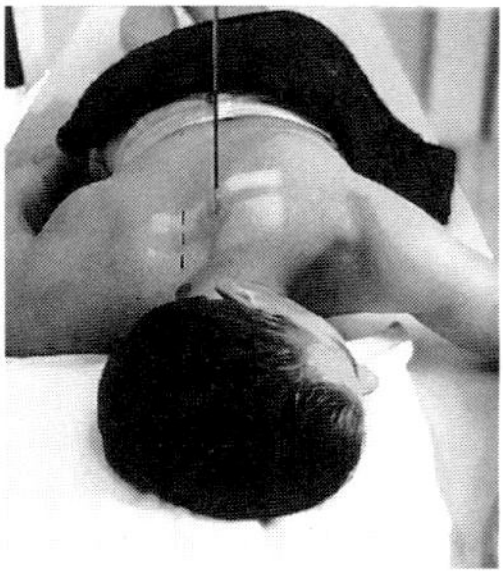

RAO, 10-15° oblique, CR ⊥
(Both obli's commonly taken for comparison)

Position

PA:

- Prone or erect, midsagittal plane to centerline of CR.
- Turn head to side, no rotation of thorax.
- Center film to CR.

Oblique: Rotate thorax 10-15° to shift vertebrae away from sternum (visualizes upside joint).[3]

Central Ray: PA - CR ⊥, to MSP and ≈ 3" or 7 cm distal to vertebra prominens. (1.5" or 2.5 cm inferior to jugular notch.)
Oblique - CR ⊥, to ≈ 2" (5 cm) lateral to MSP (toward elevated side) and ≈ 3" or 7 cm distal to vertebra prominens.

SID: 40–48" (102–122 cm)

Collimation: To area of sternoclavicular joints.

Respiration: Expose after expiration.

Technique: kVp: (65±5) _____ mrad, two projections

S 80	G NDC M
ML 28	<0.1F

	cm	kVp	mA	Time	mAs	SID	Film–Screen	Grid	F.S.
Model Room	20	65			10	44"	Kodak 400	12:1	S
S									
M									
L									
InSight									

AP or PA Ribs-Above Diaphragm

Generally taken as AP for posterior ribs, and PA for anterior ribs.

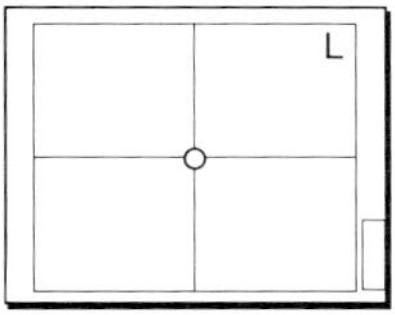

- 14 x 17" C.W. or L.W. (35 x 43 cm)
- Grid

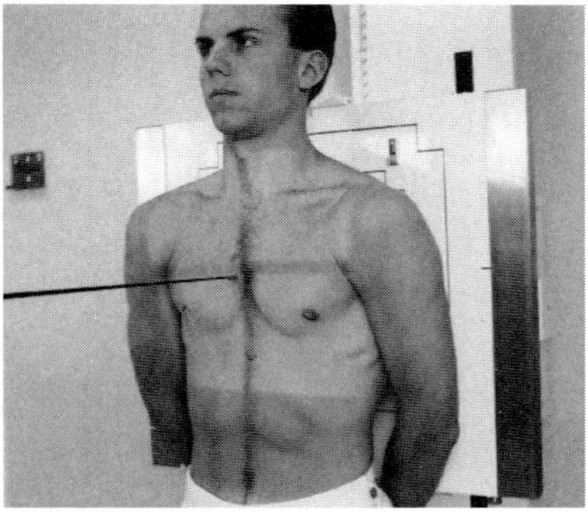

AP bilateral ribs (above diaphragm)

Position

- Erect, or recumbent, midsagittal plane to centerline and CR.
- Top of cassette ≈ 1 1/2" (4 cm) above shoulders.
- Roll shoulders forward, no rotation.
- Ensure that thorax is centered to film laterally.

Central Ray

- CR ⊥, to center of film (level of T7).

SID: 72" (183 cm) erect; 40–48" (102–122 cm) recumbent.

Collimation: To rib margins on all sides.

Respiration: Expose on **inspiration** (diaphragm down).

Technique: kVp: (70±5) _____

mrad

S 66	G<0.01 M
ML 13	0.1 F

	cm	kVp	mA	Time	mAs	SID	Film–Screen	Grid	F.S.
Model	21	70			32	72"	Kodak 400	12:1	S
Room									
S									
M									
L									
InSight									

AP Ribs – Below Diaphragm

For injury to lower ribs

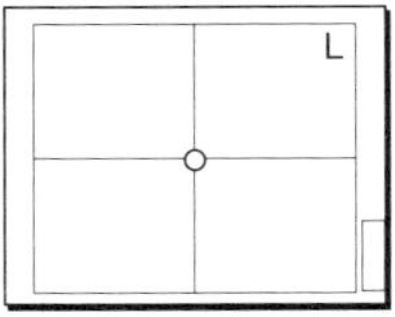

- 14 x 17" C.W. (35 x 43 cm)
- Grid

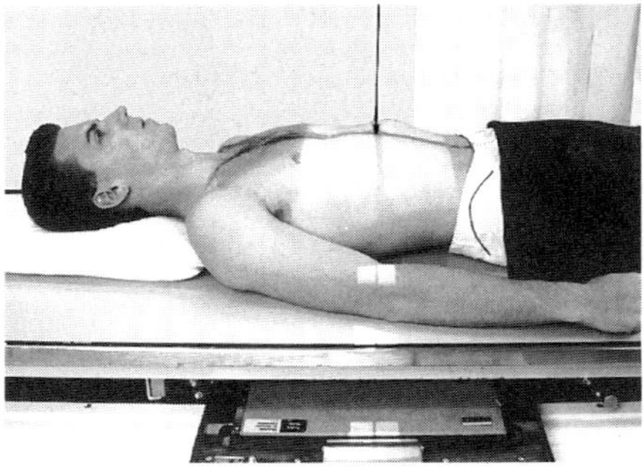

AP bilateral ribs (below diaphragm)

Position

- Erect, or recumbent, MSP to centerline of table and film (and CR).
- Inferior margin of film at iliac crest or slightly below.
- Ensure that both lateral margins of thorax are included.
- **Shield gonads** for male and female. (See gonadal doses as shown below without shields due to scatter and secondary.)

Note: Some routines include only unilateral ribs of affected side.

Central Ray

- CR ⊥, centered to film (level of ≈ T10, xiphoid tip).

SID: 72" (183 cm) erect; 40–48" (102–122 cm) recumbent.

Collimation: To rib margins or area of interest.

Respiration: Expose on **expiration** (diaphragm up).

Technique: kVp: (75±5) _____ mrad

S 120	G	2 M
ML 26		23 F

	cm	kVp	mA	Time	mAs	SID	Film–Screen	Grid	F.S.
Model	18	75			15	44"	Kodak 400	12:1	S
Room									
S									
M									
L									
InSight									

Bontrager Textbook, 3rd ed., p. 308

Anterior Oblique Ribs – PA

Side of interest **away from film**; or both R & L obliques to include entire rib cage.

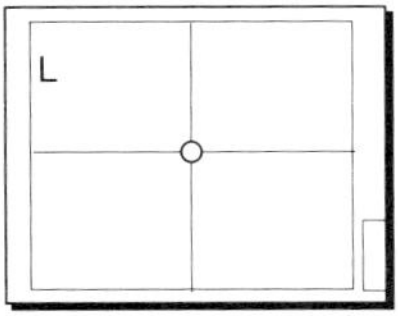

- 14 x 17" C.W. (35 x 43 cm)
- Grid

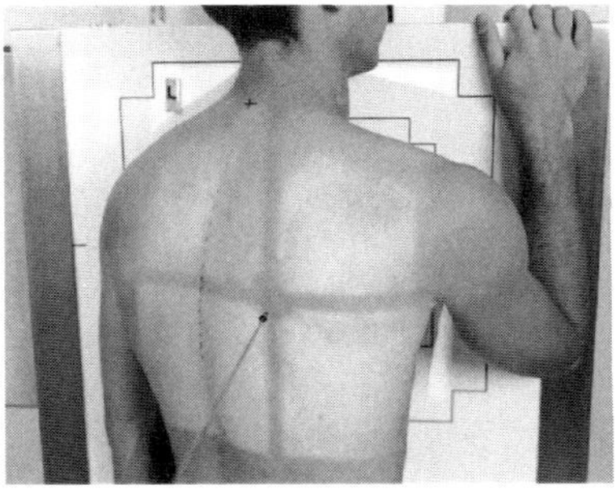

45° LAO above diaphragm – bilateral, right anterior injury (to shift spine away from injury)

Position

- Erect, or recumbent if needed.
- Oblique 45°, rotate spine away from area of interest.
- Entire thorax is centered to film bilaterally, with top of cassette ≈1 1/2" (4 cm) above shoulders.

Note: Some routines indicate unilateral oblique only of affected side, with smaller film L.W.

Central Ray

- CR ⊥, to center of film (level of T7).

SID: 72 (183 cm) erect, 40–48" (102–122 cm) recumbent.

Collimation: To area of interest.

Respiration: Above diaphragm - expose on inspiration.

Technique: kVp: (70±5) _____

mrad

S 91	G<0.01 M
ML 15	0.2 F

	cm	kVp	mA	Time	mAs	SID	Film–Screen	Grid	F.S.
Model Room	23	70			40	72"	Kodak 400	12:1	S
S									
M									
L									
InSight									

Posterior Oblique Ribs – AP

Side of interest **closest to film**; or both R & L obliques, to include entire rib cage. (Oblique to shift spine away from area of injury.)

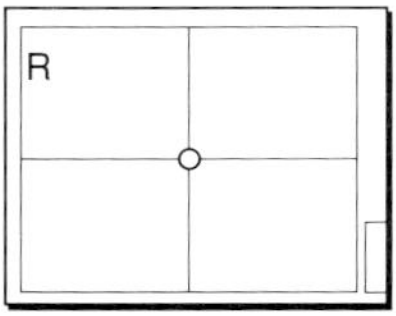

- 14 x 17" C.W. (35 x 43 cm)
- Grid

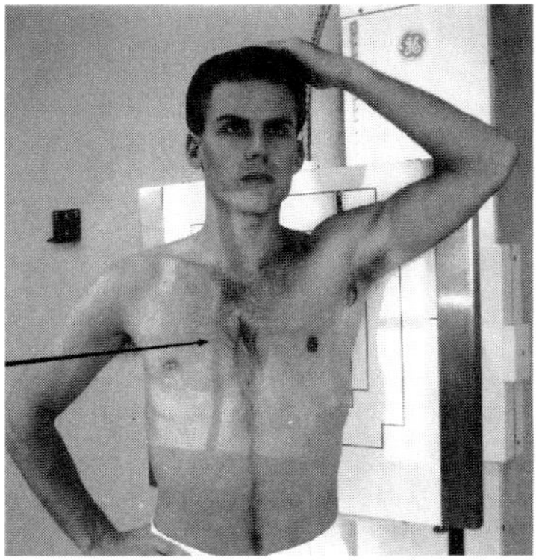

45° LPO (above diaphragm)

Position

- Erect, or recumbent (erect preferred).
- Top of cassette ≈ 1 1/2" (4 cm) above shoulders.
- Rotate 45° from AP, arm closest to film up, resting on head; opposite hand on waist with arm away from body.

Central Ray: CR ⊥, centered to film (level of T7).

SID: 72" (183 cm) erect, 40–48" (102–122 cm) recumbent.

Collimation: To area of interest.

Respiration: Above diaphragm - expose on inspiration.

Technique: kVp (70±5) _____ mrad

S 85	G<0.01 M
ML 14	0.2 F

	cm	kVp	mA	Time	mAs	SID	Film–Screen	Grid	F.S.
Model	23	70			40	72"	Kodak 400	12:1	S
Room									
S									
M									
L									
InSight									

Bontrager Textbook, 3rd ed., p. 310

Chest or Bony Thorax

Position:

Central Ray:

SID:

Collimation:

Respiration:

Technique:

	Room	cm	kVp	mA	Time	mAs	SID	Film–Screen	Grid	F.S.
S										
M										
L										
InSight										

Chest or Bony Thorax

Position:

Central Ray:

SID:

Collimation:

Respiration:

Technique:

	Room	cm	kVp	mA	Time	mAs	SID	Film–Screen	Grid	F.S.
S										
M										
L										
InSight										

Bontrager Textbook, 3rd ed., p.

Chapter 3

Upper Limb (Extremity)

3

Upper Limb

Upper Limb (Extremity)

Technical Factors

The following technical factors are important for all upper and lower limb procedures to maximize the sharpness, or the recorded detail of radiographs:

a. 40–48" (102–122 cm) SID, minimum OID
b. Small focal spot
c. TT (Table Top), detail (extremity) screens
d. Short exposure time
e. Immobilization (when needed)

Techniques provided are with Kodak lanex™ extremity screens and TMG film at 100 speed.

Radiation Protection

Collimation

Close collimation to the area of interest is important without "cutting off" essential anatomy. (Close collimation is the most effective practice for preventing unnecessary radiation exposure to the patient.)

Gonadal Shields

Erect patients: Patients seated at the end of the table should **always have a shield over their pelvic region** to prevent exposure from scatter radiation, and from the divergent primary beam.

Recumbent patients: A good practice to follow for upper limb exams for patients on a stretcher or table is to **always** have gonadal shields in place if the gonads are near the primary beam.

Patient Dose

Calculated patient doses based on the suggested "model" exposure factors for each projection are listed as skin (S), midline (ML) and gonads (G) doses for male and female. These doses assume gonadal shielding was in place (across patient's pelvic region) if patient is seated at the end of the table.

PA Fingers

Alternate routine: Include entire hand on PA finger projection for possible secondary trauma to other parts of hand (see PA hand).

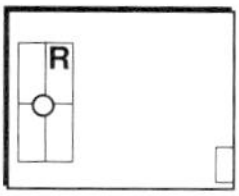

- 8 x 10" C.W. (20 x 24 cm)
- TT (detail screens)

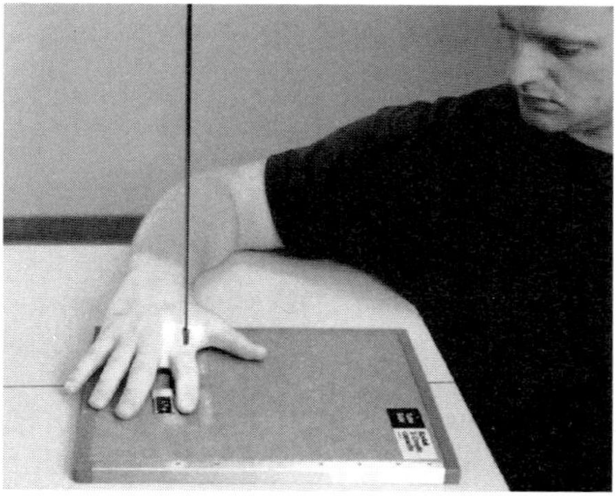

PA, 2nd digit

Position

- Patient seated at end of table, elbow flexed 90° (lead shield over lap).
- Pronate hand, separate fingers.
- Center and align long axis of affected finger(s) to portion of film being exposed.

Central Ray

- CR ⊥, centered to PIP joint.

SID: 40–48" (102–122 cm)

Collimation: On four sides to area of interest.

Technique: kVp (55±5) _____

mrad

S 6	G .NDC M
ML 6	<0.1 F

	cm	kVp	mA	Time	mAs	SID	Film–Screen	Grid	F.S.
Model Room	2	60			2	40"	Kodak 100	–	S
S									
M									
L									

Bontrager Textbook, 3rd ed., p. 112

Oblique Fingers

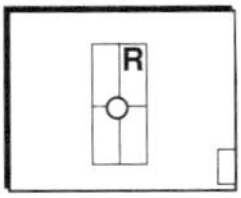

- 8 x 10" C.W. (20 x 24 cm)
- TT (detail screens)

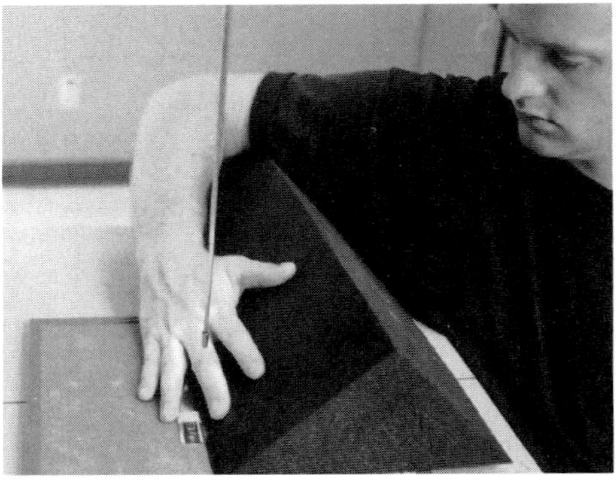

Oblique, 3rd digit (parallel to film)

Position

- Patient seated, hand on table, elbow flexed 90° (lead shield over lap).
- Align fingers to long axis of portion of film being exposed.
- Rotate hand 45°, resting on 45° angle support block.
- Separate fingers, ensure that affected finger(s) is (are) parallel to film.

Central Ray

- CR ⊥, centered to PIP joint.

SID: 40–48" (102–122 cm)

Collimation: On four sides to area of affected finger(s).

Technique: kVp (55±5) _____

mrad

S	6	G NDC M
ML	6	<0.1 F

	cm	kVp	mA	Time	mAs	SID	Film–Screen	Grid	F.S.
Model Room	2	60			2	40"	Kodak 100	–	S
S									
M									
L									

Bontrager Textbook, 3rd ed., p. 113

Lateral Fingers

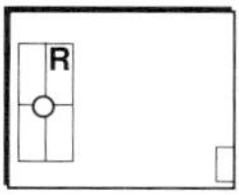

- 8 x 10" C.W. (20 x 24 cm)
- TT (detail screens)

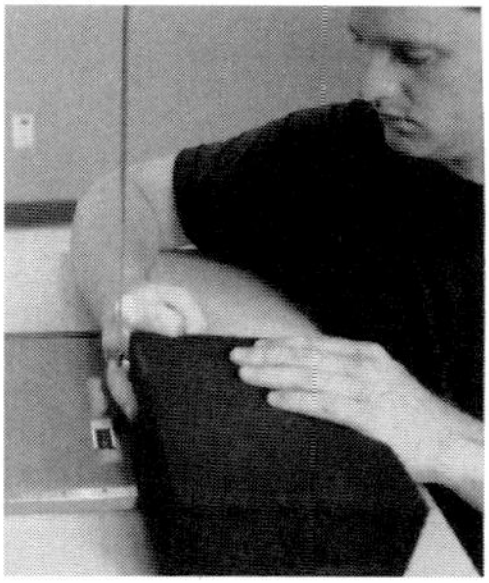

4th digit

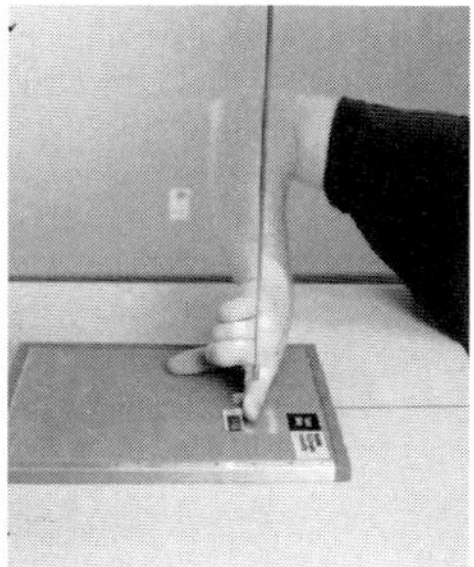

2nd digit

(digit parallel to film)

Position

- Patient seated, hand on table (lead shield over lap).
- Hand in lateral position, thumb side up for 3rd –5th digits, thumb side down for 2nd digit.
- Align finger to long axis of portion of film being exposed.

Central Ray

- CR ⊥, centered to PIP joint.

SID: 40–48" (102–122 cm)

Collimation: On four sides to area of affected finger.

Technique: kVp (55±5) _____

mrad		
	S 6	G NDC M
	ML 6	<0.1 F

	cm	kVp	mA	Time	mAs	SID	Film–Screen	Grid	F.S.
Model	2	60			2	40"	Kodak 100	–	S
Room									
S									
M									
L									

Bontrager Textbook, 3rd ed., p. 114

AP Thumb

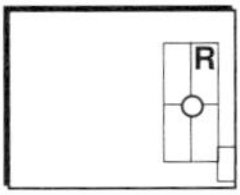

- 8 x 10" C.W. (20 x 24 cm)
- TT (detail screens)

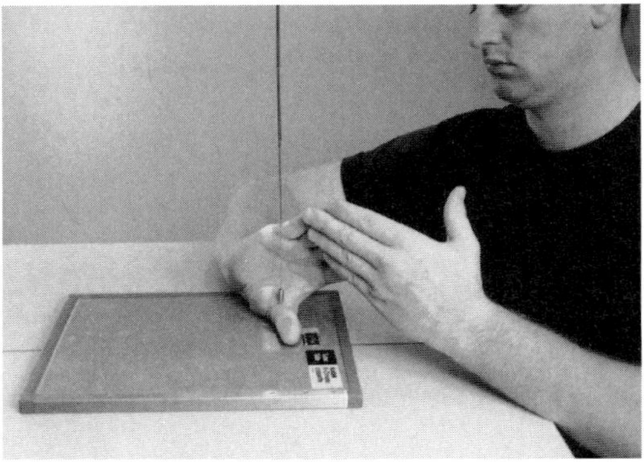

AP thumb, CR to 1st MP joint

Position

- Patient standing or seated, hand rotated internally with palm out to bring the posterior surface of thumb in direct contact with cassette.
- Align thumb to long axis of portion of film being exposed.

Central Ray

- CR ⊥, centered to 1st MP joint.

SID: 40–48" (102–122 cm)

Collimation: Collimate closely to area of thumb (include entire 1st metacarpal extending to carpals).

Technique: kVp (55±5) _____

mrad		
S	10	G NDC M
ML	10	<0.1 F

	cm	kVp	mA	Time	mAs	SID	Film–Screen	Grid	F.S.
Model Room	3	60			3	40"	Kodak 100	–	S
S									
M									
L									

Bontrager Textbook, 3rd ed., p. 115

Oblique Thumb

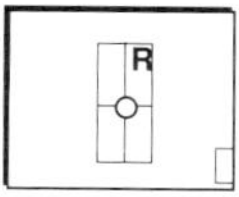

- 8 x 10" C.W. (20 x 24 cm)
- TT (detail screens)

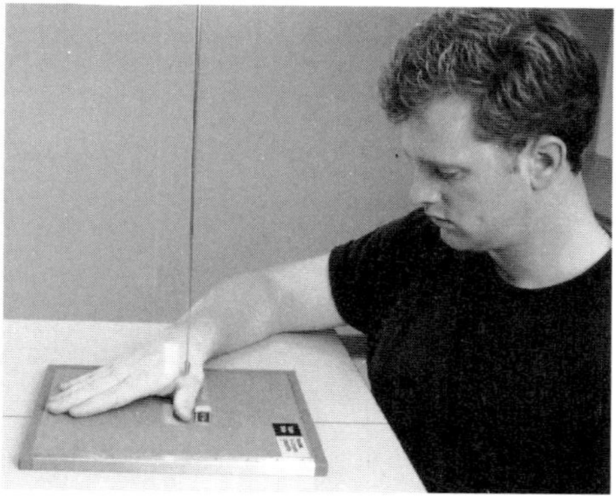

Oblique thumb, CR to 1st MP joint

Position

- Patient seated, hand on table, elbow flexed (shield over lap).
- Align thumb to long axis of portion of film being exposed.
- With hand pronated, abduct thumb slightly. This position tends to naturally rotate thumb into 45° oblique.

Central Ray

- CR ⊥, centered to 1st MP joint.

SID: 40–48" (102–122 cm)

Collimation: Collimate closely to area of thumb (include entire 1st metacarpal extending to carpals).

Technique: kVp (55±5) _____

mrad

S	10	G	NDC M
ML	10		<0.1 F

	cm	kVp	mA	Time	mAs	SID	Film–Screen	Grid	F.S.
Model Room	3	60			3	40"	Kodak 100	–	S
S									
M									
L									

Bontrager Textbook, 3rd ed., p. 117

Lateral Thumb

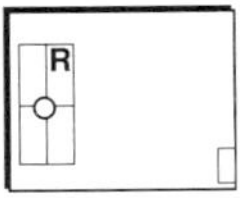

- 8 x 10" C.W. (20 x 24 cm)
- TT (detail screens)

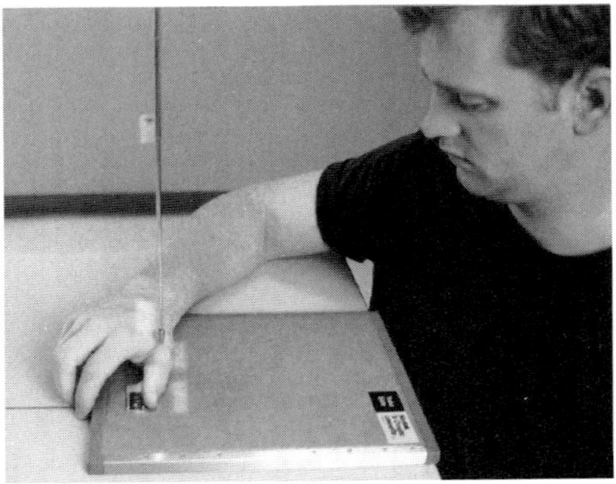

Lateral thumb, CR to 1st MP joint

Position

- Patient seated, hand on table, elbow flexed (shield across lap).
- Align thumb to long axis of portion of film being exposed.
- With hand pronated and slightly arched, rotate hand medially until thumb is in true lateral position.

Central Ray

- CR ⊥, centered to 1st MP joint.

SID: 40–48" (102–122 cm)

Collimation: Collimate closely to area of thumb (include entire 1st metacarpal extending to carpals).

Technique: kVp (55±5) _____

mrad

S	10	G	NDC M
ML	10		<0.1 F

	cm	kVp	mA	Time	mAs	SID	Film–Screen	Grid	F.S.
Model	3	60			3	40"	Kodak 100	–	S
Room									
S									
M									
L									

Bontrager Textbook, 3rd ed., p. 116

PA Hand

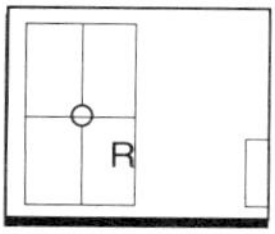

Small Hand
- 10 x 12" C.W.
  (24 x 30 cm)

or

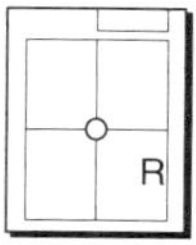

Large hand
- 8 x 10" L.W.
  (20 x 24 cm)

- TT (detail screens)

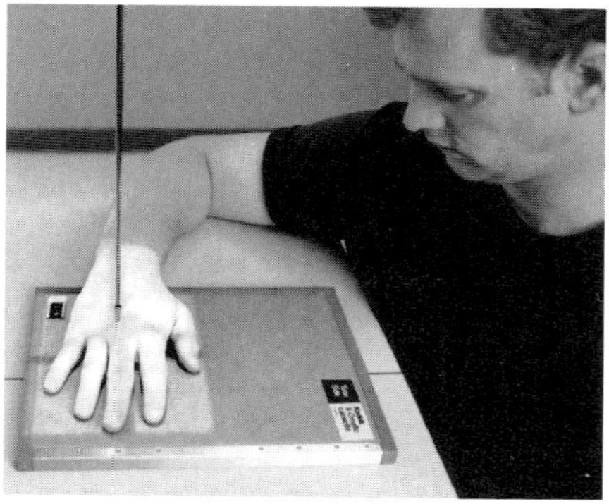

PA hand

Position

- Patient seated, hand on table, elbow flexed (shield across lap).
- Align long axis of hand and wrist parallel to edge of cassette.
- Hand fully pronated, digits slightly separated.

Central Ray

- CR ⊥, centered to 3rd MP joint.

SID: 40–48" (102–122 cm)

Collimation: Include entire hand and wrist.

Technique: kVp (60±5) _____

mrad		
	S 11	G NDC M
	ML 11	<0.1 F

	cm	kVp	mA	Time	mAs	SID	Film–Screen	Grid	F.S.
Model Room	4	62			3	40"	Kodak 100	–	S
S									
M									
L									

Bontrager Textbook, 3rd ed., p. 118

Oblique Hand

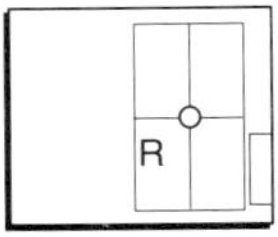

Small hand
- 10 x 12" C.W. (24 x 30 cm)

or

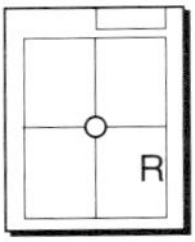

Large hand
- 8 x 10" L.W. (20 x 24 cm)

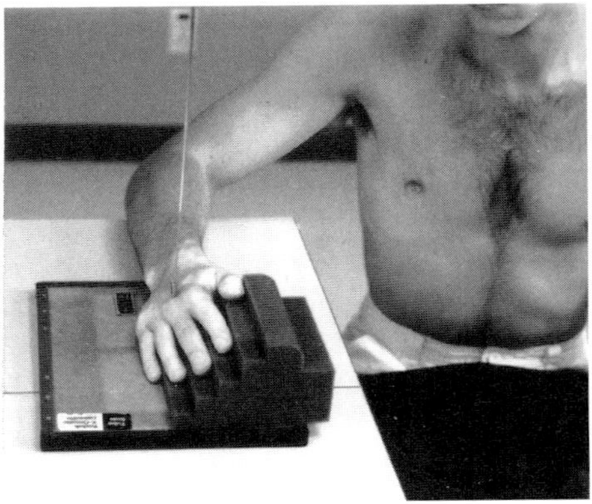

Oblique hand (digits parallel to film)

- TT (detail screens)

Position
- Patient seated, hand on table, elbow flexed (shield across lap).
- Rotate entire hand and wrist laterally 45°, support with wedge or step block. Align hand and wrist to cassette.
- Ensure that all digits are slightly separated and parallel to film.

Central Ray
- CR ⊥, centered to 3rd MP joint.

SID: 40–48" (102–122 cm)

Collimation: Include entire hand and wrist.

Technique: kVp (60±5) _____

mrad

S	12	G NDC M
ML	12	<0.1 F

	cm	kVp	mA	Time	mAs	SID	Film–Screen	Grid	F.S.
Model	4	64			3	40"	Kodak 100	–	S
Room									
S									
M									
L									

Bontrager Textbook, 3rd ed., p. 119

Lateral Hand

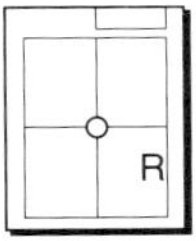

- 8 x 10" L.W. (20 x 24 cm)
- TT (detail screens)

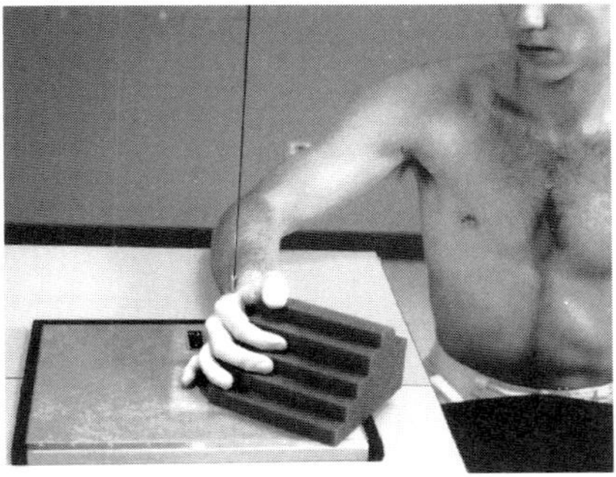

"'Fan" lateral hand (digits not superimposed)

Position

- Patient seated, hand on table, elbow flexed (shield across lap).
- Hand in lateral position, thumb side up, digits separated and spread into "fan" position and supported by radiolucent step block or similar type support.

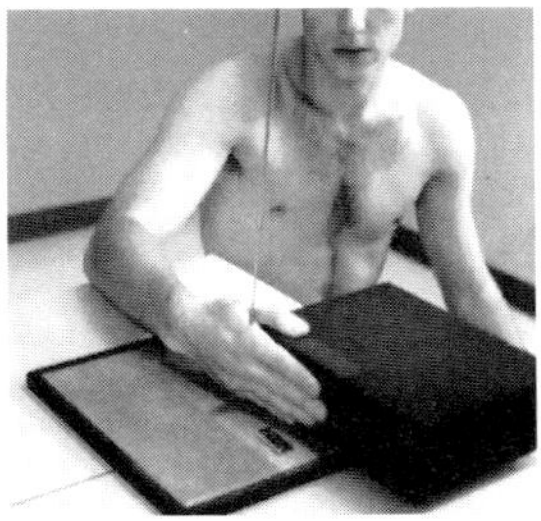

Alternate: lateral in extension (for possible foreign body & metacarpal injury)

Central Ray

- CR ⊥, centered to 2nd MP joint.

SID: 40–48" (102–122 cm)

Collimation: Include hand and wrist.

Technique: kVp (60±5) _____
(+ 4-6 kVp from PA and obli. hand)

mrad

S	14	G	NDC M
ML	8		<0.1 F

	cm	kVp	mA	Time	mAs	SID	Film–Screen	Grid	F.S.
Model	4	66			3	40"	Kodak 100	–	S
Room									
S									
M									
L									

Bontrager Textbook, 3rd ed., p. 120, 121

PA Wrist

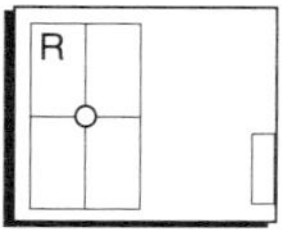

- 10 x 12" C.W. (24 x 30 cm)
- TT (detail screens)

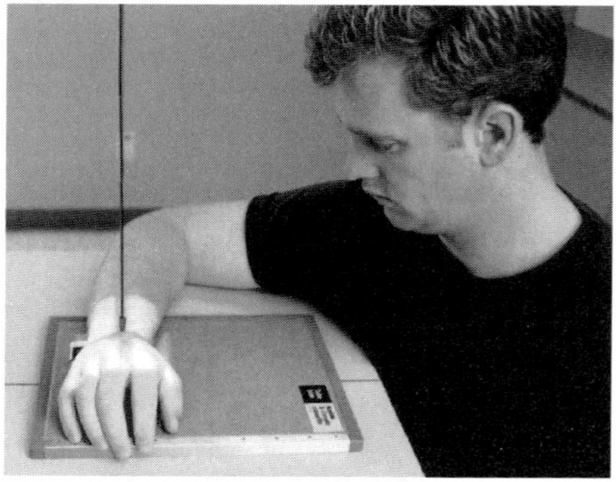

PA wrist (hand arched slightly)

Position

- Patient seated, arm on table (shield across lap).
- Align hand and wrist parallel to edge of cassette.
- Lower shoulder, rest arm on table to ensure no rotation of wrist.
- Hand pronated, fingers flexed and hand arched slightly to place wrist in direct contact with surface of cassette.

Central Ray

- CR ⊥, centered to mid carpals.

SID: 40–48" (102–122 cm)

Collimation: Include at least proximal 2/3 of metacarpals and the distal 1/3 of forearm.

Technique: kVp (60±5) _____

mrad

S 14	G	NDC M
ML 14		<0.1 F

	cm	kVp	mA	Time	mAs	SID	Film–Screen	Grid	F.S.
Model Room	4	62			4	40"	Kodak 100	–	S
S									
M									
L									

Oblique Wrist

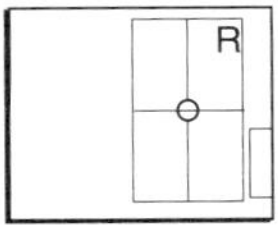

- 10 x 12" C.W. (24 x 30 cm)
- TT (detail screens)

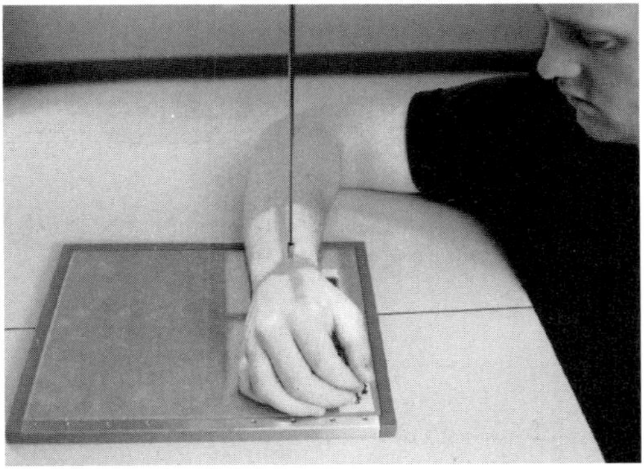

45° oblique wrist

Position

- Patient seated, arm on table, elbow flexed (shield across lap).
- Align hand and wrist parallel to edge of cassette.
- Rotate hand and wrist into 45° oblique position.
- Flex fingers to support hand in this position, or use 45° support block.

Central Ray

- CR ⊥, centered to mid carpals.

SID: 40–48" (102–122 cm)

Collimation: Include at least proximal 2/3 of metacarpals and distal 1/3 of forearm.

Technique: kVp (60±5) _____

mrad

S 16	G NDC M
ML 14	<0.1 F

	cm	kVp	mA	Time	mAs	SID	Film–Screen	Grid	F.S.
Model Room	5	64			4	40"	Kodak 100	–	S
S									
M									
L									

Lateral Wrist

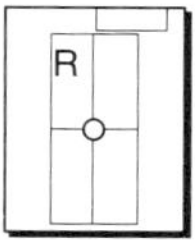

- 8 x 10" L.W. (20 x 24 cm)
- TT (detail screens)

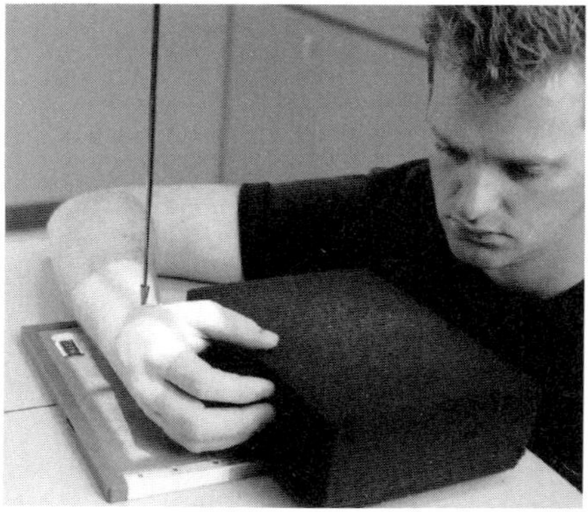

Lateral wrist

Position

- Patient seated, arm on table, elbow flexed, shoulder dropped to place humerus, forearm and wrist on same horizontal plane.
- Align hand and wrist parallel to edge of cassette.
- Place hand and wrist into a true lateral position, use support to maintain this position if needed.

Central Ray

- CR ⊥, centered to mid carpals.

SID: 40–48" (102–122 cm)

Collimation: Include at least proximal 2/3 of metacarpals and distal 1/3 of forearm.

Technique: kVp (60±5) _____
(+ ≈4 kVp from PA and obli. wrist)

mrad

S 22	G NDC M
ML 16	<0.1 F

	cm	kVp	mA	Time	mAs	SID	Film–Screen	Grid	F.S.
Model Room	7	66			5	40"	Kodak 100	–	S
S									
M									
L									

Bontrager Textbook, 3rd ed., p. 124

PA Wrist - Ulnar Flexion

Warning: The ulnar flexion view should only be attempted with possible wrist trauma after a routine wrist series rules out gross fractures to wrist or distal forearm.

These are special projections for the **scaphoid**.

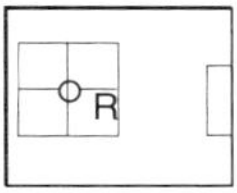

- 8 x 10" C.W. (20 x 24 cm)
- TT (detail screens)

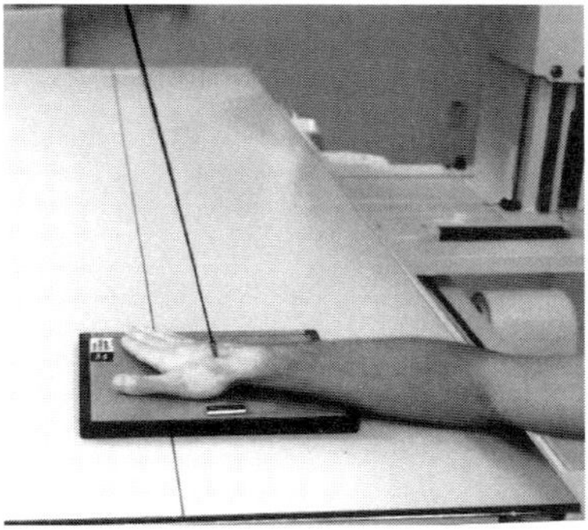

Ulnar flexion, CR 10–15° angle toward elbow

Position

- From PA wrist position, gently evert or flex wrist toward ulnar side as far as patient can tolerate.

Central Ray: Angle CR 10–15° toward elbow, centered to scaphoid (thumb side of carpal area).

Note: Additional CR angle of 20-30° may aid in demonstrating scaphoid fractures.[1]

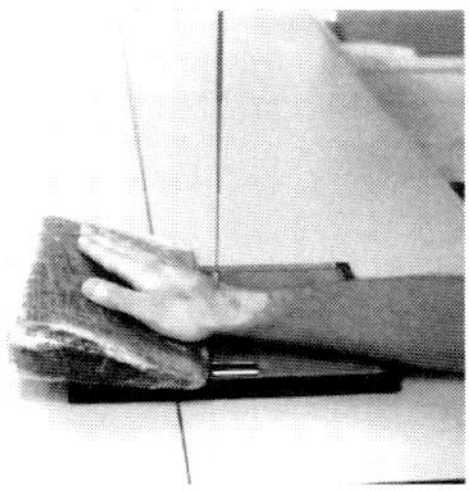

Modified Stecher method[2]
Elevate hand on 20° sponge, CR ⊥ to floor, ulnar flexion if poss.

SID: 40–48" (102–122 cm)

Collimation: To carpal region.

Technique: kVp (60±5) _____

mrad

S 16	G NDC M
ML 16	<0.1 F

	cm	kVp	mA	Time	mAs	SID	Film–Screen	Grid	F.S.
Model Room	4	64			4	40"	Kodak 100	–	S
S									
M									
L									

Bontrager Textbook, 3rd ed., p. 125

PA Wrist - Radial Flexion

Warning: This position should be attempted for possible wrist trauma only after a routine wrist series rules out gross fractures to wrist or distal forearm.

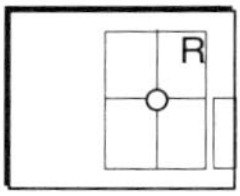

- 8 x 10" C.W. (20 x 24 cm)
- TT (detail screens)

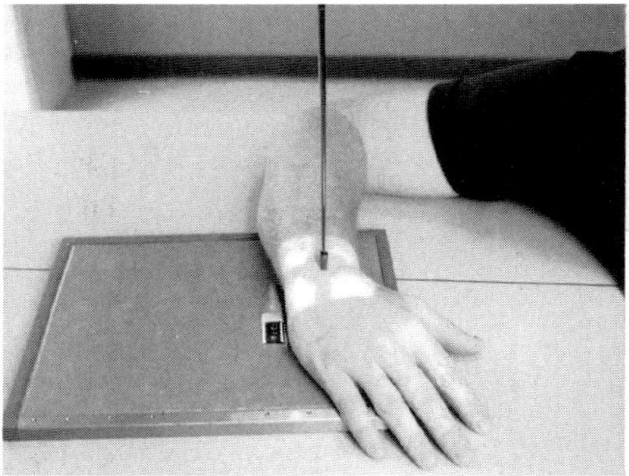

Radial flexion, CR perpendicular (demonstrates ulnar side carpals)

Position

- From PA wrist position, gently invert or flex wrist toward radial side as far as patient can tolerate (shield across lap).

Central Ray

- CR ⊥, to mid carpals.

SID: 40–48" (102–122 cm)

Collimation: Collimate closely to carpal area (≈3" or 7.5 cm square).

Technique: kVp (55±5) _____

mrad

S	16	G NDC M
ML	16	<0.1 F

	cm	kVp	mA	Time	mAs	SID	Film–Screen	Grid	F.S.
Model	4	64			4	40"	Kodak 100	–	S
Room									
S									
M									
L									

Wrist - Carpal Canal
(Gaynor-Hart Tangential Projection)

Warning: This position is sometimes called the "tunnel view" and should be attempted for possible wrist trauma only after a routine wrist series rules out gross fractures to wrist or distal forearm.

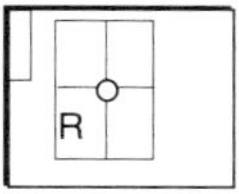

- 8 x 10" C.W. (20 x 24 cm)
- TT (detail screens)

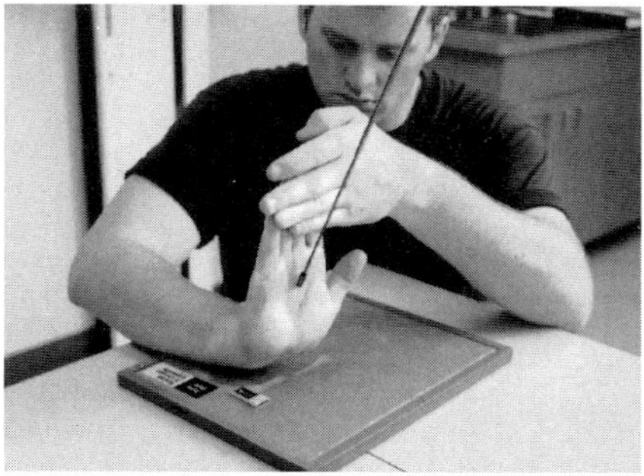

Carpal canal (tunnel) projection
(CR 25–30° to long axis of hand)

Position
- Patient seated, hand on table (shield across lap).
- Hyperextend (dorsiflex) wrist as far as patient can tolerate with patient using other hand to hold fingers back.
- Rotate hand and wrist internally slightly (≈ 5-10°).
- Work quickly as this may be painful for patient.

Central Ray
- CR 25–30° to long axis of the palmar surface of hand, centered to ≈1 1/2" (3 cm) distal to base of 3rd metacarpal.

SID: 40–48" (102–122 cm)

Collimation: Collimate closely to carpal area (≈3" square).

Technique: kVp (60±5) _____

mrad

S 20	G NDC M
ML 19	<0.1 F

	cm	kVp	mA	Time	mAs	SID	Film–Screen	Grid	F.S.
Model Room	5	65			5	40"	Kodak 100	–	S
S									
M									
L									

Bontrager Textbook, 3rd ed., p. 127

AP Forearm

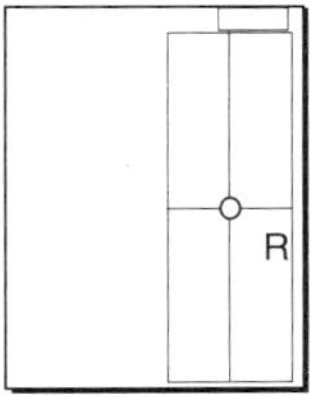

- 14 x 17" L.W. (35 x 43 cm)
- TT (detail screens)

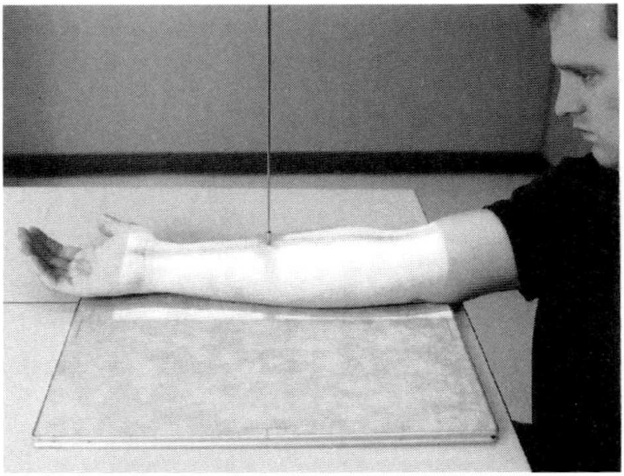

AP forearm (to include both joints)

Position

- Patient seated at end of table with arm extended, and hand supinated (shield across lap).
- Ensure that both wrist and elbow joints are included unless contraindicated.
- Have patient lean laterally as needed for a true AP of forearm.

Central Ray

- CR ⊥, centered to midpoint of forearm.

SID: 40–48" (102–122 cm)

Collimation: Collimate on four sides, include a minimum of 1" (2.5 cm) beyond both wrist and elbow joints.

Technique: kVp (60±5) _____

mrad

S	24	G NDC M
ML	13	<0.1 F

	cm	kVp	mA	Time	mAs	SID	Film–Screen	Grid	F.S.
Model	8	62			6	40"	Kodak 100	–	S
Room									
S									
M									
L									

Bontrager Textbook, 3rd ed., p. 130

Lateral Forearm

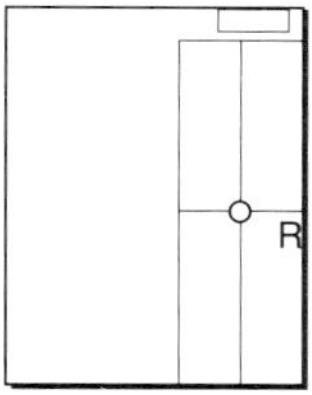

- 14 x 17" L.W. (35 x 43 cm)
- TT (detail screens)

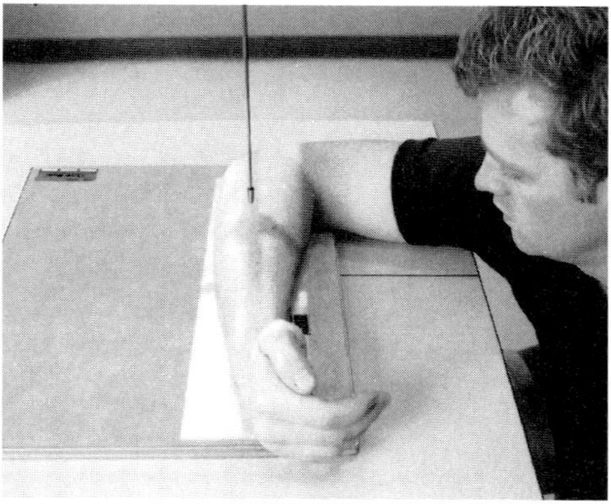

Lateral forearm (to include both joints)

Position

- Patient seated at end of table (shield across lap).
- Elbow should be flexed 90°.
- Hand and wrist must be in a true lateral position (distal radius and ulna should be directly superimposed).
- Ensure that both wrist and elbow joints are included unless contraindicated.

Central Ray: CR ⊥, centered to midpoint of forearm.

SID: 40–48" (102–122 cm)

Collimation: Collimate on four sides, include a minimum of 1" (2.5 cm) beyond both wrist and elbow joints.

Technique: kVp (64±5) _____
(+4 kVp from AP)

mrad

S	28	G NDC M
ML	16	<0.1 F

	cm	kVp	mA	Time	mAs	SID	Film–Screen	Grid	F.S.
Model Room	8	66			6	40"	Kodak 100	–	S
S									
M									
L									

Bontrager Textbook, 3rd ed., p. 131

AP Elbow

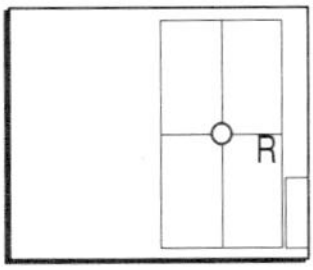

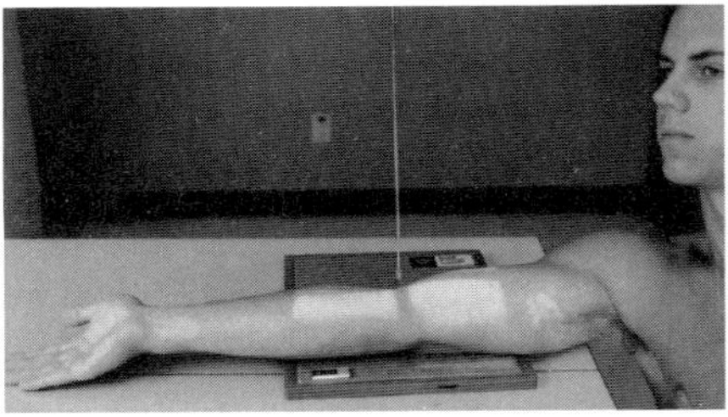

AP, fully extended

- 10 x 12" C.W. (24 x 30 cm)
- TT (detail screens)

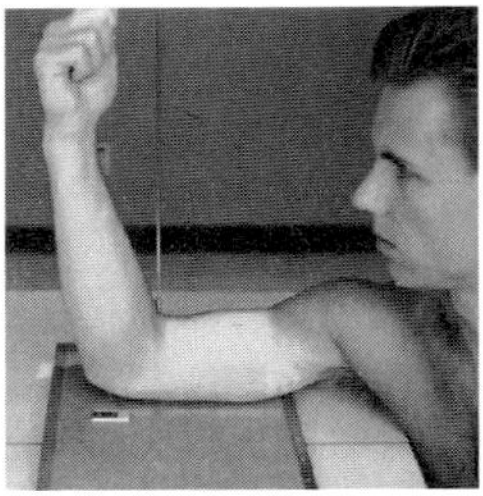

CR ⊥ humerus

Position

- Elbow extended and hand supinated (shield across lap).
- Lean laterally as needed for true AP (palpate epicondyles).
- If elbow cannot be fully extended, take two AP projections as shown with CR perpendicular to humerus on one, and perpendicular to forearm on another.

Central Ray

- CR ⊥, centered to mid elbow joint.

SID: 40–48" (102–122 cm)

Collimation: To area of interest.

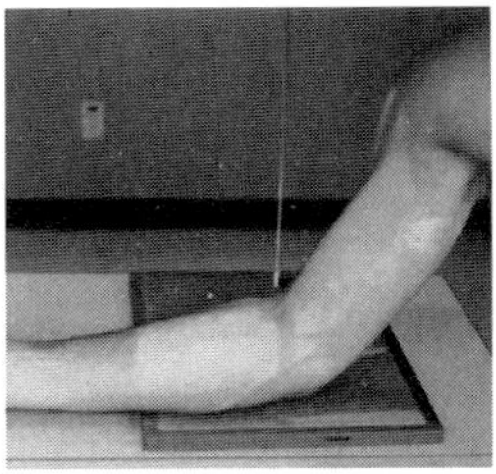

CR ⊥ forearm

Technique: kVp (60±5) _____

mrad		
	S 25	G NDC M
	ML 17	<0.1 F

	cm	kVp	mA	Time	mAs	SID	Film–Screen	Grid	F.S.
Model Room	7	64			6	40"	Kodak 100	–	S
S									
M									
L									

Bontrager Textbook, 3rd ed., p. 134

Oblique Elbow

Internal oblique best visualizes **coronoid process** (most common)
External oblique best visualizes **radial head** and **neck**

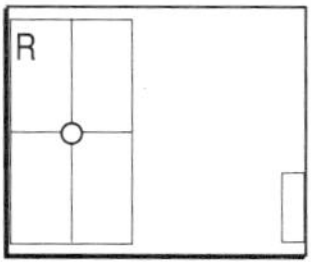

- 10 x 12" C.W. (24 x 30 cm)
- TT (detail screens)

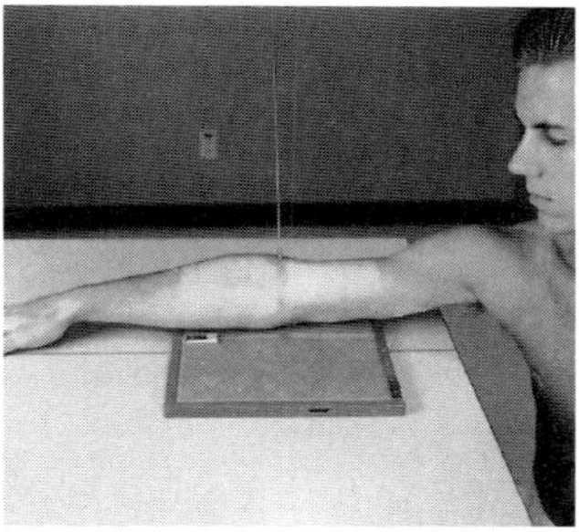

Internal obli. (45°)

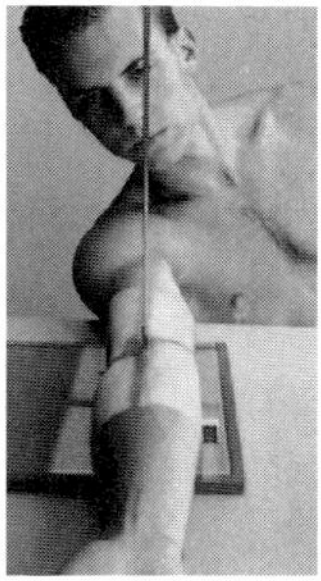

External Obli. (40-45°)

Position (Internal Oblique)

- Elbow extended, hand pronated (shield across lap).
- Palpate epicondyles to check for 45° internal rotation.

External Oblique: Similar position except supinate hand and rotate elbow 40–45° externally. This is more difficult for patient to achieve; lean entire upper body laterally as needed.

Central Ray

- CR ⊥, centered to mid elbow joint.

SID: 40–48" (102–122 cm)

Collimation: To area of interest.

Technique: kVp (60±5) _____

mrad per projection

S 25	G NDC M
ML 17	<0.1 F

	cm	kVp	mA	Time	mAs	SID	Film–Screen	Grid	F.S.
Model	7	64			6	40"	Kodak 100	–	S
Room									
S									
M									
L									

Bontrager Textbook, 3rd ed., p. 135, 136

Lateral Elbow

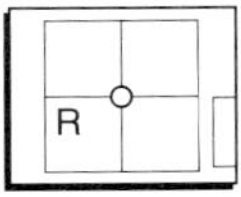

- 8 x 10" C.W. (20 x 24 cm)
- TT (detail screens)

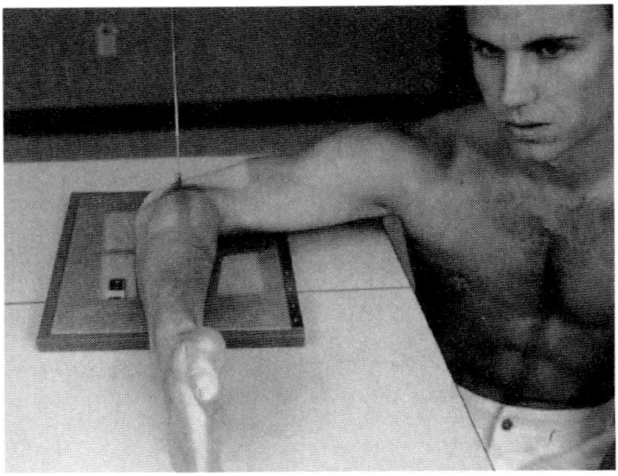

Lateral elbow, flexed 90°

Position

- Elbow flexed 90°, shoulder dropped as needed to rest forearm and humerus on table and cassette (shield across lap).
- Center elbow to center of cassette or to portion of film being exposed, with forearm aligned parallel to edge of cassette.
- Place hand and wrist in a true lateral position.

Central Ray

- CR ⊥, centered to mid elbow joint.

SID: 40–48" (102–122 cm)

Collimation: Collimate on four sides, include a minimum of ≈2" (5 cm) of forearm and humerus.

Technique: kVp (60±5) _____

mrad

S 25	G NDC M
ML 17	<0.1 F

	cm	kVp	mA	Time	mAs	SID	Film–Screen	Grid	F.S.
Model	7	64			6	40"	Kodak 100	–	S
Room									
S									
M									
L									

Bontrager Textbook, 3rd ed., p. 137

Axiolateral Elbow
(Coyle Trauma Method)[1]

Special views to demonstrate radial head and coronoid process.

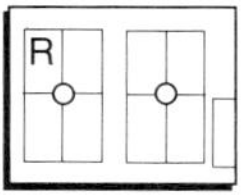

- 8 x 10" C.W. (20 x 24 cm)
- TT (detail screens)

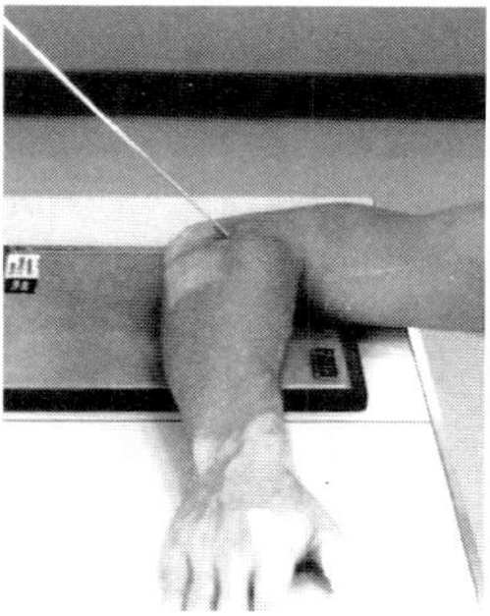

For radial head and neck, elbow flexed **90°**

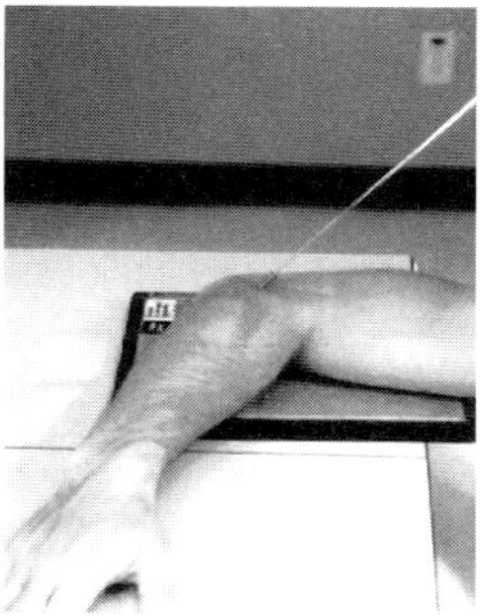

For coronoid process, elbow flexed <u>**80°**</u>**.** (Flexion of more than 80° will obscure coronoid process)

Position and Central Ray

Radial Head and Neck:
- Elbow flexed 90° if possible, with hand pronated.
- Angle CR 45° toward thorax, centered to radial head and neck. (CR to enter at mid elbow joint.)

Coronoid Process:
- Elbow flexed **only 80°**, with hand pronated.
- Angle CR 45° away from thorax, centered to coronoid process. (CR to enter at mid elbow joint.)

SID: 40–48" (102–122 cm)

Collimation: Collimate closely to area of interest.

Technique: kVp (65±5) ____
(+ 4 kVp from lateral elbow)

mrad per projection

S 29	G NDC M
ML 18	<0.1 F

	cm	kVp	mA	Time	mAs	SID	Film–Screen	Grid	F.S.
Model Room	8	68			6	40"	Kodak 100	–	S
S									
M									
L									

Bontrager Textbook, 3rd ed., p. 139

AP Humerus

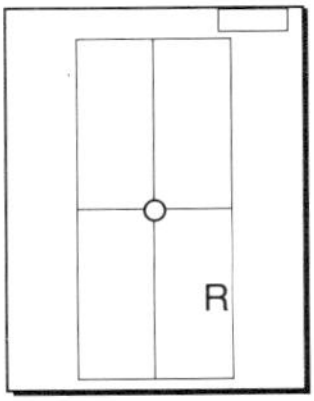

- 14 x 17" L.W. (35 x 43 cm)
  or for small patient
  11 x 14" L.W. (30 x 35 cm)
- Grid >10 cm, Screen <10 cm

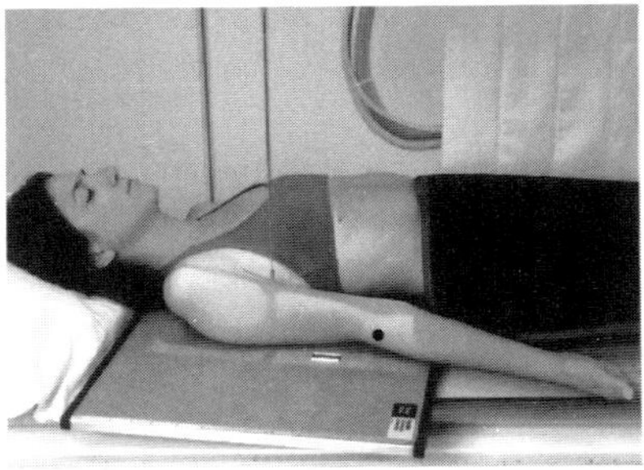

AP supine

Position

- Erect or supine with humerus aligned to long axis of cassette (unless diagonal placement is needed to **include both elbow and shoulder joints**). Place shield over gonads.
- Abduct arm slightly, supinate hand for true AP. (Epicondyles parallel to film.)

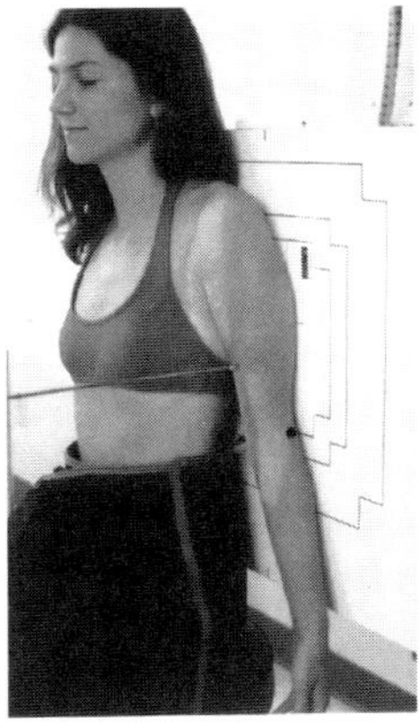

AP erect

Central Ray

- CR ⊥, to mid humerus.

SID: 40–48" (102–122 cm)

Collimation: Collimate on four sides to area of interest.

Technique: kVp, grid, (70±5) _____
screen, (60±5) _____

mrad

S	33	G NDC M
ML	16	<0.1 F

	cm	kVp	mA	Time	mAs	SID	Film–Screen	Grid	F.S.
Model	9	70			6	40"	Kodak 100	–	S
Room									
S									
M									
L									

Bontrager Textbook, 3rd ed., p. 141

Rotational Lateral Humerus

Warning: Do not attempt to rotate arm if fracture or dislocation is suspected (see following page for trauma lateral).

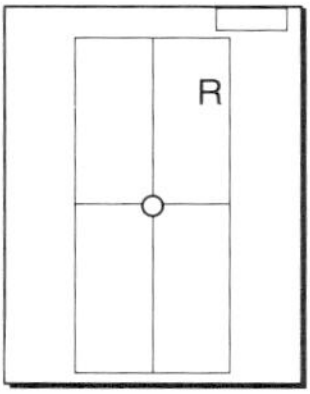

- 14 x 17" L.W. (35 x 43 cm) or 11 x 14" L.W.
- Grid >10 cm, Screen <10

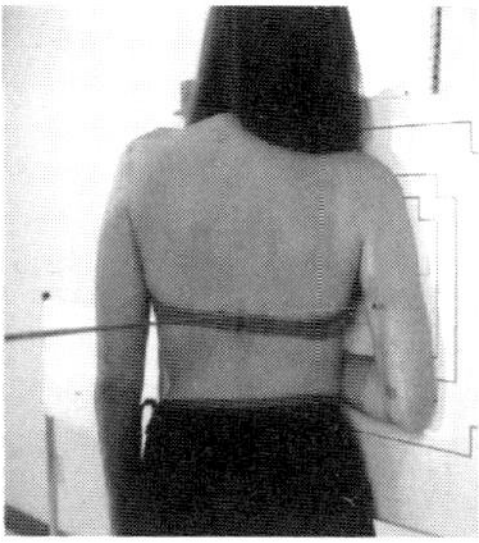

Erect lateral (PA)

or

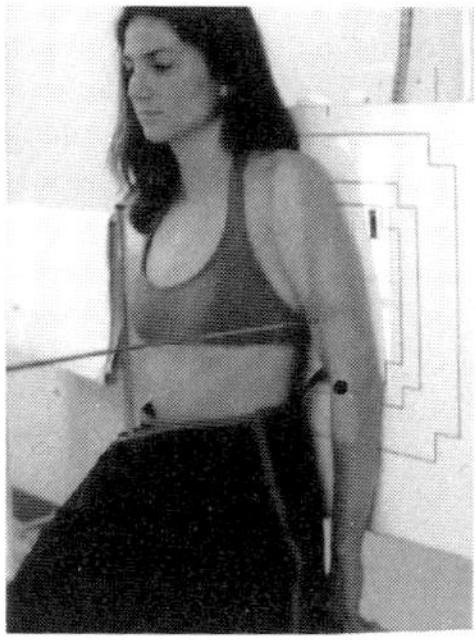

Erect lateral (AP)

Position (may be taken erect AP or PA, or supine)

- **Erect (PA):** Elbow flexed 90°, patient rotated 15–20° from PA or as needed to bring humerus and shoulder in contact with film holder (epicondyles ⊥ to film for true lateral).
- **Erect or Supine AP:** Elbow slightly flexed, arm and wrist rotated for lateral position (palm back), epicondyles ⊥ to film.
- Film centered to **include both elbow and shoulder joints**.

Central Ray: CR ⊥, to mid humerus.

SID: 40–48" (102–122 cm)

Collimation: To area of interest.

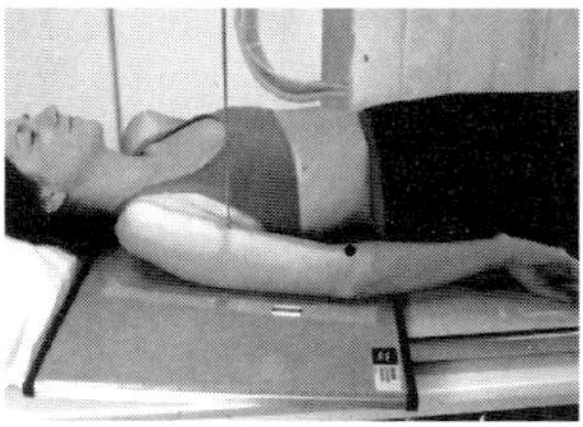

Supine lateral

Technique: kVp, grid, (70±5) _____
screen, (60±5) _____

	cm	kVp	mA	Time	mAs	SID	Film–Screen	Grid	F.S.
Model	9	70			6	40"	Kodak 100	–	S
Room									
S									
M									
L									

mrad		
	S 33	G NDC M
	ML 16	<0.1 F

Bontrager Textbook, 3rd ed., p. 142

Trauma Lateral Humerus
(mid and distal humerus)

For proximal humerus see transthoracic lateral or scapular Y in following chapter.

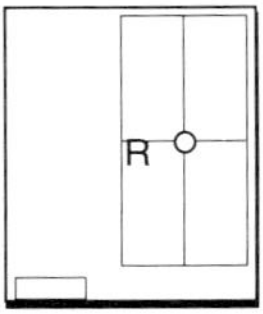

- 11 x 14" L.W. (30 x 35 cm) or 10 x 12" L.W. (24 x 30 cm)
- TT (detail screens)

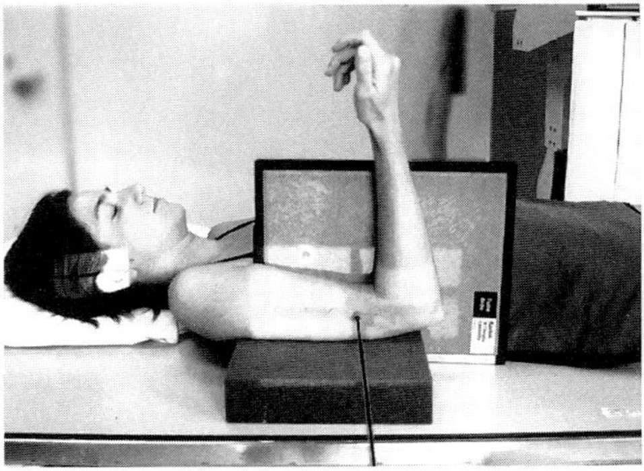

Lateral cross table, mid and distal humerus

Position

- Gently lift arm and place support block under arm, rotate hand into lateral position if possible for true lateral elbow projection.
- Place cassette vertically between arm and thorax with top of cassette at axilla (place shield between cassette and patient).

Central Ray

- CR horizontal and ⊥ to film, centered to distal 1/3 of humerus.

SID: 40–48" (102–122 cm)

Collimation: On four sides, include elbow joint and proximal forearm.

Technique: kVp (65±5) _____

mrad

S	28	G	NDC M
ML	16		<0.1 F

	cm	kVp	mA	Time	mAs	SID	Film–Screen	Grid	F.S.
Model	8	66			6	40"	Kodak 100	–	S
Room									
S									
M									
L									

Bontrager Textbook, 3rd ed., p. 144

Pediatric AP Upper Limb

With possible trauma, handle limb very gently with minimal movement. Take a single exposure to rule out gross fractures before additional radiographs are taken.

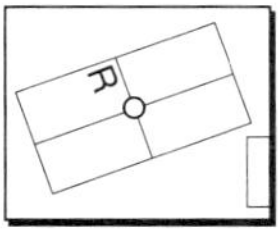

- Film size determined by patient age and size
- TT (detail screens)

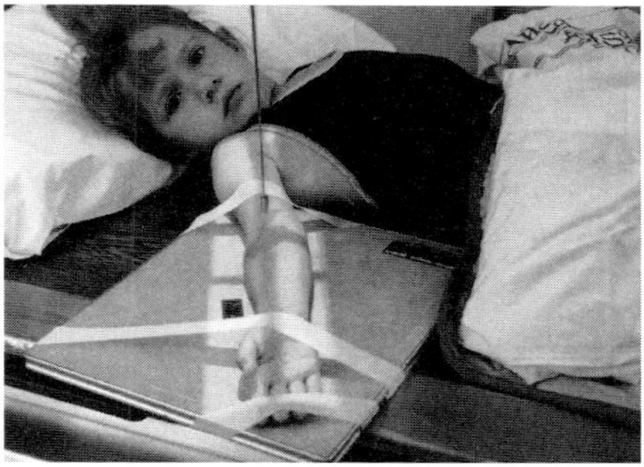

AP, upper limb

Position

- Supine position, arm abducted away from body, lead shield over pelvic area.
- Include entire limb unless a specific joint or bone is indicated.
- Immobilize with clear flexible type retention band and sandbags, or with tape.
- Use parental assistance only if necessary, provide lead gloves and apron.

Central Ray: CR ⊥, centered to midlimb.

SID: 40–48" (102–122 cm)

Collimation: On four sides to area of interest.

Technique: kVp (50±5) _____

mrad		
	S 13	G NDC M
	ML 13	<0.1 F

	cm	kVp	mA	Time	mAs	SID	Film–Screen	Grid	F.S.
Model	4	60			4	40"	Kodak 100	–	S
Room									
S									
M									
L									

Bontrager Textbook, 3rd ed., p. 560

Pediatric Lateral Upper Limb

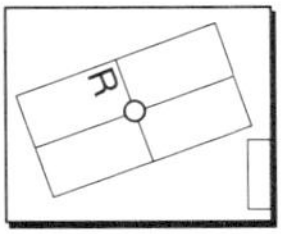

- Film size determined by patient age and size
- TT (detail screens)

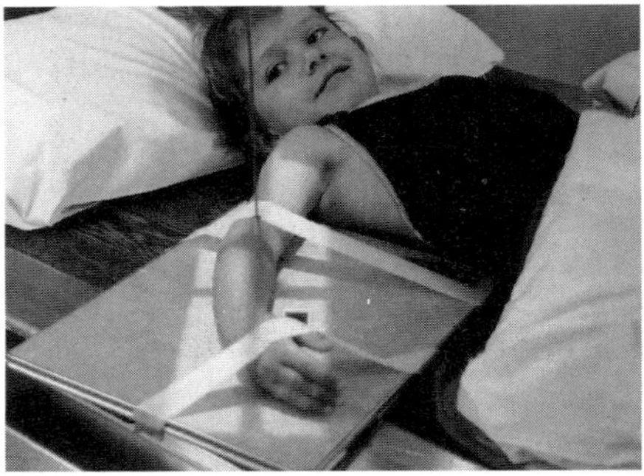

Lateral, upper limb

Position

- Supine position with arm abducted away from body, lead shield over pelvic area.
- Include entire limb unless a specific joint or bone is indicated.
- Immobilize with clear flexible type retention band and/or with sandbags or with tape.
- Flex elbow and rotate entire arm into a lateral position.
- Use parental assistance only if necessary, provide lead gloves and apron.

Central Ray

- CR ⊥, centered to mid limb.

SID: 40–48" (102–122 cm)

Collimation: On four sides to area of interest.

Technique: kVp (50±5) _____

mrad		
	S 13	G NDC M
	ML 13	<0.1 F

	cm	kVp	mA	Time	mAs	SID	Film–Screen	Grid	F.S.
Model Room	4	60			4	40"	Kodak 100	–	S
S									
M									
L									

Bontrager Textbook, 3rd ed., p. 560

Upper Limb

Position:

Central Ray:

SID:

Collimation:

Respiration:

Technique:

	Room	cm	kVp	mA	Time	mAs	SID	Film–Screen	Grid	F.S.
S										
M										
L										

Upper Limb

Position:

Central Ray:

SID:

Collimation:

Respiration:

Technique:

	cm	kVp	mA	Time	mAs	SID	Film–Screen	Grid	F.S.
Model									
Room									
S									
M									
L									

Chapter 4

Shoulder Girdle
Shoulder, Clavicle, Scapula, & AC Joints

AP Shoulder
Ext. and Int. Rotation

Warning: Do not attempt if fracture or dislocation is suspected.

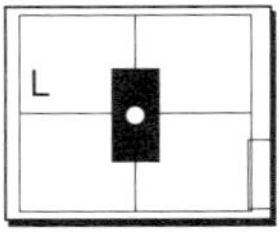

- 10 x 12" C.W. (24 x 30 cm)
- Grid

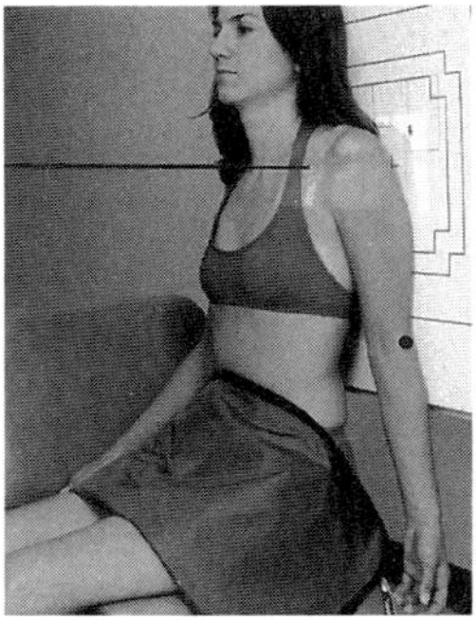
External (AP humerus)

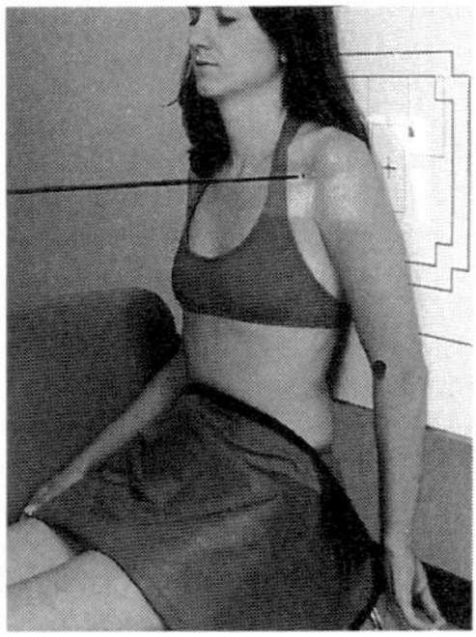
Internal (lat. humerus)

Position

- Erect (seated or standing) or supine, arm slightly abducted.
- Rotate thorax as needed to place posterior shoulder against film holder. • Center of cassette to glenohumeral joint and CR.

  External Rotation: Rotate arm externally until hand is supinated and epicondyles are parallel to film.

  Internal Rotation: Rotate arm internally until hand is pronated and epicondyles are perpendicular to film.

Central Ray: CR ⊥, to mid glenohumeral joint (≈1" (2.5 cm) inferior and lateral to coracoid process).

SID: 40–48" (102–122 cm)

Collimation: On four sides to area of interest.

Respiration: Suspend during exposure.

Technique: kVp (70±5) ______ mrad, two projections

S 70	G NDC M
ML 24	<0.1 F

	cm	kVp	mA	Time	mAs	SID	Film–Screen	Grid	F.S.
Model Room	12	70			6	44"	Kodak 400	12:1	S
S									
M									
L									

Bontrager Textbook, 3rd ed., pp. 155-156

Axiolateral Shoulder

Inferosuperior Projection (Lawrence Method)

Warning: Do not attempt if fracture or dislocation is suspected

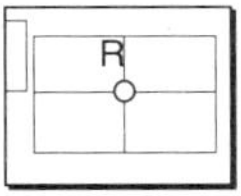

- 8 x 10" C.W. (20 x 24 cm)
- Stationary grid; grid lines horizontal and CR to centerline of grid.

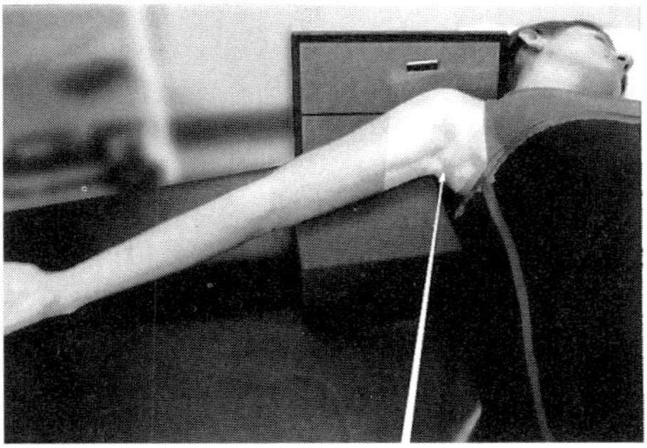

Inferosuperior (axiolateral)

Position (Inferosuperior)

- Patient supine, to front edge of table or stretcher, with support under shoulder to center part to center line of cassette, head turned away from cassette.
- Arm abducted 90° from body.
- Rotate arm externally, hand supinated.

Central Ray: CR horizontal, directed to axilla (place tube next to table or stretcher at same level as axilla).

SID: 40–48" (102–122 cm)

Collimation: To area of interest.

Respiration: Suspend during exposure.

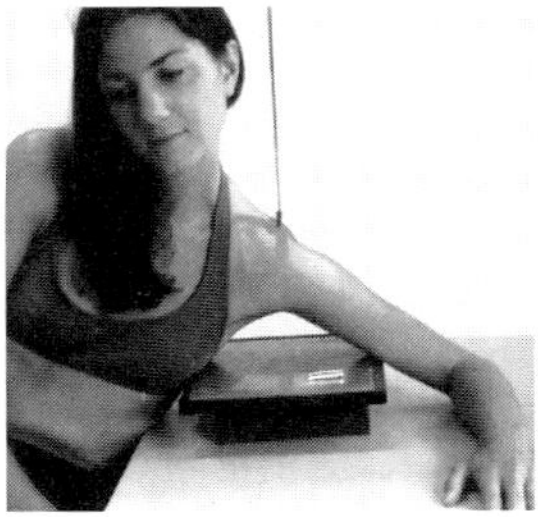

Alternate erect supero-inferior projection.[1,2]
- Abduct arm, flex elbow 90°.
- CR 5-10° toward elbow.

Technique: kVp (70±5) ______

	cm	kVp	mA	Time	mAs	SID	Film–Screen	Grid	F.S.
Model	15	65			10	40"	Kodak 400	6:1	S
Room									
S									
M									
L									

mrad

S 39	G NDC M
ML 12	<0.1 F

Bontrager Textbook, 3rd ed., p. 157

Posterior Oblique Shoulder
Glenoid Cavity (Grashey Method)

Special projection for visualizing glenoid cavity in profile with open joint space.

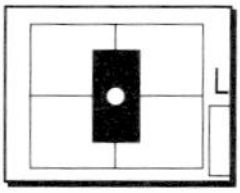

- 8 x 10" C.W. (20 x 24 cm)
- Grid

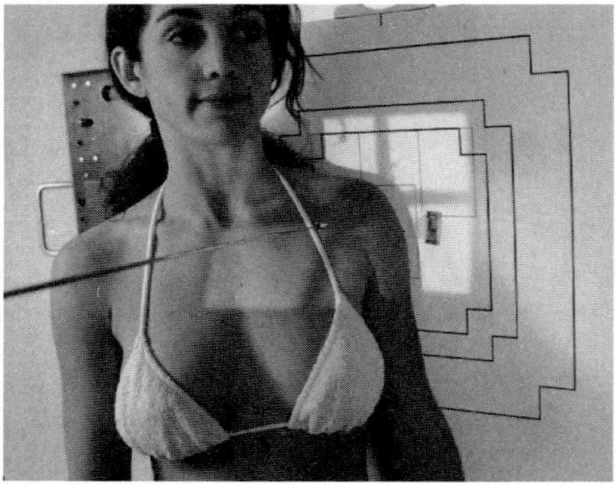

Glenoid cavity (35–45° post. oblique)

Position
- Erect or supine (erect preferred).
- Oblique 35–45° toward side of interest (body of scapula should be parallel with film), hand and arm in neutral rotation.
- Center glenohumeral joint and cassette to CR.

Central Ray
- CR ⊥, to mid glenohumeral joint.

SID: 40–48" (102–122 cm)

Collimation: Collimate closely to area of interest.

Respiration: Suspend during exposure.

Technique: kVp (75±5) ______

mrad

S 51	G NDC M
ML 14	<0.1 F

	cm	kVp	mA	Time	mAs	SID	Film–Screen	Grid	F.S.
Model Room	13	75			7	44"	Kodak 400	12:1	S
S									
M									
L									

Bontrager Textbook, 3rd ed., p. 158

Shoulder

Intertubercular (Bicipital) Groove

(Tangential Projection– Fisk Method)

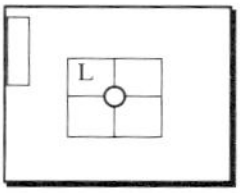

- 8 x 10" C.W. (20 x 24 cm)
- TT (detail screen)

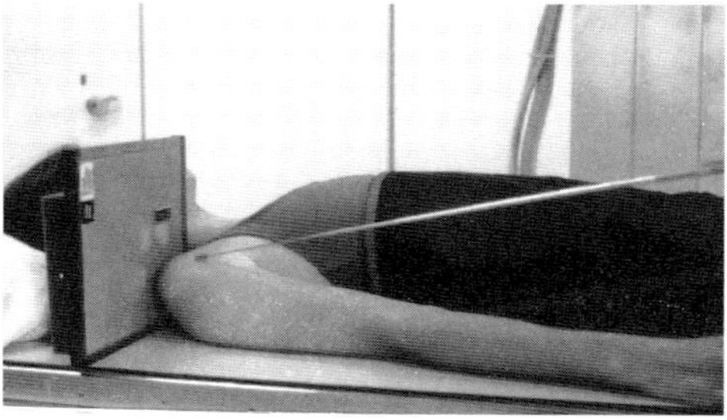

Supine inferosuperior projection (CR 15–20° from horizontal)

Position

- Supine or erect. Palpate anterior humeral head to locate groove.

Supine: Abduct arm slightly, supinate hand.

- Center cassette and groove to CR.
- CR 10-15° down from horizontal, to groove, cassette vertical against top of shoulder, perpendicular to CR.

Alternate Erect: Patient leans forward 15-20°, CR vertical, ⊥ to film.

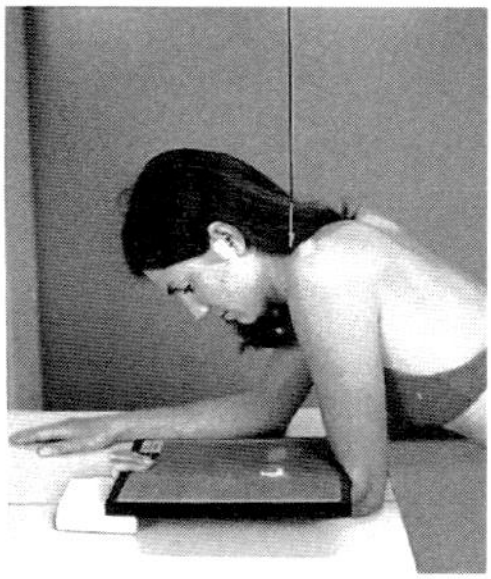

Erect superoinferior (Humerus 15–20° from vertical, CR ⊥ to film)

SID: 40–48" (102–122 cm)

Collimation: Collimate closely.

Respiration: Suspend during exposure.

Technique: kVp (60±5) ______

mrad

S	16	G	NDC M
ML	8		<0.1 F

	cm	kVp	mA	Time	mAs	SID	Film–Screen	Grid	F.S.
Model Room	–	65			4	44"	Kodak 100	–	S
S									
M									
L									

Lateral Shoulder

Scapular Y Lateral (and Neer Method)

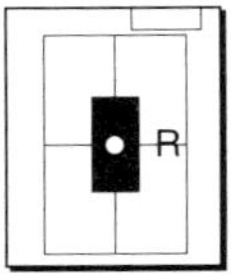

- 10 x 12" L.W. (24 x 30 cm)
- Grid

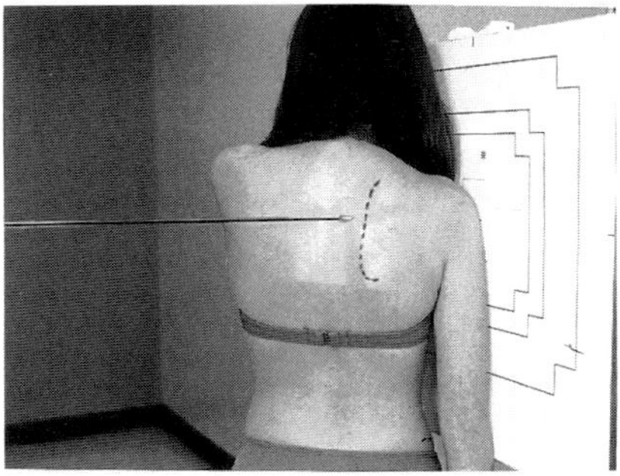

Scapular Y lateral position, – CR ⊥

Position

- Erect or recumbent (erect preferred).
- Rotate patient into an ≈60° anterior oblique (≈30° from lateral) as for a lateral scapula. (Body of scapula perpendicular to film.)
- Unaffected arm up in front of patient, affected arm down.
- Center glenohumeral joint and cassette to CR.

Central Ray: CR ⊥ to glenohumeral joint.
Neer method[1,2] Angle CR 10-15° caudad to better demonstrate the acromio-humeral space (supraspinatus outlet), CR to superior margin of humeral head.

SID: 40–48" (102–122 cm)

Collimation: To area of interest.

Respiration: Suspend during exposure.

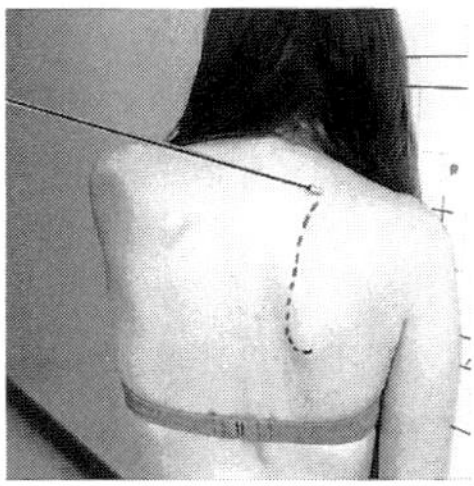

Neer method
- CR 10-15° caudad

Technique: kVp (75±5) ______

	cm	kVp	mA	Time	mAs	SID	Film–Screen	Grid	F.S.
Model	16	75			15	44"	Kodak 400	12:1	S
Room									
S									
M									
L									

Bontrager Textbook, 3rd ed., p. 161

mrad		
	S 112	G NDC M
	ML 28	<0.1 F

AP Shoulder Trauma Projection
Neutral Rotation

Warning: Do not attempt to rotate arm if fracture or dislocation is suspected without special orders by a physician.

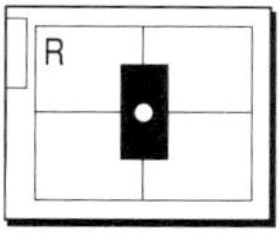

- 10 x 12" C.W. (24 x 30 cm) or 11 x 14" L.W. (30 x 35 cm) to include more of humerus
- Grid

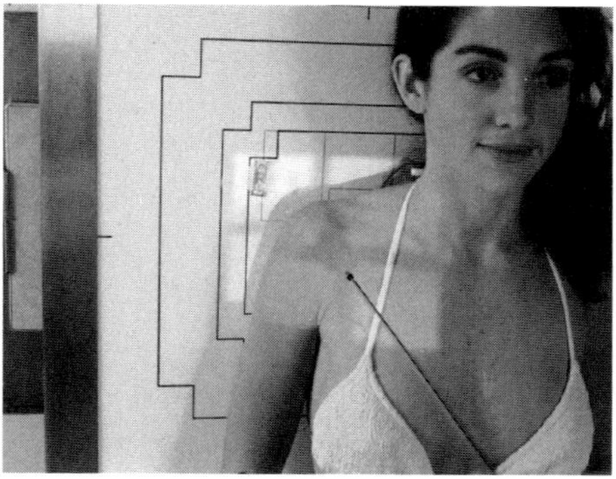

AP– neutral rotation

Position
- Erect (seated or standing) or supine, arm slightly abducted.
- Rotate thorax slightly as needed to place posterior shoulder against film.
- Arm in neutral position (generally this is with palm inward).

Central Ray
- CR ⊥, to ≈1"(2.5 cm) inferior to coracoid process.

SID: 40–48" (102–122 cm)

Collimation: On four sides to area of interest.

Respiration: Suspend during exposure.

Technique: kVp (70±5) ______

mrad

S	35	G	NDC M
ML	12		<0.1 F

	cm	kVp	mA	Time	mAs	SID	Film–Screen	Grid	F.S.
Model Room	12	70			6	44"	Kodak 400	12:1	S
S									
M									
L									

Bontrager Textbook, 3rd ed., p. 159

Lat. Shoulder Trauma Projection

Transthoracic Lateral

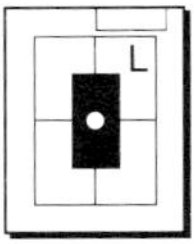

- 10 x 12" L.W. (24 x 30 cm)
- Grid

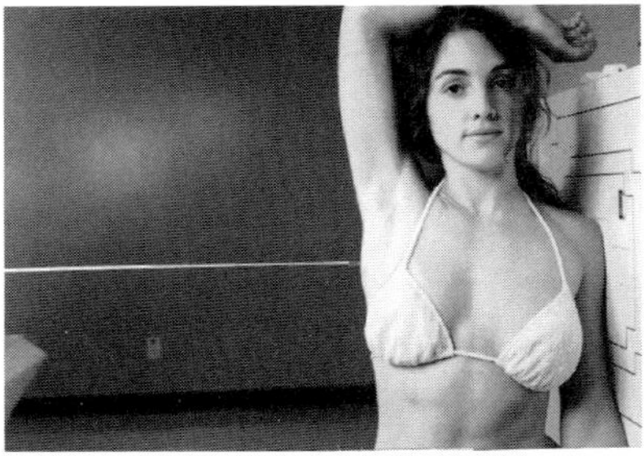

Erect transthoracic lateral

Position

- Erect or supine, affected arm against cassette, arm at side in neutral position.
- Raise unaffected arm above head.
- Elevate unaffected shoulder, **or** angle CR 10–15° cephalad to prevent superimposition of unaffected shoulder.
- True lateral, or slight anterior rotation of unaffected shoulder.
- Center grid cassette to CR.

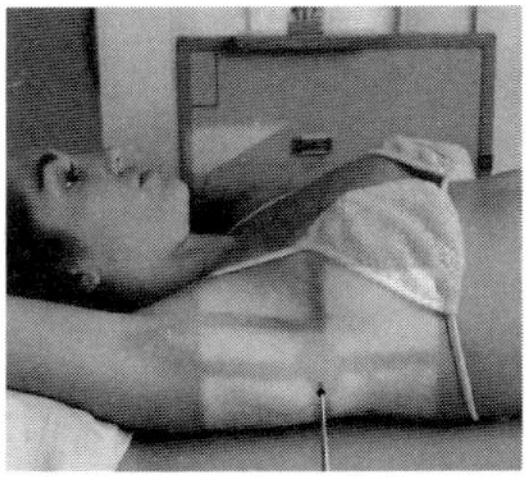

Supine transthoracic lateral

Central Ray: CR ⊥ through thorax to surgical neck.

SID: 40–48" (102–122 cm)

Collimation: On four sides to area of interest.

Respiration: Gentle, shallow breathing during exposure.

Technique: kVp with grid (75±5) ____; 3-4 sec. with breathing technique

mrad

S 1310	G NDC M
ML 169	<0.1 F

	cm	kVp	mA	Time	mAs	SID	Film–Screen	Grid	F.S.
Model Room	37	75			100	44"	Kodak 400	12:1	S or L
S									
M									
L									

Bontrager Textbook, 3rd ed., p. 160

Apical Oblique Shoulder
(Garth Method)

A good projection for acute shoulder trauma, demonstrating shoulder dislocations, glenoid fractures and Hill-Sachs lesions.[3,4]

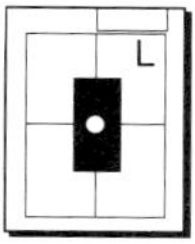

- 8 x 10" L.W. (20 x 24 cm)
- Grid

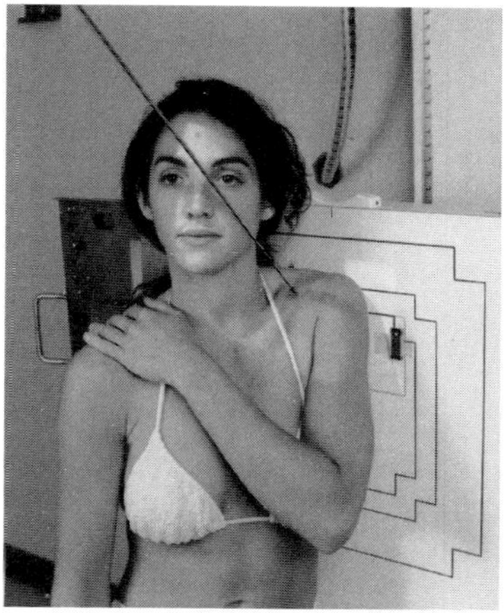

Erect apical oblique
(45° posterior obli., CR 45° caudad)

Position

- Erect preferred (recumbent if necessary).
- Rotate thorax 45° with affected shoulder against cassette.
- Flex affected elbow and place hand on opposite shoulder.
- Center film to exiting CR.

Central Ray

- CR 45° caudad, to media aspect of glenohumeral joint.

SID: 40–48" (102–122 cm)

Collimation: On four sides to area of interest.

Respiration: Suspend during exposure.

Technique: kVp (75±5) _____

mrad

S 85	G NDC M
ML 26	<0.1 F

	cm	kVp	mA	Time	mAs	SID	Film–Screen	Grid	F.S.
Model Room	14	75			12	44"	Kodak 400	12:1	S
S									
M									
L									

Bontrager Textbook, 3rd ed., p. 162

AP (PA) and Axial Clavicle

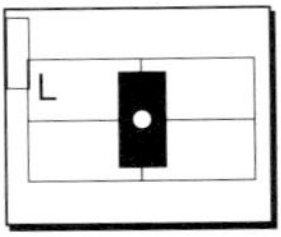

- 10 x 12" C.W. (24 x 30 cm)
- Grid

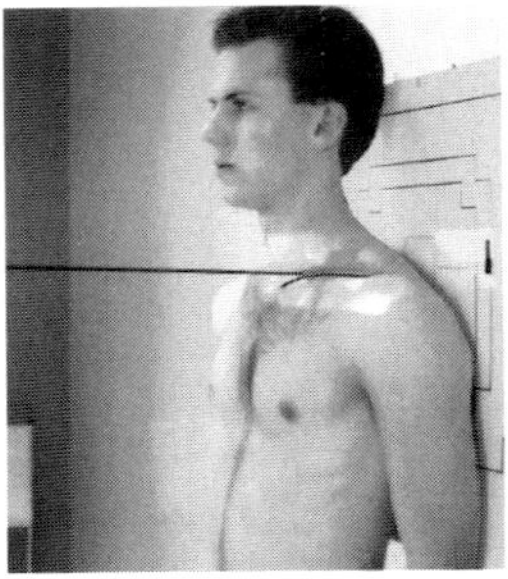

AP, 0°

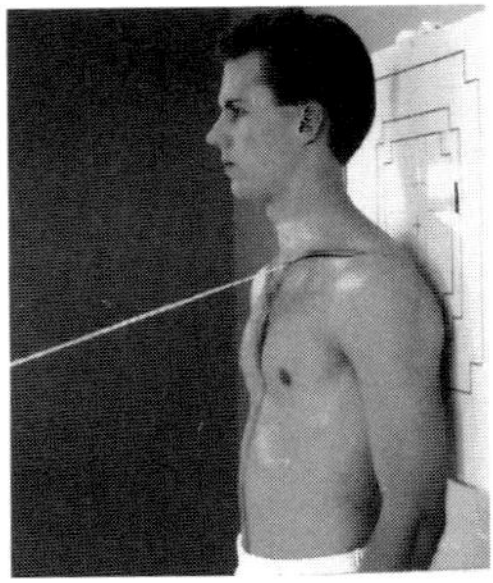

AP axial, 20° **cephalad**

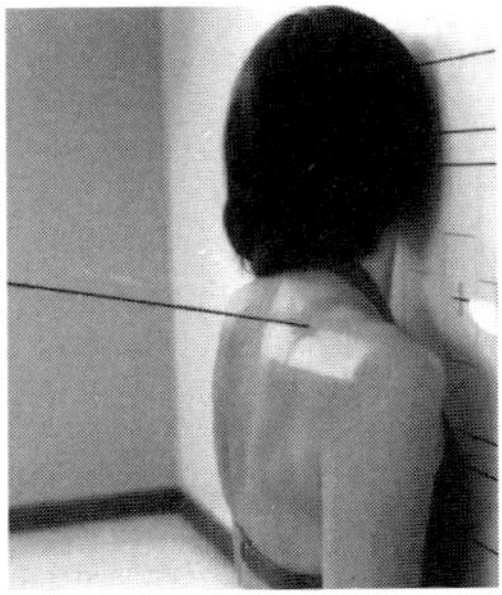

Alternate PA, 10-20° **caudad**

Position

- Erect or recumbent.
- Center clavicle and film to CR (midway between jugular notch medially and AC joint laterally).

Central Ray

- CR to mid clavicle.
  AP: CR ⊥, to mid-clavicle.
  AP axial: 15 to 30° cephalad (thin shoulders require 5-10° more angle than thick shoulders).

Note: Departmental routines may include AP 0°, or axial AP, or both.

SID: 40–48" (102–122 cm)

Collimation: Collimate closely to area of clavicle.

Respiration: Expose upon expiration.

Technique: kVp (70±5) ______ (+4 kVp for axial)

mrad, per projection		
	S 47	G NDC M
	ML 15	<0.1 F

	cm	kVp	mA	Time	mAs	SID	Film–Screen	Grid	F.S.
Model	14	70			8	44"	Kodak 400	12:1	S
Room									
S									
M									
L									

Bontrager Textbook, 3rd ed., p. 163

AP Scapula

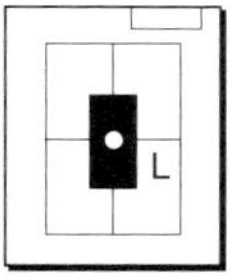

- 10 x 12" L.W. (24 x 30 cm)
- Grid

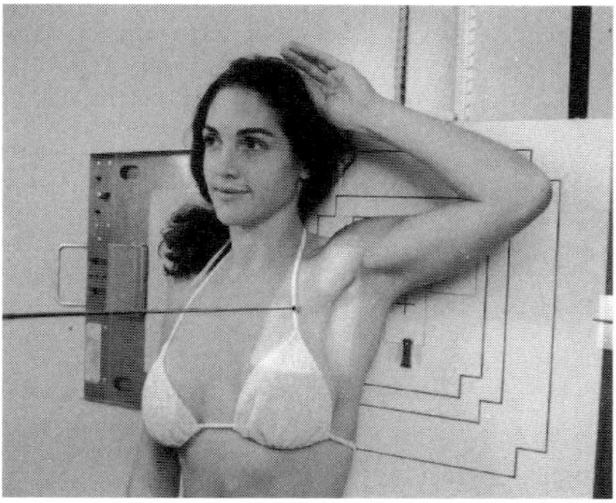

AP scapula

Position

- Erect or supine (erect preferred with pain in scapula area).
- Gently abduct arm 90° if possible, supinate hand (abduction results in less superimposition of scapula by ribs).
- Center cassette and entire scapula to CR.

Central Ray

- CR ⊥, to mid scapula (≈2" or 5 cm inferior to coracoid process and ≈ 1" (2.5 cm) medial to lateral border).

SID: 40–48" (102-122 cm)

Collimation: On four sides to scapula borders.

Respiration: Suspend during exposure.

Technique: kVp (75±5) _____

mrad

S 51	G NDC M
ML 14	<0.1 F

	cm	kVp	mA	Time	mAs	SID	Film–Screen	Grid	F.S.
Model Room	15	75			7	44"	Kodak 400	12:1	S
S									
M									
L									

Bontrager Textbook, 3rd ed., p. 166

Lateral Scapula

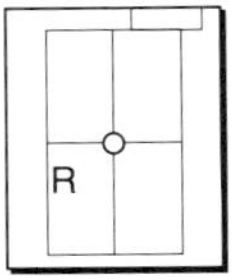

- 10 x 12" L.W. (24 x 30 cm)
- Grid

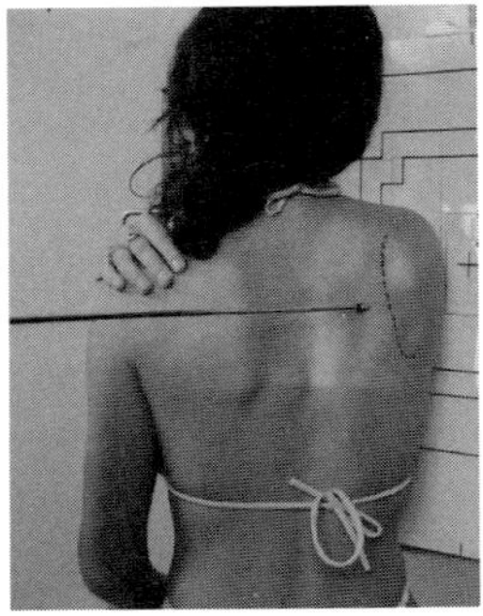

Lateral for body of scapula

Position

- Erect or recumbent (erect preferred).
- Palpate borders of scapula and rotate thorax until body of scapula is perpendicular to film (will vary from 45-60° rotation from PA).

Area of interest is body of scapula: Arm up, patient reaches across and grasps opposite shoulder.

Area of interest is superior scapula: Arm down and back, place affected arm behind back, flex elbow, palm out.

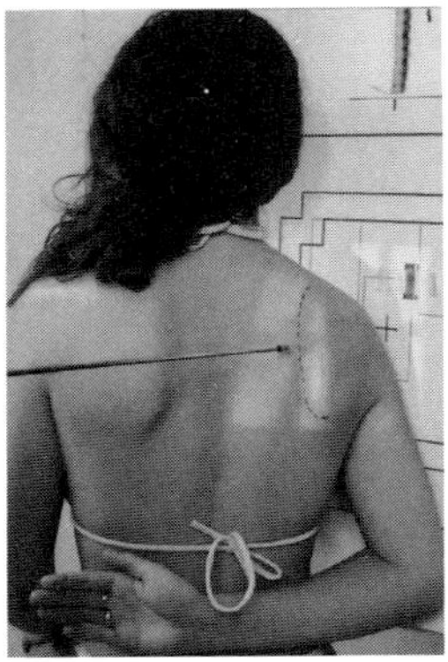

Lateral for acromion or coracoid process

Central Ray

- CR ⊥, to mid medial (vertebral) border of scapula.

SID: 40–48" (102–122 cm)

Collimation: To scapular region.

Respiration: Suspend during exposure.

Technique: kVp (75±5) _____

mrad

S 112	G NDC M
ML 29	<0.1 F

	cm	kVp	mA	Time	mAs	SID	Film–Screen	Grid	F.S.
Model	16	75			13	44"	Kodak 400	12:1	S
Room									
S									
M									
L									

Bontrager Textbook, 3rd ed., p. 167

Acromioclavicular (AC) Joints
AP – Bilateral with and without weights

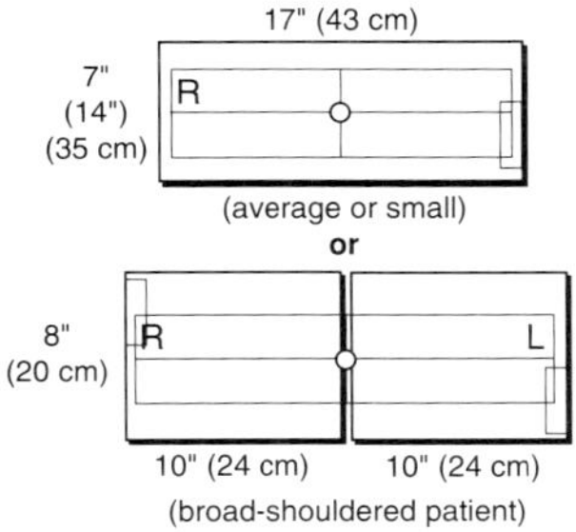

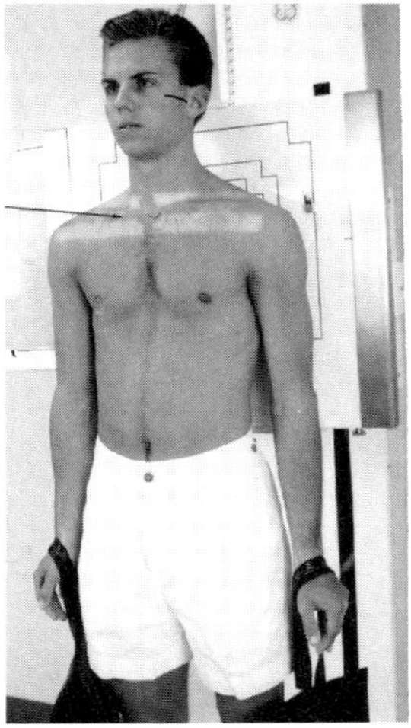
Bilateral with weights

- Detail screens
- Use markers "with weights" and "without weights"

Position
- Erect, standing if possible, or may be seated on chair.
- Arms at sides, one exposure for bilateral without weights, and a second exposure bilateral with 10-15 lb. weights tied to wrists,[5,6] shoulders and arms relaxed, center cassette to CR.

Central Ray: CR ⊥, to jugular notch.

SID: 72–120" (183–305 cm)

Collimation: Long narrow horizontal exposure field.

Respiration: Suspend during exposure.

Technique: kVp (65±5) _____

mrad

S 37	G NDC M
ML 8	<0.1 F

	cm	kVp	mA	Time	mAs	SID	Film–Screen	Grid	F.S.
Model	15	65			20	72"	Kodak 400	12:1	S
Room									
S									
M									
L									

Bontrager Textbook, 3rd ed., p. 164

Shoulder Girdle

Position:

Central Ray:

SID:

Collimation:

Respiration:

Technique:

	Room	cm	kVp	mA	Time	mAs	SID	Film–Screen	Grid	F.S.
S										
M										
L										

Bontrager Textbook, 3rd ed.,

Chapter 5

Lower Limb (Extremity)

Lower Limb (Extremity)

Technical Factors

kVp Range

A 55–65 kVp range is commonly used for the lower limbs for body parts distal to the knee which measure less than 10 cm for which grids are not used. An exception is the **foot** where an **increase of kVp to 70–75 is suggested** due to the large difference in part thickness between the phalanges and the metatarsal region. This higher kVp creates a longer scale contrast with greater exposure latitude resulting in more uniform density between the phalanges, metatarsals and distal tarsals.

Detail Screens and Small Focal Spot

Detail (extremity) intensifying screens are commonly used on all exams of the upper and lower limbs along with a small focal spot for maximum definition (detail). Techniques as provided are with Kodak lanex extremity screens with TMG film at 100 speed.

Radiation Protection

Collimation and Gonad Shields

A general rule for gonadal shielding states that gonadal shields should be used whenever radiation sensitive areas lie within or near (2" or 2.5 cm) the primary beam.[1] However a good practice to follow is in addition to **close collimation** to the area of interest, also use **gonadal shields** on childbearing age patients for **all** lower limb procedures. This provides assurance to the patient that they are being protected from unnecessary exposure.

Patient Dose

Calculated patient doses as included for each projection are based on the suggested exposure factors as listed for skin (S), midline (ML) and gonad (G) doses for male and female. These gonadal doses as listed are without gonadal shielding, and by reviewing these, one can determine when shielding is especially important. Examples of this are the AP and lateral femur due to the proximity of the gonads to the exposure field.

AP Toes

Alternate Routine: Include entire foot on AP toe projection for possible secondary trauma to other parts of foot (see AP foot).

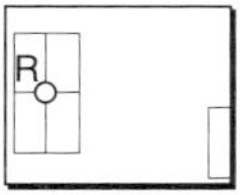

- 8 x 10" C.W. (20 x 24 cm)
- TT (detail screens)

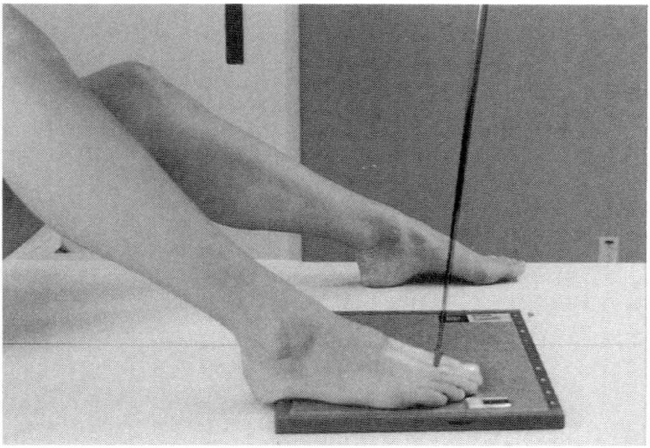

AP 2nd digit, CR 10–15° posteriorly

Position

- Supine or seated on table with knee flexed, plantar surface of foot resting on cassette.
- Align long axis of affected toe(s) to portion of film being exposed.

Central Ray

- CR angled 10–15° posteriorly (⊥ to long axis of digits).
- CR centered to MP joint(s) of interest.

SID: 40–48" (102–122 cm)

Collimation: To digits of interest.

Technique: kVp (55±5) ______

mrad		
S	6	G NDC M
ML	6	<0.1 F

	cm	kVp	mA	Time	mAs	SID	Film–Screen	Grid	F.S.
Model Room	2	60			2	40"	Kodak 100	–	S
S									
M									
L									

Bontrager Textbook, 3rd ed., p. 187

Oblique Toes

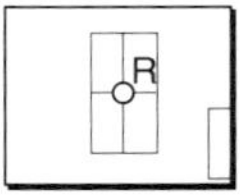

- 8 x 10" C.W. (20 x 24 cm)
- TT (detail screens)

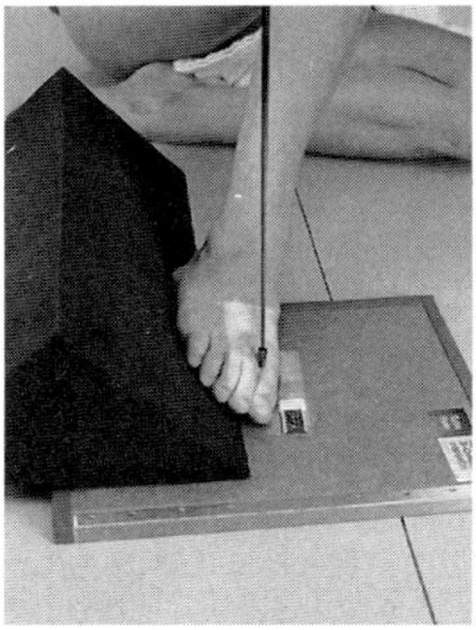

Medial oblique (1st digit)

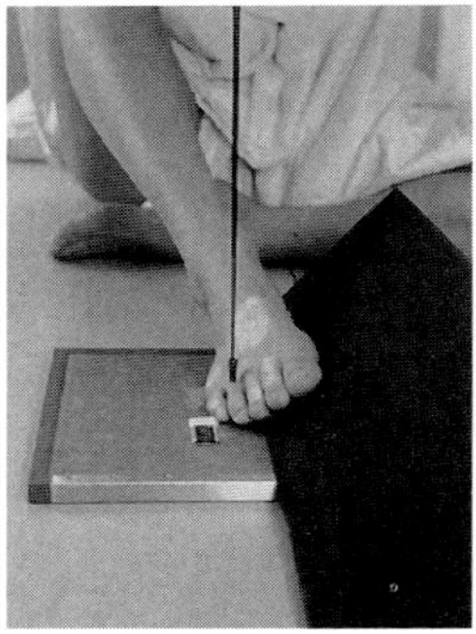

Lateral oblique (4th digit)

Position

- Supine or seated on table, foot resting on cassette.
- Align long axis of affected toe(s) to portion of film being exposed.
- Oblique foot 30–45° medially for 1st–3rd digits, and laterally for 4th and 5th digits. Place support under foot as shown.

Central Ray

- CR ⊥, centered to MP joint(s) of interest.

SID: 40–48" (102–122 cm)

Collimation: Four sides to digits of interest.

Technique: kVp (55±5) ______

mrad

S	6	G	NDC M
ML	6		<0.1 F

	cm	kVp	mA	Time	mAs	SID	Film–Screen	Grid	F.S.
Model	3	60			2	40"	Kodak 100	–	S
Room									
S									
M									
L									

Bontrager Textbook, 3rd ed., p. 188

Lateral Toes

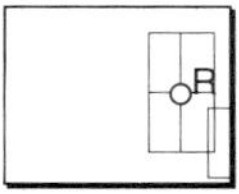

- 8 x 10" C.W. (20 x 24 cm)
- TT (detail screens)

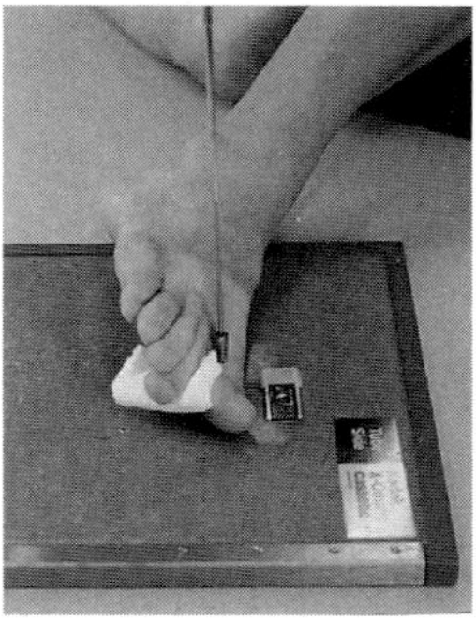

Lateromedial (1st digit)

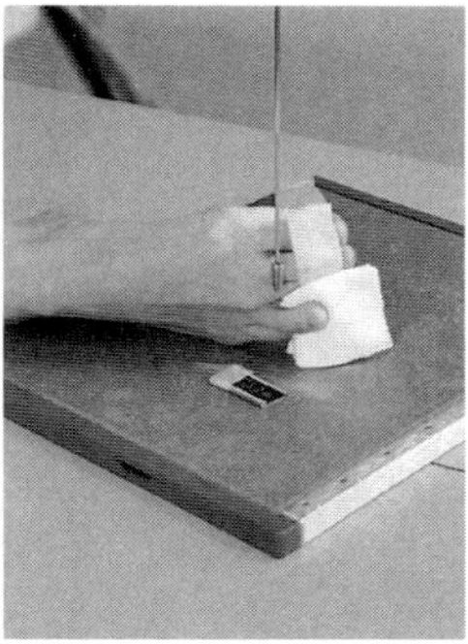

Mediolateral (4th digit)

Position

- Seated or recumbent on table top.
- Carefully use tape, and/or radiolucent gauze to help isolate unaffected digits as shown:

  1st–3rd digits – lateromedial projection (1st digit down).

  4th–5th digits – mediolateral projection (1st digit up).

Central Ray

- CR ⊥, to IP joint for 1st digit, and to PIP joint for 2nd–5th digits.

SID: 40–48" (102–122 cm)

Collimation: Collimate closely to area of interest.

Technique: kVp (55±5) ______

mrad

S	6	G NDC M	
ML	6	<0.1 F	

	cm	kVp	mA	Time	mAs	SID	Film–Screen	Grid	F.S.
Model Room	3	60			2	40"	Kodak 100	–	S
S									
M									
L									

Bontrager Textbook, 3rd ed., p. 189

Toes – Sesamoids
Tangential Projection

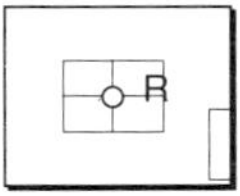

- 8 x 10" C.W. (20 x 24 cm)
- TT (detail screens)

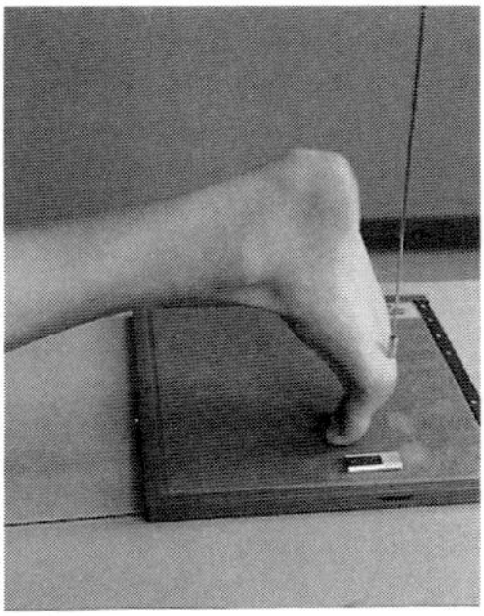

Patient prone

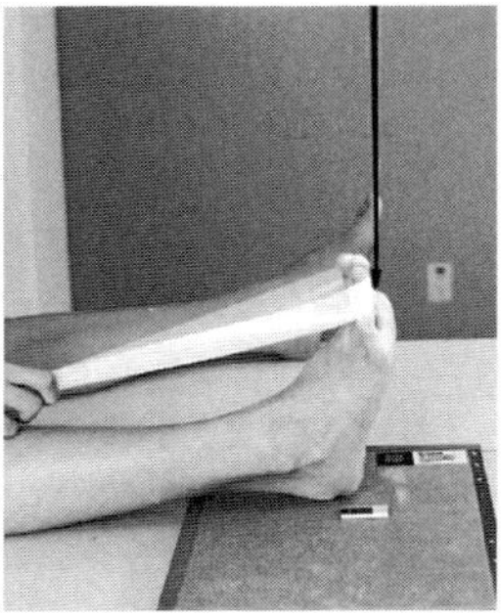

Alternate supine position

Position
- Patient prone with foot and great toe carefully dorsiflexed so the plantar surface forms a 15–20° angle from vertical if possible (adjust CR angle as needed).

Alternate supine position: This may be a more tolerable position for patient to maintain if in great pain.

Central Ray
- CR ⊥, or angled as needed to be 15–20° from plantar surface of foot, centered to head of first metatarsal.

SID: 40–48" (102–122 cm)

Collimation: Collimate closely to area of interest; include distal 2nd and 3rd metatarsals for possible sesamoids.

Technique: kVp (55±5) ______

mrad

S 13	G NDC M
ML 13	<0.1 F

	cm	kVp	mA	Time	mAs	SID	Film–Screen	Grid	F.S.
Model	4	60			4	40"	Kodak 100	–	S
Room									
S									
M									
L									

Bontrager Textbook, 3rd ed., p. 190

AP Foot
(Dorsoplantar Projection)

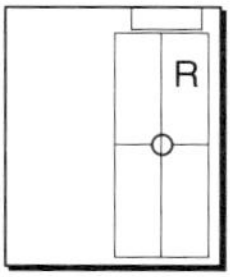

- 10 x 12" L.W. (24 x 30 cm)
- TT (detail screens)

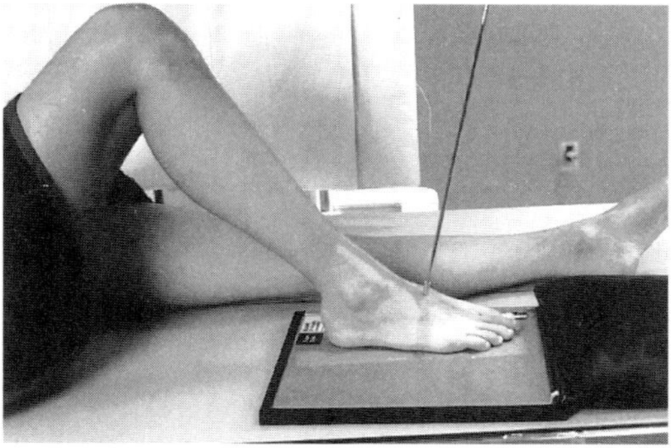

AP foot, CR 10° posteriorly

Position
- Supine or seated with plantar surface of foot flat on cassette, aligned lengthwise to portion of film being exposed.
- Extend (plantar flex) foot by sliding foot and cassette distally while keeping plantar surface flat on cassette. (Support with sandbags to keep foot and cassette from sliding farther.)

Central Ray
- CR ⊥ to metatarsals, which is about 10° posteriorly (toward heel), centered to base of 3rd metatarsal.

SID: 40–48" (102–122 cm)

Collimation: Four sides to margins of foot.

mrad @70 kVp

S	10	G	NDC M
ML	8		<0.1 F

Technique: kVp (60±5) _____, or 70–75 kVp with reduced mAs for more uniform density throughout foot.[2]

	cm	kVp	mA	Time	mAs	SID	Film–Screen	Grid	F.S.
Model Room	6	70/60			2/4	40"	Kodak 100	–	S
S									
M									
L									

Bontrager Textbook, 3rd ed., p. 191

Oblique Foot

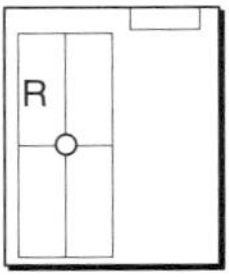

- 10 x 12" L.W. (24 x 30 cm)
- TT (detail screens)

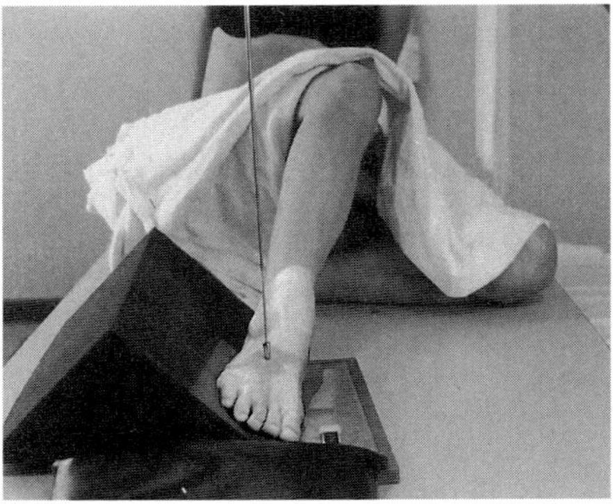

30-45° medial oblique

Position

- Supine or seated with foot centered lengthwise to portion of film being exposed.
- Oblique foot 30-45° medially[3,4], support with 45° radiolucent angle block and sandbags to prevent slippage.

Note: Some departments prefer a routine of only 30° oblique and some prefer nearer 45°.

Central Ray

- CR ⊥, centered to base of 3rd metatarsal.

SID: 40–48" (102–122 cm)

Collimation: Four sides to margins of foot.

mrad @ 70 kVp

S 11	G NDC M
ML 8	<0.1 F

Technique: kVp (60±5) _____, or 70–75 kVp with reduced mAs for more uniform density throughout foot.

	cm	kVp	mA	Time	mAs	SID	Film–Screen	Grid	F.S.
Model	7	70/60			2/4	40"	Kodak 100	–	S
Room									
S									
M									
L									

Bontrager Textbook, 3rd ed., p. 192

Lateral Foot

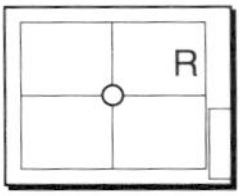

- 8 x 10" C.W. (20 x 24 cm)
  or
- 10 x 12" (24 x 30 cm) for large foot
- TT (detail screens)

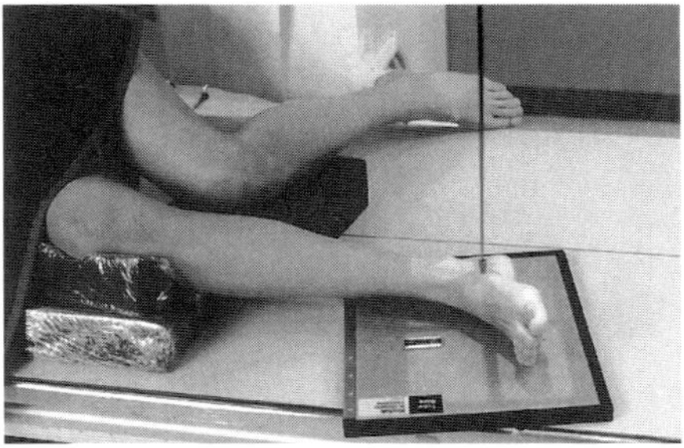

Mediolateral foot

Position (Mediolateral)

- Recumbent, turned on affected side, knee flexed with unaffected leg behind to prevent over rotation.
- Place support under affected knee and leg as needed to place plantar surface of foot perpendicular to film for a true lateral.

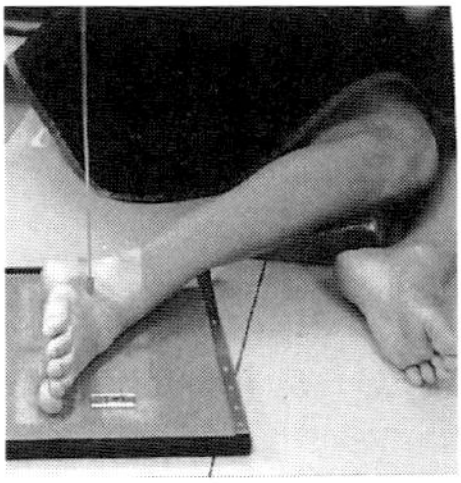

Lateromedial foot

Lateromedial projection: May be easier to achieve a true lateral if patient's condition allows this position.[5]

Central Ray

- CR ⊥, centered to mid area of base of metatarsals.

SID: 40–48" (102–122 cm)

Collimation: Four sides to margins of foot.

Technique: kVp (60±5) _____

mrad

S 22	G NDC M
ML 13	<0.1 F

	cm	kVp	mA	Time	mAs	SID	Film–Screen	Grid	F.S.
Model	8	66			4	40"	Kodak 100	–	S
Room									
S									
M									
L									

Bontrager Textbook, 3rd ed., p. 193

Weight-Bearing Feet
AP and Lateral

Lateral is most common for longitudinal arch (flat feet), AP demonstrates alignment of metatarsals and phalanges.

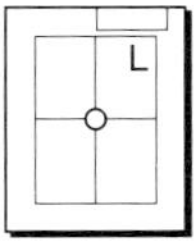

- 10 x 12" L.W. (24 x 30 cm)
- TT (detail screens)

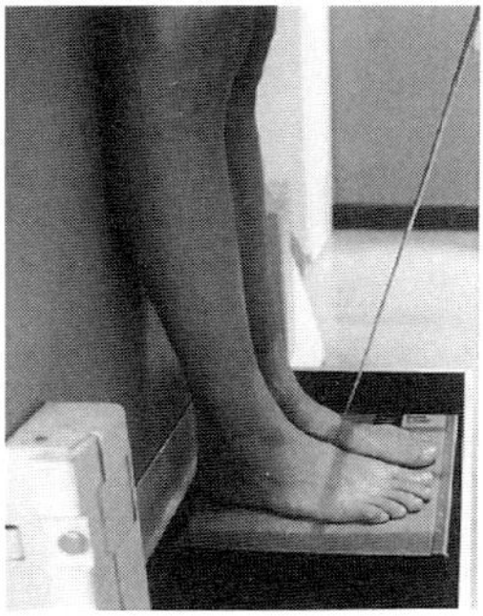

AP - both feet

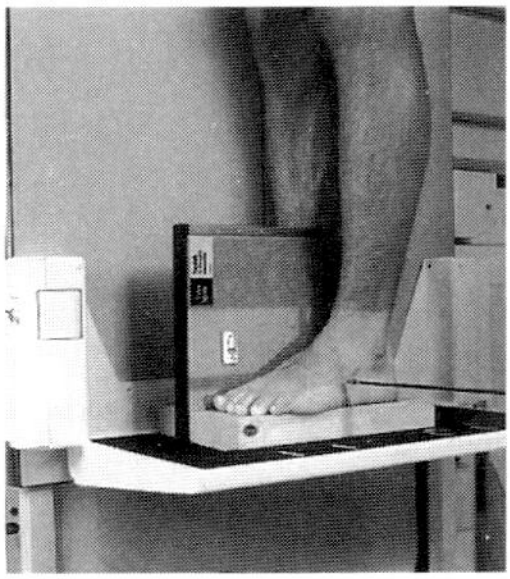

Lateral - left foot

Position

- **AP:** Erect, weight evenly distributed on both feet, on one film.
- **Lateral:** Erect, full weight on both feet, vertical cassette between feet, standing on blocks, high enough from floor for horizontal CR. (R and L feet taken for comparison.)

Central Ray: **AP** - CR 15° posteriorly, CR to level of base of 3rd metatarsal, midway between feet.[6,7]
Lateral - CR horizontal, to base of 5th metatarsal.

SID: 40–48" (102–122 cm)

Collimation: Four sides to area of foot.

Technique: kVp (65±5) _____

mrad

S 22	G NDC M
ML 13	<0.1 F

	cm	kVp	mA	Time	mAs	SID	Film–Screen	Grid	F.S.
Model Room	6	70			2.5	48"	Kodak 100	–	S
S									
M									
L									

Bontrager Textbook, 3rd ed., p. 194 (Laterals)

Plantodorsal Calcaneus
Axial Projection

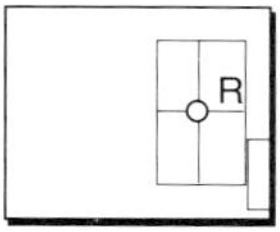

- 10 x 12" C.W. (24 x 30 cm)
- TT (detail screens)

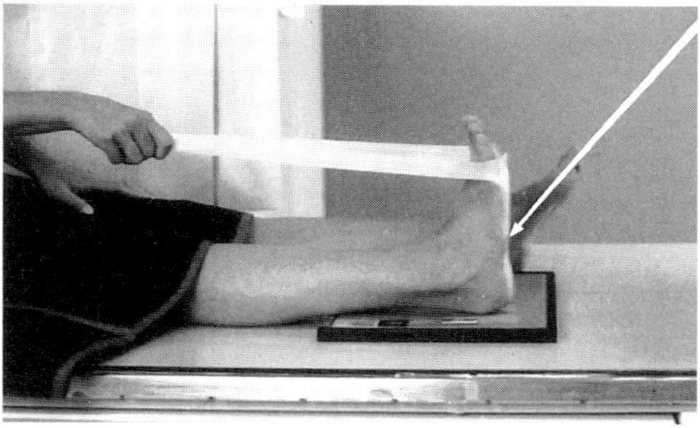

CR 40° to long axis of foot

Position
- Supine or seated, dorsiflex foot to as near vertical position as possible. If possible, have patient pull on gauze as shown. (This may be painful for patient to maintain, don't delay!)
- Center CR to part, with film centered to projected CR.

Central Ray
- CR 40° to long axis of plantar surface (may require more than 40° from vertical if foot is not dorsiflexed a full 90°).
- CR centered to base of 3rd metatarsal, to emerge just distal and inferior to ankle joint.

SID: 40–48" (102–122 cm)

Collimation: Four sides to area of interest.

Technique: kVp (70±5) _____

mrad

S 27	G NDC M
ML 14	<0.1 F

	cm	kVp	mA	Time	mAs	SID	Film–Screen	Grid	F.S.
Model Room	10	70			5	40"	Kodak 100	–	S
S									
M									
L									

Bontrager Textbook, 3rd ed., p. 195

Lateral Calcaneus

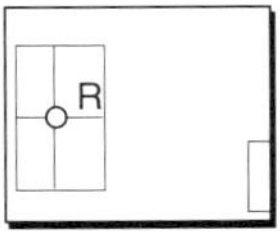

- 10 x 12" C.W. (24 x 30 cm)
- TT(detail screens)

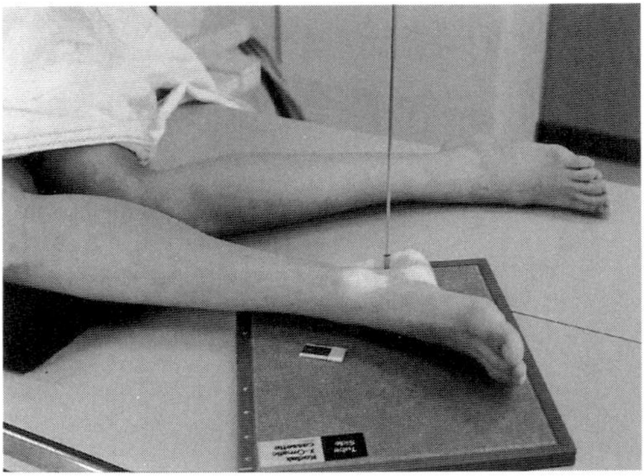

Lateral calcaneus

Position

- Recumbent, on affected side, knee flexed with unaffected limb behind, to prevent over rotation.
- Place support under knee and leg as needed for a true lateral.
- Dorsiflex foot so the plantar surface is near 90° to leg if possible.

Central Ray

- CR ⊥, to mid calcaneus, about 3/4" (2 cm) distal to medial malleolus.

SID: 40–48" (102–122 cm)

Collimation: Four sides to area of calcaneus, include ankle joint at upper margin.

Technique: kVp (60±5) _____

mrad

S 16	G NDC M
ML 16	<0.1 F

	cm	kVp	mA	Time	mAs	SID	Film–Screen	Grid	F.S.
Model	5	65			4	40"	Kodak 100	–	S
Room									
S									
M									
L									

Bontrager Textbook, 3rd ed., p. 196

AP Ankle

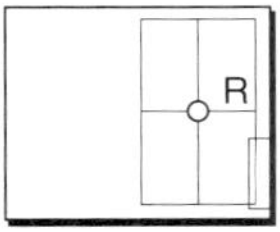

- 10 x 12" C.W. (24 x 30 cm)
- TT (detail screens)

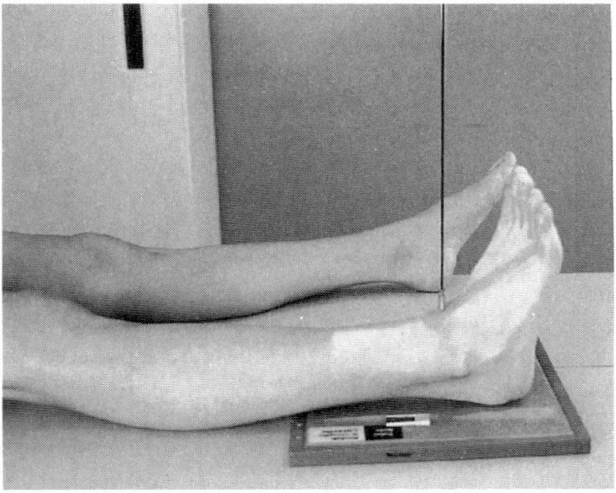

AP ankle

Position

- Supine or seated on table, leg extended, support under knee.
- Align leg and ankle parallel to edge of cassette.
- Dorsiflex foot so long axis of foot is perpendicular to film (if possible).
- True AP, ensure no rotation (lateral malleolus will be about 15° more posterior than medial malleolus).

Central Ray

- CR ⊥, to midway between malleoli.

SID: 40–48" (102–122 cm)

Collimation: Collimate to ankle region.

Technique: kVp (60±5) _____

mrad		
	S 27	G NDC M
	ML 16	<0.1 F

	cm	kVp	mA	Time	mAs	SID	Film–Screen	Grid	F.S.
Model	8	65			6	40"	Kodak 100	–	S
Room									
S									
M									
L									

Bontrager Textbook, 3rd ed., p. 197

AP Mortise Oblique Ankle

This is a frontal view of the entire ankle mortise and generally should not be a substitute for the routine AP or 45° oblique ankle.[8]

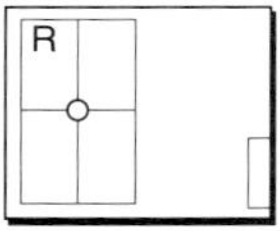

- 10 x 12" C.W. (24 x 30 cm)
- TT (detail screens)

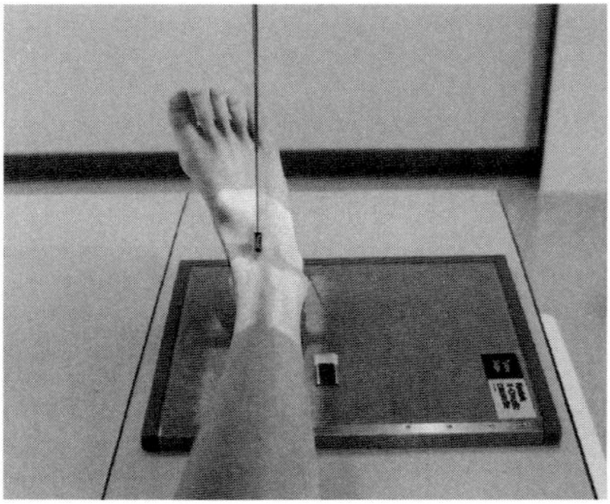

AP, to visualize entire ankle mortise (15–20° int. obli.)

Position

- Supine or seated on table, leg extended, support under knee.
- Dorsiflex foot 90° to leg if patient can tolerate.
- Rotate leg and foot internally 15–20° so **intermalleolar line is parallel to table top.**

Central Ray

- CR ⊥, to midway between malleoli.

SID: 40–48" (102–122 cm)

Collimation: Collimate to ankle region.

Technique: kVp (60±5) _____

mrad

S 27	G NDC M
ML 16	<0.1 F

	cm	kVp	mA	Time	mAs	SID	Film–Screen	Grid	F.S.
Model	8	65			6	40"	Kodak 100	–	S
Room									
S									
M									
L									

Bontrager Textbook, 3rd ed., p. 198

AP Oblique Ankle

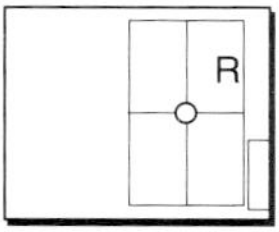

- 10 x 12" C.W. (24 x 30 cm)
- TT (detail screens)

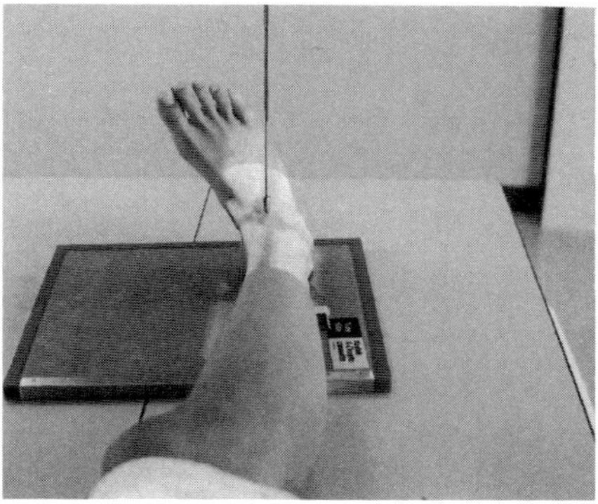

45° medial oblique ankle

Position

- Supine or seated, leg extended, support under knee.
- Dorsiflex foot 90° to leg if patient can tolerate.
- Rotate leg and foot 45° internally (long axis of foot is 45° to film).

Central Ray

- CR ⊥, to midway between the malleoli.

SID: 40–48" (102–122 cm)

Collimation: Collimate to ankle region.

Technique: kVp (65±5) _____

mrad

S 27	G NDC M
ML 16	<0.1 F

	cm	kVp	mA	Time	mAs	SID	Film–Screen	Grid	F.S.
Model Room	8	65			6	40"	Kodak 100	–	S
S									
M									
L									

Bontrager Textbook, 3rd ed., p. 199

Lateral Ankle

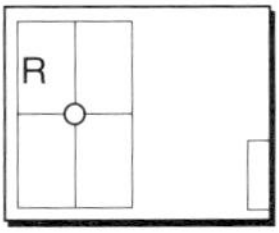

- 10 x 12" C.W. (24 x 30 cm)
- TT (detail screens)

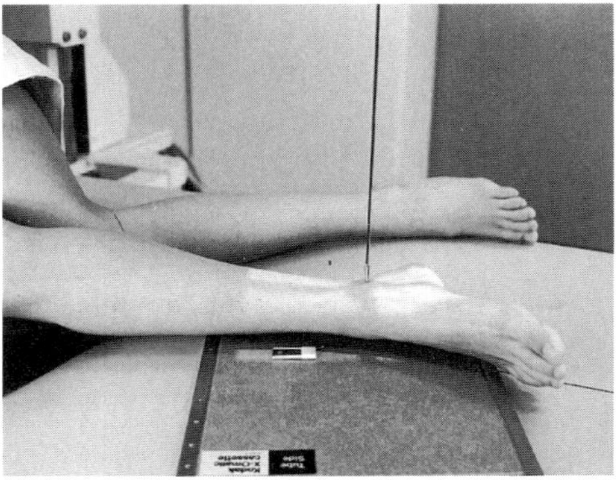

Mediolateral ankle

Position

- Recumbent, affected side down, affected knee partially flexed.
- Dorsiflex foot 90° to leg if patient can tolerate.
- Place support under knee as needed for true lateral of foot and ankle (lateral malleolus will be 15–20° posterior to medial malleolus).

Note: May also be taken as a lateromedial projection if patient condition allows, may be easier to achieve a true lateral.

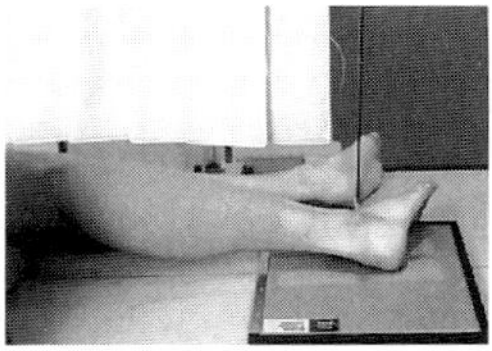

Lateromedial ankle

Central Ray: CR ⊥, to medial malleolus.

SID: 40–48" (102–122 cm)

Collimation: Four sides to ankle region.

Technique: kVp (65±5) _____

mrad

S 21	G NDC M
ML 16	<0.1 F

	cm	kVp	mA	Time	mAs	SID	Film–Screen	Grid	F.S.
Model	6	65			5	40"	Kodak 100	–	S
Room									
S									
M									
L									

Bontrager Textbook, 3rd ed., p. 200

AP Ankle - Stress Views

Warning: Stress must be applied very carefully, either by a long gauze held by patient or hand held with lead gloves and apron. (May require injection of local anesthetic by a physician.)

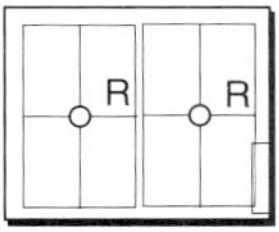

- 10 x 12" C.W. (24 x 30 cm)
- TT (detail screens)

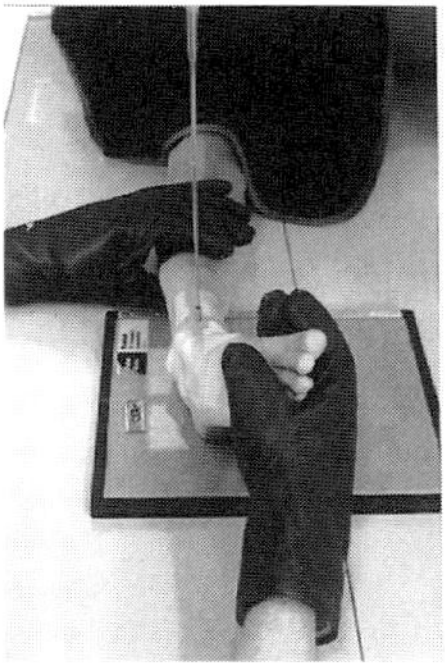

Inversion stress

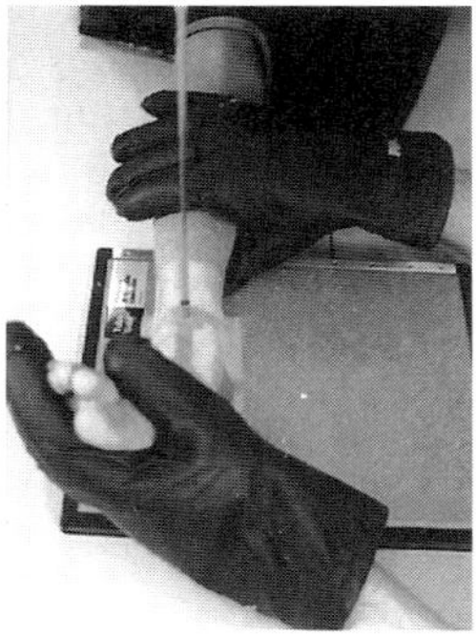

Eversion stress

Position

- Supine or seated on table, leg extended.
- Without rotating leg or ankle (true AP), stress is applied to ankle joint by first turning plantar surface of foot inward (inversion stress), then outward (eversion stress). Two projections on one film.

Central Ray

- CR ⊥, to midway between malleoli.

SID: 40–48" (102–122 cm)

Collimation: Collimate closely to ankle region.

Technique: kVp (65±5) _____

mrad, two projections		
	S 54	G NDC M
	ML 32	<0.1 F

	cm	kVp	mA	Time	mAs	SID	Film–Screen	Grid	F.S.
Model	8	65			6	40"	Kodak 100	–	S
Room									
S									
M									
L									

Bontrager Textbook, 3rd ed., p. 201

AP Leg (Tibia–Fibula)

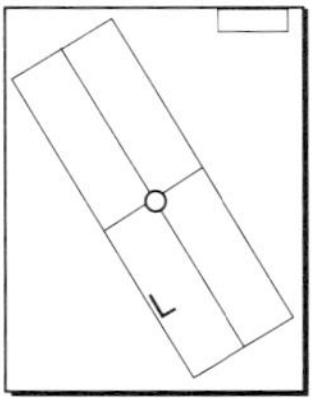

Diagonal if needed to include both ankle and knee joints. (With smaller patients, place leg lengthwise to film with AP and lateral on same 14 x 17" film.)

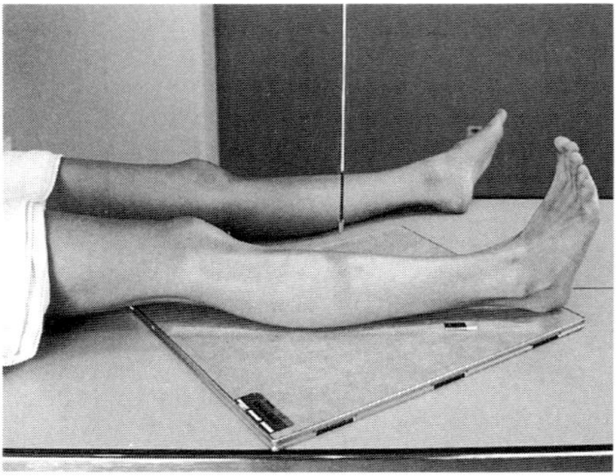

AP leg

- 14 x 17" (35 x 43 cm)
- Table top
- Knee at cathode end (anode–heel effect)

Position

- Supine, leg extended, ensure no rotation of knee, leg or ankle.
- Include 1–1.5" (≈3 cm) minimum beyond knee and ankle joints considering divergent rays.

Central Ray

- CR ⊥, to mid shaft of leg (to midfilm).

SID: 40–48" (102–122 cm)

Collimation: On four sides, to include knee and ankle joints.

Technique: kVp (70±5) _____

mrad

S	34	G NDC M
ML	16	<0.1 F

	cm	kVp	mA	Time	mAs	SID	Film–Screen	Grid	F.S.
Model	10	70			6	48"	Kodak 100	–	S
Room									
S									
M									
L									

Bontrager Textbook, 3rd ed., p. 202

Lateral Leg (Tibia–Fibula)

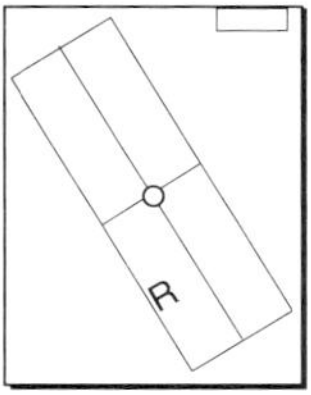

Diagonal if needed

- 14 x 17" (35 x 43 cm)
- Table top
- Knee at cathode end (anode–heel effect)

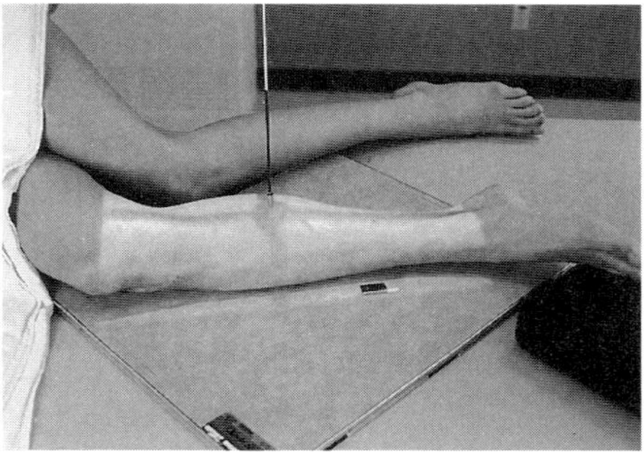

Lateral leg

Position

- Recumbent, affected side down, flex affected knee ≈45°.
- Place unaffected limb behind patient to prevent over rotation.
- Place support under distal portion of affected foot as needed to ensure a true lateral position of foot, ankle, and knee.
- Include 1–1.5" (≈3 cm) minimum beyond knee and ankle joints considering divergent rays.

Central Ray

- CR ⊥, to mid shaft of leg (to midfilm).

SID: 40–48" (102–122 cm)

Collimation: On four sides, to include knee and ankle joints.

Technique: kVp (70±5) _____

mrad

S	33	G NDC M
ML	19	<0.1 F

	cm	kVp	mA	Time	mAs	SID	Film–Screen	Grid	F.S.
Model	9	70			6	48"	Kodak 100	–	S
Room									
S									
M									
L									

Bontrager Textbook, 3rd ed., p. 203

AP Knee

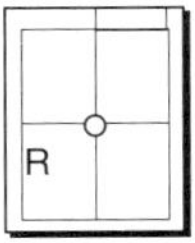

- 8 x 10" (20 x 24 cm)
- Grid >10 cm
  Screen <10 cm

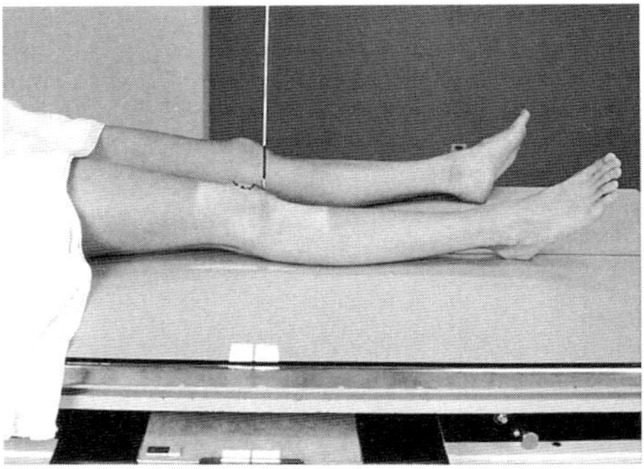

AP knee (CR ⊥ to film for average patient)

Position

- Supine, or seated on table, leg extended and centered to CR and midline of table or cassette.
- Rotate leg slightly inward as needed to place knee and leg into a true AP. Center cassette to CR.

Central Ray: CR centered to 3/4" (2 cm) distal to apex of patella.

- CR **parallel to tibial plateau**. (Measure distance from ASIS to TT to determine CR angle.)[9]
  - Thin thighs and buttocks (<19 cm ASIS to TT), **3-5° caudad**.
  - Average to thick thighs and buttocks (19-24 cm), **0° ⊥ film**.
  - Thick thighs and buttocks (>24 cm), **3-5° cephalad**.

Note: This author found that the tibial plateau normally slopes 7-11° downward from anterior to posterior with respect to the long axis of the tibia, others suggest 10-20°.[10]

SID: 40–48" (102–122 cm)

Collimation: Sides to skin borders, ends to film borders.

Technique: kVp for grid (70±5) _____

	cm	kVp	mA	Time	mAs	SID	Film–Screen	Grid	F.S.
Model	11	70			5	44"	Kodak 400	12:1	S
Room									
S									
M									
L									

Bontrager Textbook, 3rd ed., p. 204

mrad		
	S 28	G NDC M
	ML 12	<0.1 F

AP Oblique Knee

Medial Oblique: Demonstrates fibular head and neck unobscured.
(Lateral oblique may also be taken as a second oblique of knee.)

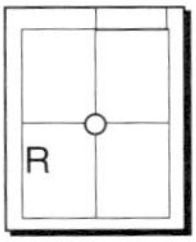

- 8 x 10" (20 x 24 cm)
- Grid >10 cm
  Screen <10 cm

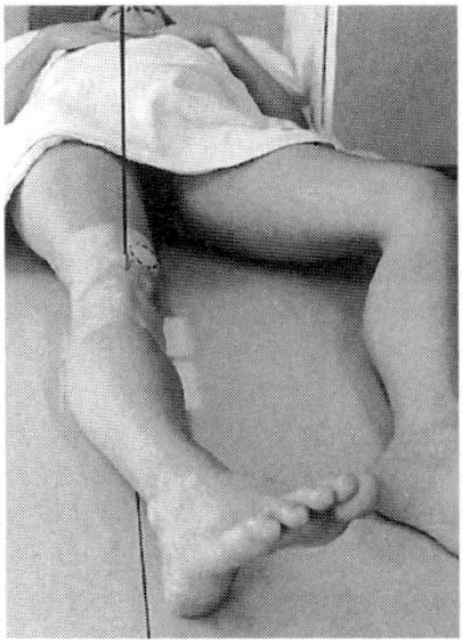

45° medial oblique

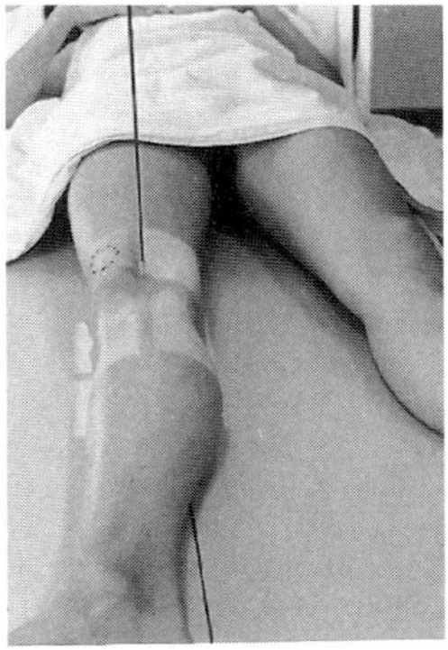

45° lateral oblique

Position

- Supine, leg extended and centered to CR and midline of table or cassette.
- Rotate entire leg including knee, ankle and foot internally 45° for medial oblique, and 45° externally for external oblique.
- Center cassette to CR.

Central Ray

- CR ⊥ to film on average patient (see AP knee).
- CR to mid joint space (3/4" or 2 cm inferior to patella).

SID: 40–48" (102–122 cm)

Collimation: Sides to skin borders, ends to film borders.

mrad per projection

S	28	G	NDC M
ML	13		<0.1 F

Technique: kVp for grid (70±5) _____

	cm	kVp	mA	Time	mAs	SID	Film–Screen	Grid	F.S.
Model	10	70			5	44"	Kodak 400	12:1	S
Room									
S									
M									
L									

Bontrager Textbook, 3rd ed., p. 205

Lateral Knee

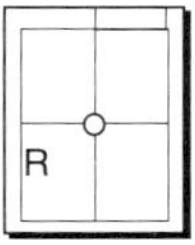

- 8 x 10" L.W. (20 x 24 cm)
- Grid >10 cm
  Screen <10 cm

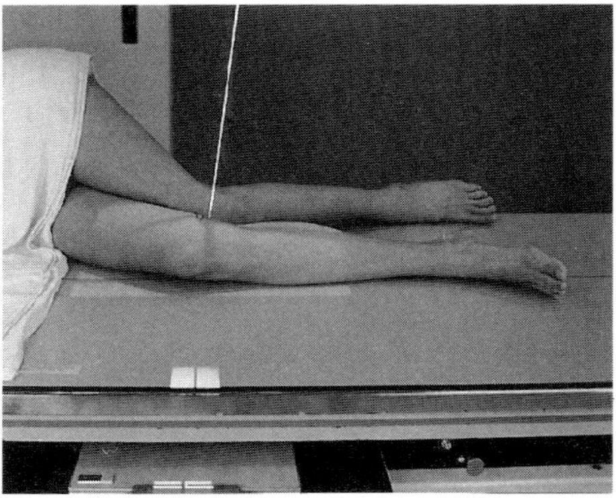

Mediolateral knee, CR 5° cephalad

Position

- Patient on affected side, knee flexed ≈20° [11], centered to CR and midline of table or cassette.
- Unaffected leg & knee placed behind to prevent over rotation.
- Place support under affected ankle and foot if needed and adjust body rotation as required for a true lateral of knee.
- Center cassette to CR.

Central Ray

- CR 5–7° cephalad.[12,13]
- CR centered to ≈ 3/4" (2 cm) distal to medial epicondyle (level of 3/4" or 2 cm distal to apex of patella).

SID: 40–48" (102–122 cm)

Collimation: Sides to skin borders, ends to borders of film.

Technique: kVp for grid (70±5) _____

mrad

S 22	G NDC M
ML 11	<0.1 F

	cm	kVp	mA	Time	mAs	SID	Film–Screen	Grid	F.S.
Model Room	10	70			4	44"	Kodak 400	12:1	S
S									
M									
L									

Bontrager Textbook, 3rd ed., p. 206

Knees - AP or PA Weight Bearing

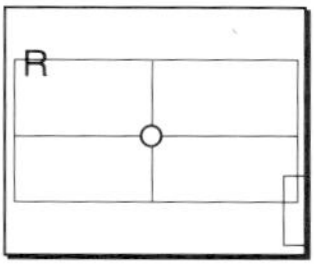

- 11 x 14" C.W. (28 x 35 cm)
- Grid

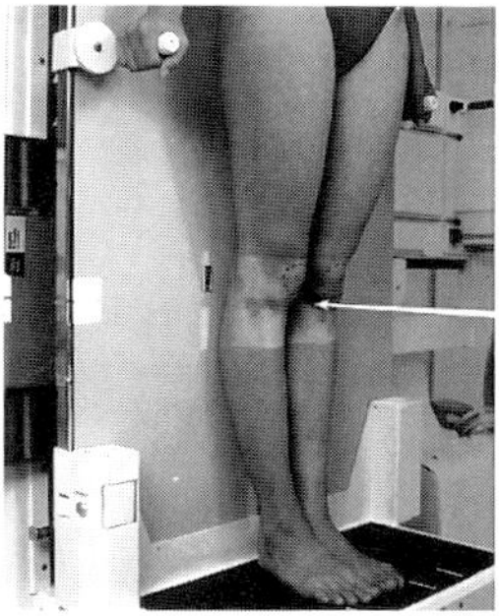

AP weight bearing - bilateral - CR ⊥ to film

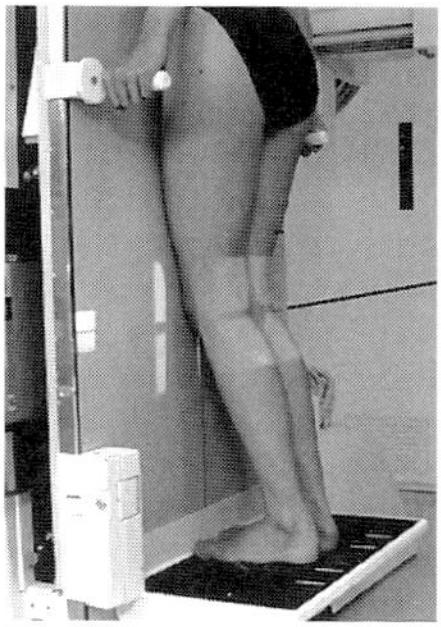

PA weight bearing - bilateral. - CR 10° caudad

Position

AP:

- Erect, standing on step stool or foot board as needed (to be high enough to get x-ray tube low for horizontal beam).
- Feet straight ahead, knees straight, weight distributed evenly on both feet. Have patient hold onto table handles for support.

Alternate PA: Patient facing the table or film holder, with knees against table or vertical film holder, knees flexed ≈20°.

Central Ray: CR to midpoint betweeen knee joints, at level of ≈ 3/4" (2 cm) distal to apex of patellae.

AP: CR horizontal, ⊥ to film on average patient (see AP knee).

PA: CR 10° caudad (if lower legs are flexed ≈20°).

SID: 40–48" (102–122 cm)

Collimation: To bilateral knee joint region.

Technique: kVp (70±5) _____

mrad

S 34	G NDC M
ML 14	<0.1 F

	cm	kVp	mA	Time	mAs	SID	Film–Screen	Grid	F.S.
Model	11	70			6	44"	Kodak 400	12:1	S
Room									
S									
M									
L									

Knee for Intercondylar Fossa
Camp Coventry and Holmblad Methods
(Tunnel View)

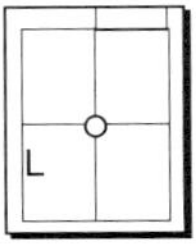

- 8 x 10" L.W. (20 x 24 cm)
- Grid

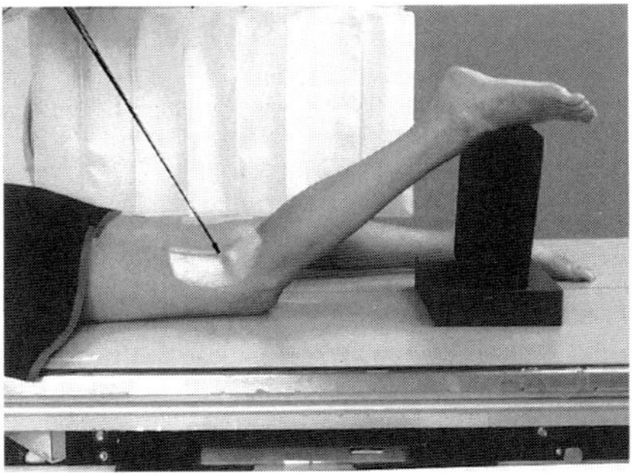

PA axial projection (Camp Coventry)

Camp Coventry:
Position

- Prone, knee flexed 40–50°, large support under ankle.
- Knee centered to CR.
- Cassette centered to projected CR.

Central Ray: CR 40–50° caudad (⊥ to lower leg), centered to knee joint, to emerge at distal margin of patella.

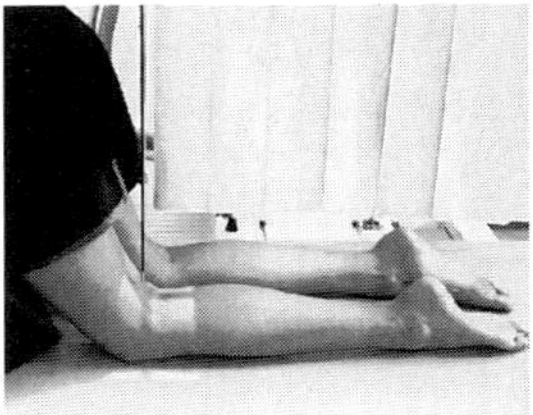

Holmblad Method
- Patient kneeling, leans forward 20-30°.
- CR ⊥ to film

Alternate Holmblad Method:

SID: 40–48" (102–122 cm)

Collimation: Four sides to area of interest.

Technique: kVp for grid (78±5) _____
(+ ≈8 kVp from PA due to CR angle)

mrad

S 36	G NDC M
ML 17	<0.1 F

	cm	kVp	mA	Time	mAs	SID	Film–Screen	Grid	F.S.
Model	11	78			5	44"	Kodak 400	12:1	5
Room									
S									
M									
L									

Bontrager Textbook, 3rd ed., p. 207

PA Patella

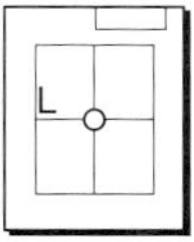

- 8 x 10" L.W. (20 x 24 cm)
- Grid

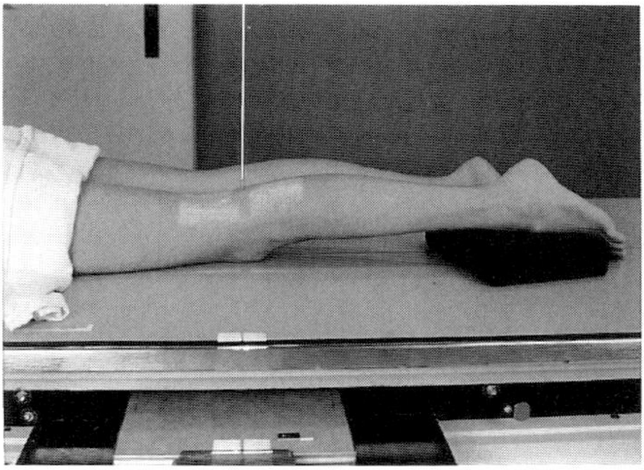

PA patella

Position

- Prone, knee centered to CR and midline of table or film.
- If patella area is painful, place pad under thigh and leg to prevent direct pressure on patella.
- Rotate anterior knee approximately 5° internally or as needed to place an imaginary line between the epicondyles parallel to the plane of the film.
- Center cassette to CR.

Central Ray

- CR ⊥, centered to central patella region (at mid-popliteal crease).

SID: 40–48" (102–122 cm)

Collimation: To area of patella and knee joint.

mrad

S 33	G NDC M
ML 17	<0.1 F

Technique: kVp (76±5) _____(+ 6–8 kVp from PA knee for better visualization of patella through the femur)

	cm	kVp	mA	Time	mAs	SID	Film–Screen	Grid	F.S.
Model Room	10	76			5	44"	Kodak 400	12:1	S
S									
M									
L									

Bontrager Textbook, 3rd ed., p. 209

Lateral Patella

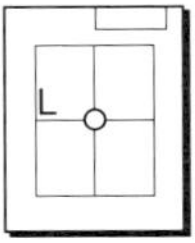

- 8 x 10" L.W. (20 x 24 cm)
- TT (detail screens - may use grid on large patient)

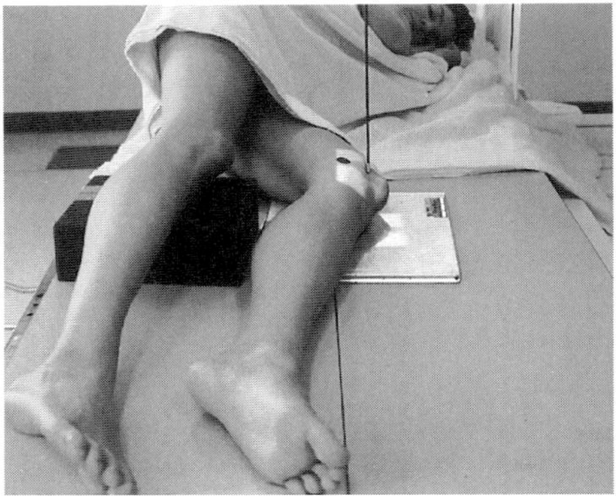

Lateral patella

Position

- Recumbent on affected side, opposite knee and leg behind to prevent over rotation.
- Flex knee ≈10°, or none at all, to prevent separation of fractured fragments if present.[14,15]
- Patellofemoral joint area centered to CR and midline of cassette.

Central Ray

- CR ⊥, centered to mid patellofemoral joint space.

SID: 40–48" (102–122 cm)

Collimation: To area of knee joint, patella and patellofemoral joint.

Technique: kVp (65±5) _____

mrad

S 20	G NDC M
ML 18	<0.1 F

	cm	kVp	mA	Time	mAs	SID	Film–Screen	Grid	F.S.
Model	5	65			4	40"	Kodak 100	–	S
Room									
S									
M									
L									

Bontrager Textbook, 3rd ed., p. 210

Patella – Tangential Projection
Merchant Bilateral Method[16]

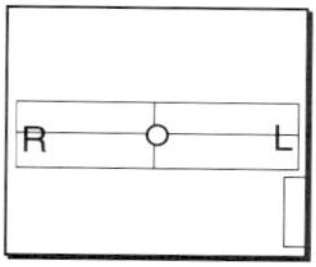

- 11 x 14" C.W. (28 x 35 cm)
- Screen (non-grid)
- Adjustable leg and cassette-holding device is required

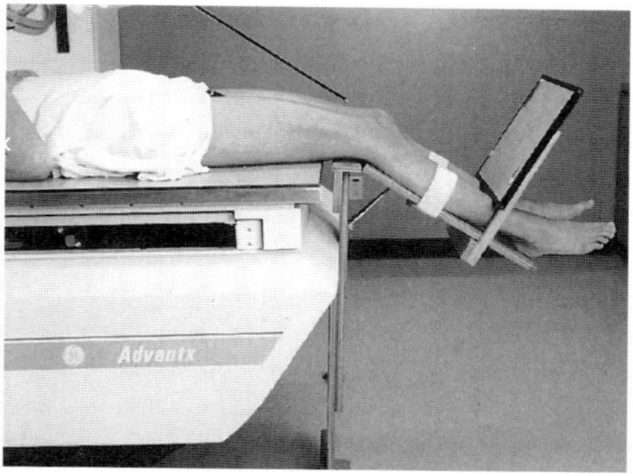

Bilateral tangential

Position
- Supine with knees flexed 45° on leg supports. (Important for patient to be comfortable with legs totally relaxed to prevent patellae from being drawn into intercondylar sulcus.)[17]
- Place cassette on supports against legs about 12" (30 cm) distal to patellae, perpendicular to CR.
- Internally rotate both legs as needed to center patellae to mid femurs.

Central Ray: CR ≈60° caudad (30° from long axis of femora).
- CR to midpoint between patellae at patellofemoral joints.

SID: 48–72" (120–180 cm), greater SID reduces magnification.

Collimation: To bilateral patellae and patellofemoral joints.

Technique: kVp (65±5) _____

mrad

S 22	G NDC M
ML 14	<0.1 F

	cm	kVp	mA	Time	mAs	SID	Film–Screen	Grid	F.S.
Model	8	65			11	60"	Kodak 100	–	S
Room									
S									
M									
L									

Bontrager Textbook, 3rd ed., p. 211

Patella – Tangential Projection
Settegast and Hughston Methods

Generally taken bilaterally for comparison purposes.

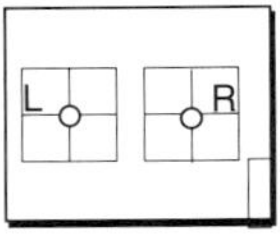

- 10 x 12" C.W. (24 x 30 cm)
- TT (detail screens)

Settegast
- Knee flexed 90°
- CR 15-20° to leg

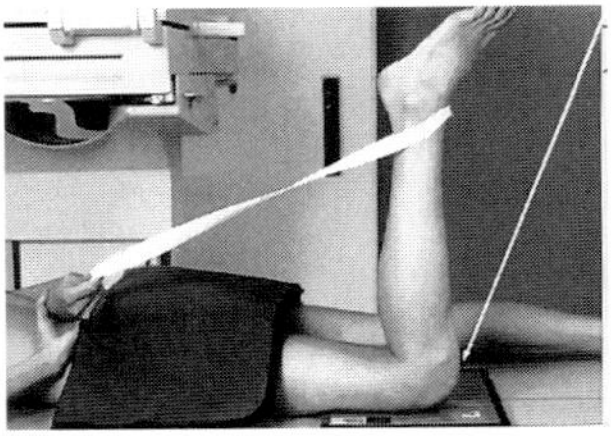

Hughston
- Knee flexed 55°
- CR 45° (10-15° to leg)

Warning - possible **hot** collimator, use pad.

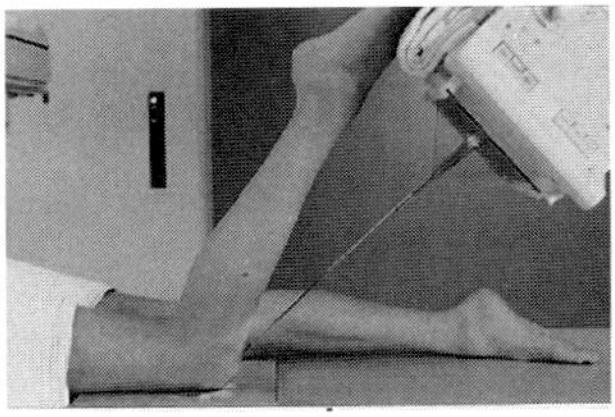

Position
- Prone, knee flexed as shown.
- Use long gauze or tape for patient to hold leg in position; for Hughston method, may support foot on collimator, use pad.

Central Ray: CR centered to patellofemoral joint space.

Settegast: CR 15-20° cephalad to long axis of leg (15-20° from vertical).

Hughston: CR 45° cephalad, 10-15° to long axis of leg.

SID: 36–40" (91–102 cm)

Collimate closely to patella region.

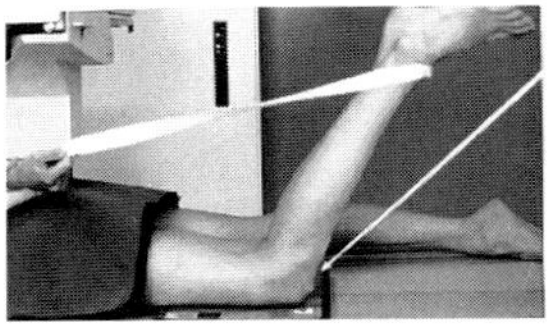

Hughston
- Using gauze or tape

Technique: kVp (65±5) _____

mrad

S	22	G NDC M
ML	14	<0.1 F

	cm	kVp	mA	Time	mAs	SID	Film–Screen	Grid	F.S.
Model	8	65			5	40"	Kodak 100	–	S
Room									
S									
M									
L									

Bontrager Textbook, 3rd ed., p. 212

AP Femur

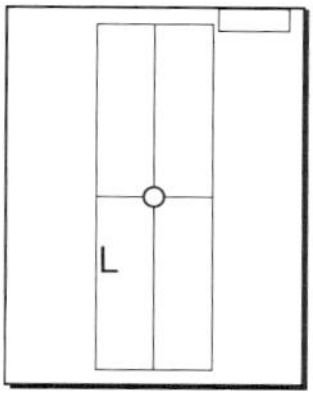

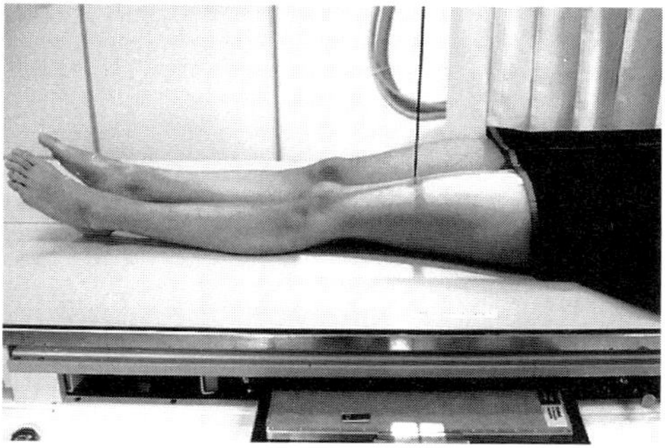

AP, mid and distal femur

- 14 x 17" L.W. (35 x 43 cm)
- Grid
- Hip at cathode end of table to maximize anode–heel effect

Note: For adults, a second smaller film of either the hip or knee should be taken on trauma patients to demonstrate both knee and hip joints to rule out possible fractures.

Position

- Supine, femur centered to midline of table or grid cassette.
- Rotate entire lower limb internally ≈5° for AP of mid and distal femur, and 15° internally for true AP to include hip.
- Lower border of cassette ≈2" (5 cm) below knee to include knee joint adequately (see AP hip for proximal femur).
- **Shield gonads** for both male and female (see gonadal doses).

Central Ray: CR ⊥, to midfilm.

SID: 40–48" (102–122 cm)

Collimation: Long narrow collimation to femur area.

Technique: kVp (75±5) _____

mrad

S 55	G 11 M
ML 20	0.2 F

	cm	kVp	mA	Time	mAs	SID	Film–Screen	Grid	F.S.
Model Room	13	75			8	44"	Kodak 400	12:1	S
S									
M									
L									

Bontrager Textbook, 3rd ed., p. 214

Lateral Femur

Warning: Take cross table lateral if fracture is suspected.

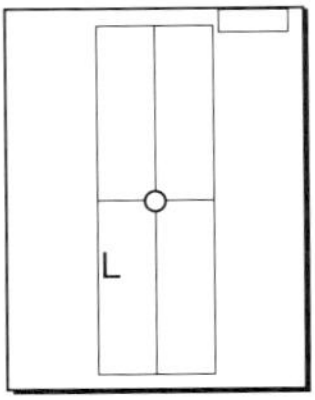

- 14 x 17" L.W. (35 x 43 cm)
- Grid
- Hip at cathode end (anode–heel effect)

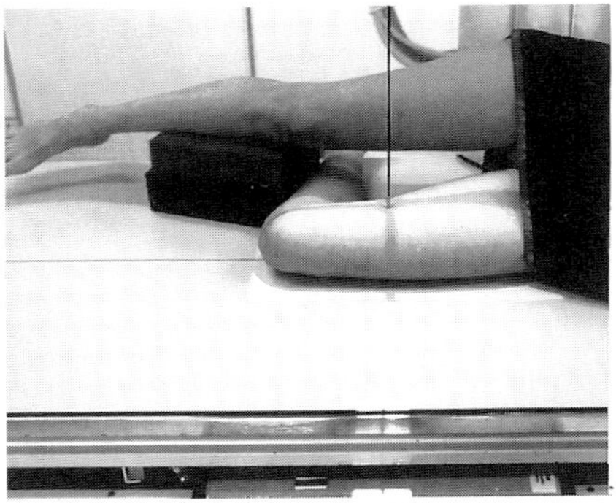

Lateral, mid and distal femur

Note: For adults, take a second smaller film of lateral hip or lateral knee if both joints are areas of interest.

Position

- Lateral recumbent, with unaffected leg placed behind to prevent over rotation.
- Include sufficient amount of either knee or hip at one end of film (see above note).
- **Shield gonads** for both male and female (see gonadal doses).

Central Ray: CR ⊥, to midfilm.

SID: 40–48" (102–122 cm)

Collimation: Long narrow collimation to femur area.

Technique: kVp (75±5) _____

mrad

S 47	G 9 M
ML 21	0.2 F

	cm	kVp	mA	Time	mAs	SID	Film–Screen	Grid	F.S.
Model	11	75			7	44"	Kodak 400	12:1	S
Room									
S									
M									
L									

Bontrager Textbook, 3rd ed., p. 215

Cross Table Lateral Femur

Trauma Mid and Distal Femur

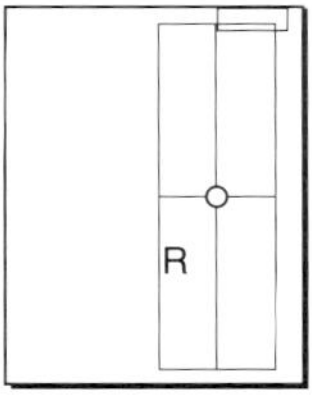

- 14 x 17" L.W. (35 x 43 cm)
- Portable grid

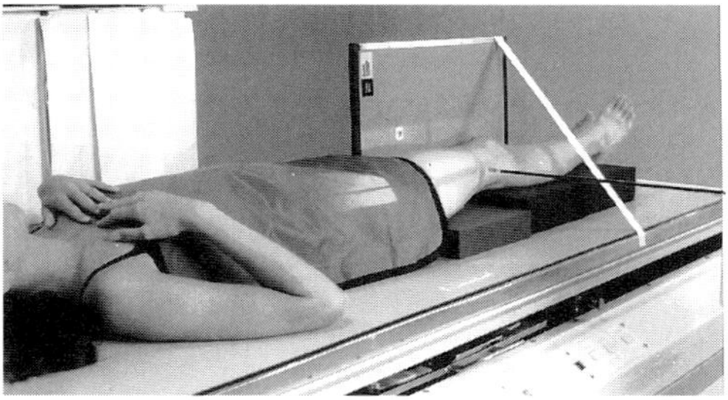

Cross table trauma projection (mid and distal femur)

Note: For proximal femur take axiolateral hip (see next chapter).

Position

- Without moving trauma patient from the supine position, gently lift injured leg and place support under knee and leg.
- Place vertical cassette between legs, as far superiorly as possible, but include knee distally. Use tape to hold grid cassette in position.
- **Shield gonads** for both male and female (see gonadal doses).

Central Ray: CR cross table, ⊥ to midfilm.

SID: 40–48" (102–122 cm)

Collimation: Four sides to area of interest.

Technique: kVp (75±5) _____

mrad

S	21	G	4 M
ML	9		0.1 F

	cm	kVp	mA	Time	mAs	SID	Film–Screen	Grid	F.S.
Model	13	72			5	48"	Kodak 400	6:1	S
Room									
S									
M									
L									

Bontrager Textbook, 3rd ed., p. 215

Pediatric AP Lower Limb

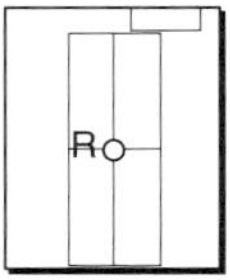

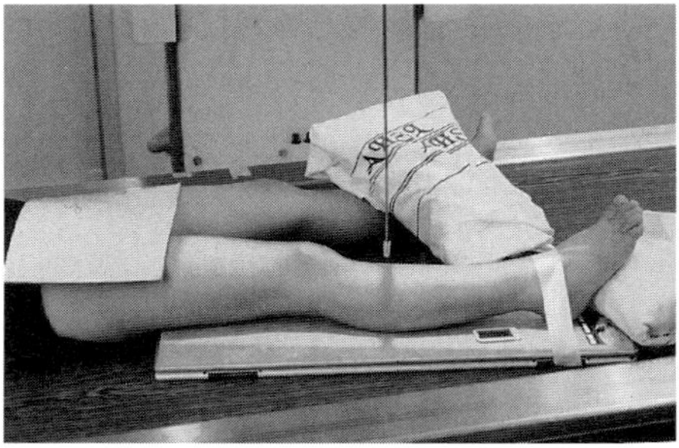

AP lower limb

- Size determined by patient size
- Table top

Note - If foot is specific area of interest, AP and lateral projections of foot only may be required (see later page). A second film of pelvis and/or proximal femur may be required.

Position - Shield gonads.
- Supine, include entire limb, shield over pelvic area.
- Immobilize arms and unaffected leg with sandbags.
- Use parental assistance only if necessary; provide lead gloves and apron.

Central Ray
- CR ⊥, centered to midlimb (midfilm).

SID: 40–48" (102–122 cm)

Collimation: Four sides to area of interest.

Technique: kVp (55–65) _____

mrad

S 17	G NDC M
ML 16	NDC F

	cm	kVp	mA	Time	mAs	SID	Film–Screen	Grid	F.S.
Model Room	5	66			4	40"	Kodak 100	–	S
S									
M									
L									

Bontrager Textbook, 3rd ed., p. 562

Pediatric Lateral Lower Limb

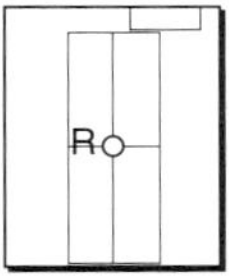

- Size determined by patient size
- Table top

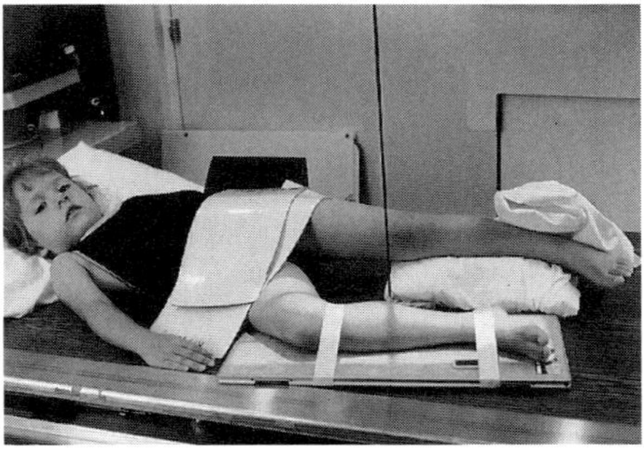

Lateral lower limb

Note - If foot is specific area of interest, AP and lateral projections of foot only may be required. A second film of proximal femur may be required.

Position - Shield gonads.

- Semi-supine, include entire limb, shield over pelvic area.
- Immobilize arms and unaffected leg with sandbags as needed.
- Abduct (frog leg) affected limb into lateral position, immobilize with tape or compression band. (Do not attempt with hip trauma or hip disease, instead turn patient on side for lateral positioning of leg.)
- If parental assistance is necessary, provide lead gloves and apron.

Central Ray: CR ⊥, centered to midlimb (midfilm).

SID: 40–48" (102–122 cm)

Collimation: Four sides to area of interest.

Technique: kVp (55–65) _____

mrad

S 17	G NDC M
ML 16	NDC F

	cm	kVp	mA	Time	mAs	SID	Film–Screen	Grid	F.S.
Model Room	5	66			4	40"	Kodak 100	–	S
S									
M									
L									

Bontrager Textbook, 3rd ed., p. 562

Pediatric-AP & Lateral Foot

(Congenital clubfoot - Kite Method) [17]

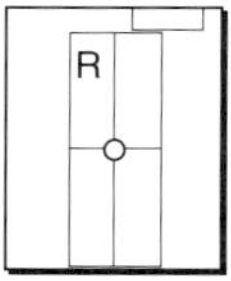

- 8 x 10 L.W. (20 x 24 cm)
- TT (detail screens)

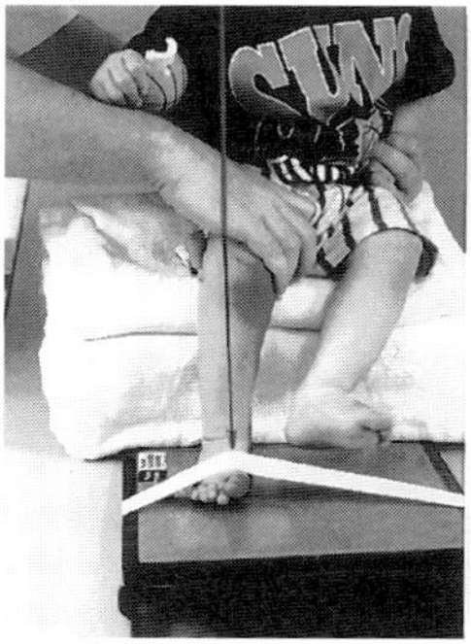

AP foot

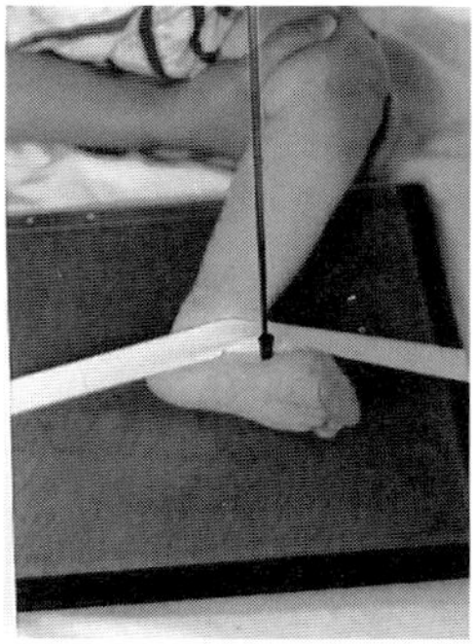

Mediolateral foot

Note: With Kite method no attempt is made to straighten foot when placing on cassette. The foot is held or immobilized for a frontal and side view (AP and lateral projections) 90° from each other. Both feet generally taken for comparison.

Position:
- **AP:** Elevate patient on support, flex knee, foot on cassette.
- **Lateral:** Patient and/or leg on side, affected side down, use tape or compression band.

Central Ray:
- **AP:** CR ⊥ to film, directed to mid tarsals (Kite suggests no angle).
- **Lateral:** CR ⊥, centered to proximal metatarsal area.

SID: 40–48" (102–122 cm)

Collimation: Closely on four sides to area of foot.

Technique: kVp (50±5) _____

mrad, two projections			
	S	5	G NDC M
	ML	5	NDC F

	cm	kVp	mA	Time	mAs	SID	Film–Screen	Grid	F.S.
Model Room	3-4	50			3	40"	Kodak 100	–	S
S									
M									
L									

Lower Limb

Position:

Central Ray:

SID:

Collimation:

Respiration:

Technique:

	Room	cm	kVp	mA	Time	mAs	SID	Film–Screen	Grid	F.S.
S										
M										
L										

Lower Limb

Position:

Central Ray:

SID:

Collimation:

Respiration:

Technique:

	cm	kVp	mA	Time	mAs	SID	Film–Screen	Grid	F.S.
Model									
Room									
S									
M									
L									

Bontrager Textbook, 3rd ed.,

Chapter 6

Proximal Femora & Pelvis

Proximal Femora and Pelvis

Radiation Protection

Male: Gonadal shields should be used on pelvis and hip procedures for **all** male children and adults of childbearing age. Contact shields should be placed over the testes with the upper edge of the shield placed at the inferior margin of the symphysis pubis.

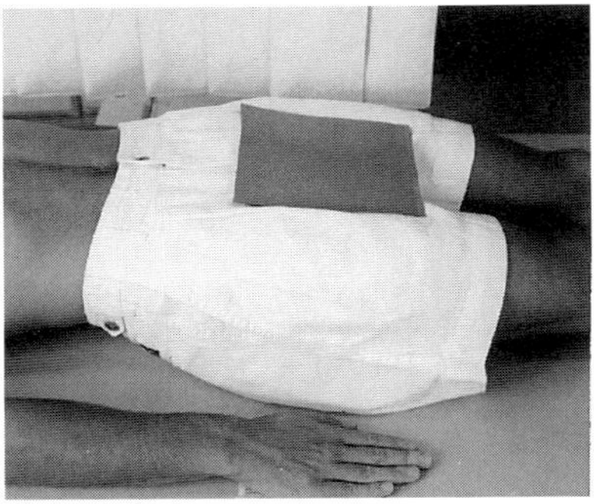

Male gonadal shielding

Female: For AP and "frog-leg" laterals of the hips, special shaped ovarian shields can be carefully placed over the area of the ovaries without obscuring essential anatomy as shown. This should be done on all children and adults of childbearing age. These ovarian shields however, may obscure essential anatomy on certain pelvic exams. Departmental policy regarding shielding and kVp range to be used should be determined.

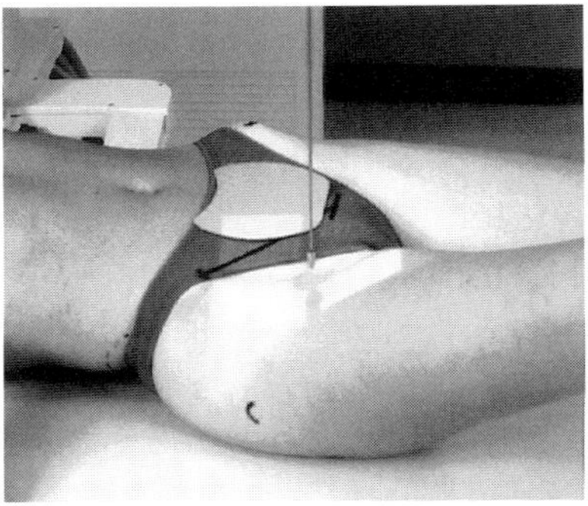

Female ovarian shielding
(Superior borders at or slightly above level of ASIS's and lower border just above pubis.)

kVp Range: A higher kVp range (90±5) may be used for exams of the hips and pelvis of adults to reduce the total radiation dose to the patient.[1] (See page 140 for patient dosage at 90 kVp compared to 80 kVp for AP bilateral hips.)

Close collimation to the area of interest is important for all procedures including the hips and pelvis, even with gonadal shields. (See Appendix E for further explanation.)

Location of Femoral Head and Neck

Location of the femoral head and neck regions can be accurately determined by first drawing an imaginary line between two landmarks, the **ASIS** and the **symphysis pubis**. The midpoint of this line is determined, from which a perpendicular imaginary line is drawn to locate the head and/or neck. The femoral head (A) is approximately 1 1/2" or 4 cm (≈2 finger widths) down on this line. The midfemoral neck (B) is about 2 1/2" or 6 cm (3 to 4 finger widths) down as shown in the photo below.

A second method for locating the femoral neck is ≈1" (2.5 cm) medial to ASIS at the level of the proximal or upper margin of the symphysis pubis.

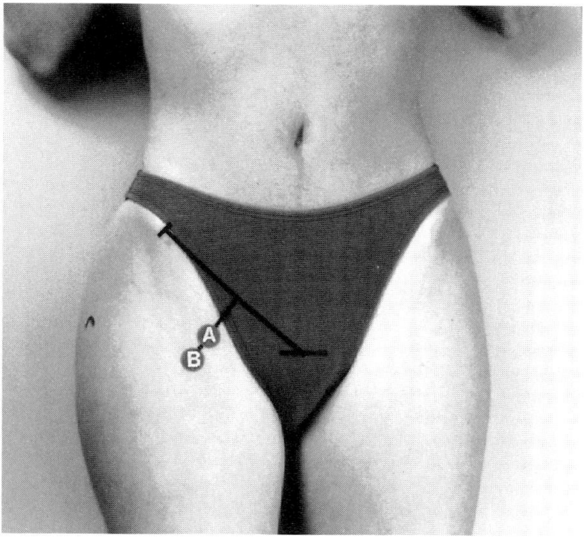

- A Femoral head
  - 1 1/2" (4 cm) or ≈2 finger widths
- B Femoral neck
  - 2 1/2" (6 cm) or 3-4 finger widths

AP Bilateral Hips

Warning: Do not attempt to rotate leg if fracture is suspected. Take "as is" bilateral hips for comparison purposes.

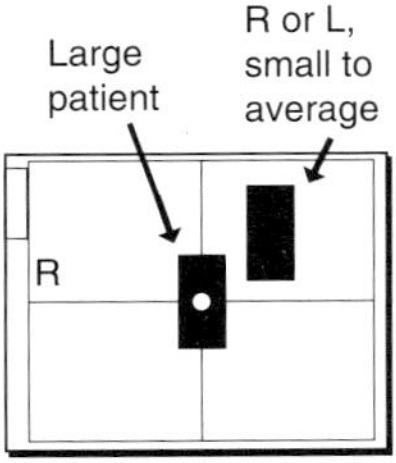

• 14 x 17" C.W. (35 x 43 cm)
• Grid

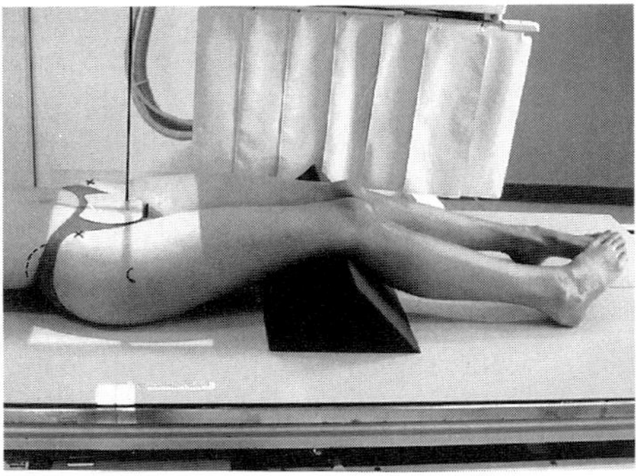

AP bilateral hips

Position

• Supine, aligned and centered to CR and cassette, both legs extended and equally rotated internally 15-20°. (See warning above.)
• Ensure no rotation of pelvis (bilateral ASIS' the same distances from table top). Support under knees for patient comfort.
• Center cassette to CR. **Shield gonads**.* (See p. 138.)

Central Ray: CR ⊥, to midpoint between femoral heads (≈1" or 2.5 cm superior to symphysis pubis).

SID: 40–48" (102–122 cm)

Collimation: To pelvic and hip borders.

Respiration: Suspend during exposure.

mrad without shields*

@ 80 kVp	S 53	G 49 M
	ML 14	18 F
@ 90 kVp	S 38	G 34 M
	ML 11	14 F

Technique: kVp (80±5) (or 90±5 for less pt. exposure) _____

	cm	kVp	mA	Time	mAs	SID	Film–Screen	Grid	F.S.
Model	16	80/90			6/4	44"	Kodak 400	12:1	S
Room									
S									
M									
L									

*Gonadal shields placed correctly will reduce these female gonadal doses to ≈ 1.0 mrad or less, and male doses to testes to <0.1.

AP Unilateral Hip

Warning: For possible fractured hip, take AP bilateral hips (preceding page) **without rotation** of injured hip for comparison purposes.

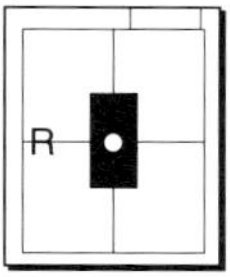

- 10 x 12" L.W. (24 x 30 cm)
- Grid

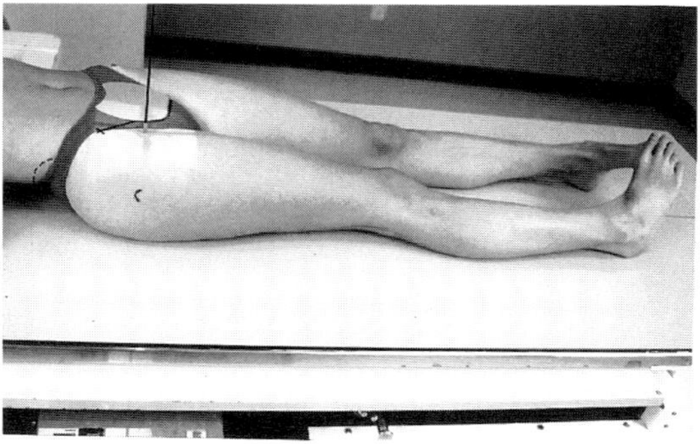

AP hip – CR to femoral neck

Position

- Supine, leg extended and rotated internally 15–20°.
- Center femoral neck to CR and center cassette (2 1/2" or 6–7 cm inferior to midpoint of line connecting ASIS and symphysis pubis). Support may be placed under knees for patient comfort.
- Center cassette to CR. **Shield gonads*** (males and females).

Central Ray

- CR ⊥, to femoral neck.

SID: 40–48" (102–122 cm)

Collimation: Four sides to area of interest.

Respiration: Suspend during exposure.

@ 80 kVp
mrad without shields*

S	52	G	33 M
ML	15		6 F

Technique: kVp (80±5) (or 90±5 for less pt. exposure) _____

	cm	kVp	mA	Time	mAs	SID	Film–Screen	Grid	F.S.
Model Room	16	80/90			6/4	48"	Kodak 400	12:1	S
S									
M									
L									

*Gonadal shields placed correctly will reduce these female gonadal doses to ≈ 1.0 mrad or less, and male doses to testes to <0.1.

Lateral Hip (Non–trauma)

Unilateral "Frog-leg"

Warning: Do **not** attempt with possible hip fracture or pathology of hip area.

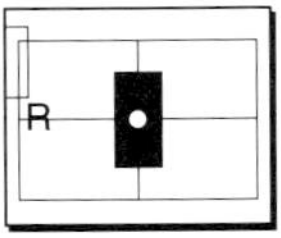

- 10 x 12" C.W. (24 x 30 cm)
- Grid

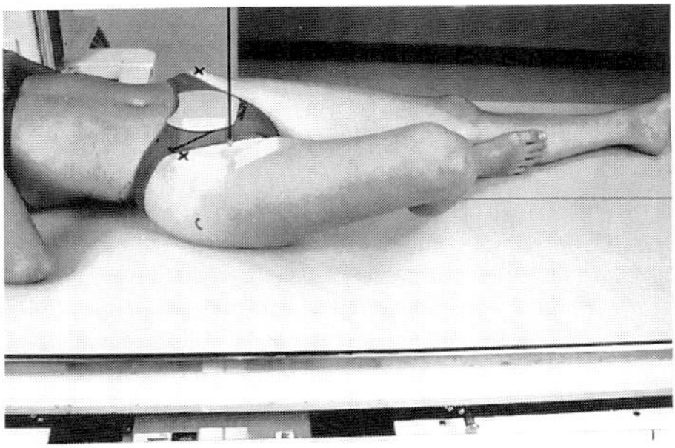
Right hip "frog-leg" lateral (for femoral neck)

Position

- Patient in supine position.
- For femoral neck, flex affected knee approx. 90°, and abduct femur 40–45° from vertical (places femoral neck parallel to film).
- For femoral head and acetabulum, oblique patient 35-45° toward affected side and abduct leg to table top if possible.
- Center hip and neck area to CR.
- Center cassette to CR. **Shield gonads*** (male and female).

Central Ray: CR ⊥, to mid femoral neck or head.

Note: CR angle of 20–25° cephalad may better demonstrate femoral neck.[2,3]

SID: 40–48" (102–122 cm)

Collimation: To proximal femur and hip.

Respiration: Suspend during exposure.

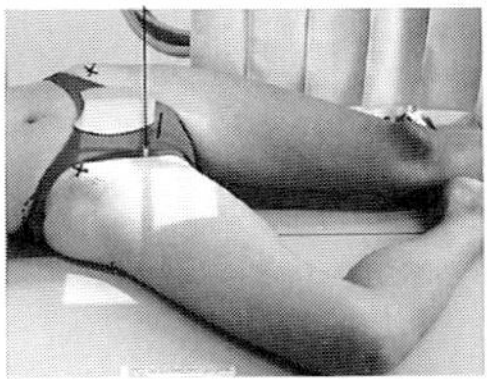
For femoral head and acetabulum

Technique:
kVp (80 or 90±5) _____

@ 80 kVp, mrad*

S	51	G	32 M
ML	16		6 F

	cm	kVp	mA	Time	mAs	SID	Film–Screen	Grid	F.S.
Model Room	16	80/90			6/4	48"	Kodak 400	12:1	S
S									
M									
L									

*Gonadal shields placed correctly will reduce these female gonadal doses to ≈ 1.0 mrad or less, and male doses to testes to <0.1.

Lateral Hips (Non–trauma)

Bilateral "Frog-leg"

Warning: Do **not** attempt with possible hip fracture or pathology of hip area.

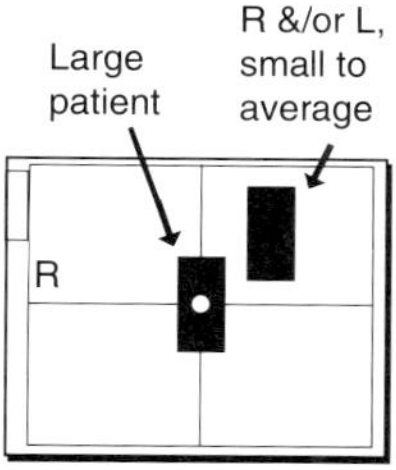

- 14 x 17" C.W. (35 x 43 cm)
- Grid

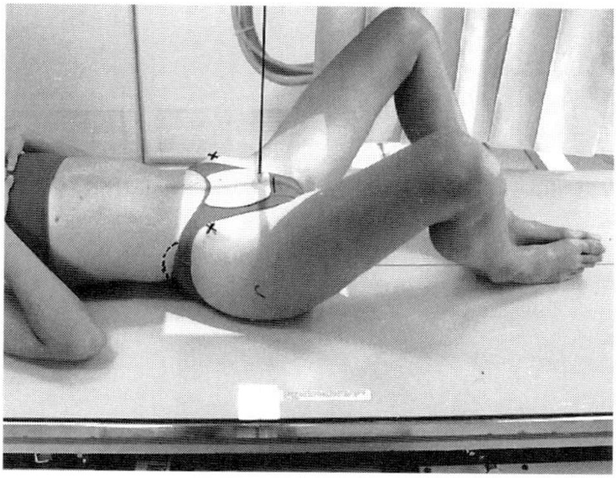

Bilateral "frog-leg" (for comparison)

Position

- Supine, centered to CR and cassette, flex hips and knees and **abduct both thighs equally** to 40–45° from vertical if possible, feet together.
- Ensure **no rotation** of pelvis (ASIS' equal distance from table).
- Center cassette to CR, **shield gonads*** (male and female).

Central Ray: CR ⊥, to level of femoral heads (≈1" or 2.5 cm superior to symphysis pubis).

SID: 40–48" (102–122 cm)

Collimation: To film borders.

Respiration: Suspend during exposure.

@ 80 kVp, mrad*

S	53	G	49 M
ML	14		18 F

Technique: kVp (80±5) (or 90±5 for reduced exposure) _____

	cm	kVp	mA	Time	mAs	SID	Film–Screen	Grid	F.S.
Model	16	80/90			6/4	48"	Kodak 400	12:1	S
Room									
S									
M									
L									

*Gonadal shields placed correctly will reduce these female gonadal doses to ≈ 1.0 mrad or less, and male doses to testes to <0.1.

Lateral Hip (Trauma Method)

Axiolateral (Cross Table) Projection (Danelius-Miller method)

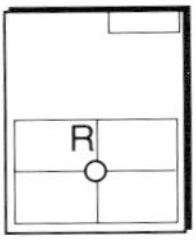

- 8 x 10" Vertical (20 x 24 cm)
- Portable grid (centered to CR)

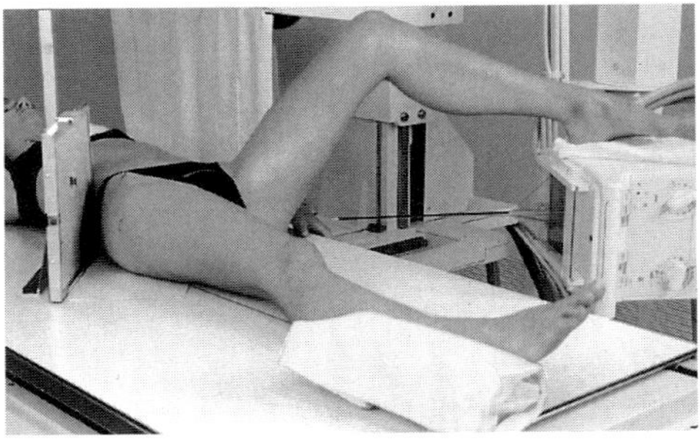

Cross table axiolateral trauma hip (pad under foot)

Position

- Supine, no rotation of pelvis.
- Flex unaffected knee and hip and provide support such as the x-ray tube (use pad or towels for possible **hot collimator**).
- Rotate affected leg internally 15° unless possible hip fracture.
- Place vertical grid cassette against patient's side just superior to iliac crest with plane of film perpendicular to CR.

Central Ray

- CR horizontal, perpendicular to femoral neck area and film.

SID: 40" (102 cm)

Collimation: On four sides to proximal femur area.

Respiration: Suspend during exposure.

Technique: kVp (80±5) _____

mrad

S 336	G 336 M
ML 56	16 F

	cm	kVp	mA	Time	mAs	SID	Film–Screen	Grid	F.S.
Model	22	75			40	40"	Kodak 400	6:1	L
Room									
S									
M									
L									

Bontrager Textbook, 3rd ed., p. 232

AP Pelvis

To include proximal femora, pelvic girdle, sacrum, and coccyx

Warning: Do not attempt to rotate legs if fractures involving hips are suspected.

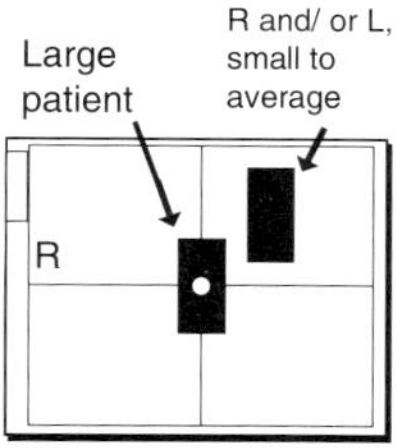

- 14 x 17" C.W. (35 x 43 cm)
- Grid

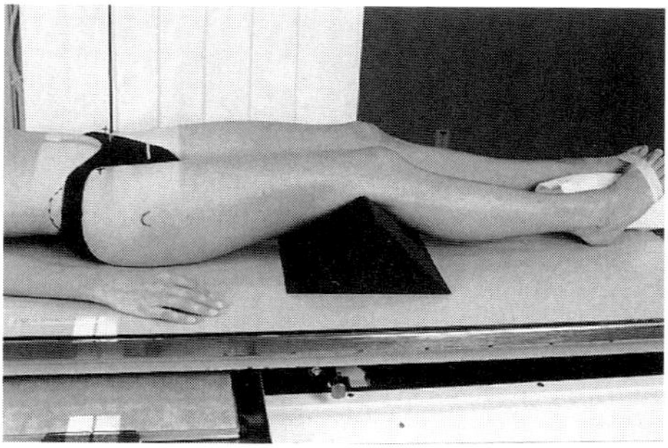

AP pelvis (entire pelvis centered to film)

Position

- Supine, pelvis centered to centerline, legs extended.
- Both feet, knees and legs equally rotated internally 15° (secure with tape if necessary). Support under knees for comfort.
- Ensure no rotation of pelvis (ASIS', equal distance from TT).
- Center cassette to entire pelvis, checking upper and lower pelvic borders. **Shield gonads for males**. (See page 138.)

Central Ray: CR ⊥, to midpoint of pelvis and film.

SID: 40–48" (102–122 cm)

Collimation: On four sides to include entire pelvis.

Respiration: Suspend during exposure.

mrad,without shields

S 61	G	6 M
ML 16		15 F

Technique: kVp (80±5) or (90±5) _____

	cm	kVp	mA	Time	mAs	SID	Film–Screen	Grid	F.S.
Model	16	80			7	40"	Kodak 400	12:1	S
Room									
S									
M									
L									

Bontrager Textbook, 3rd ed., p. 234

AP Axial Pelvis
(Anterior Pelvic Bones)

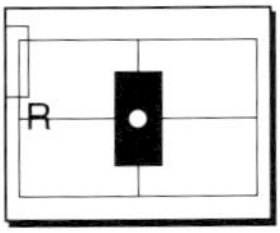

- 10 x 12" C.W. (24 x 30 cm)
- Grid

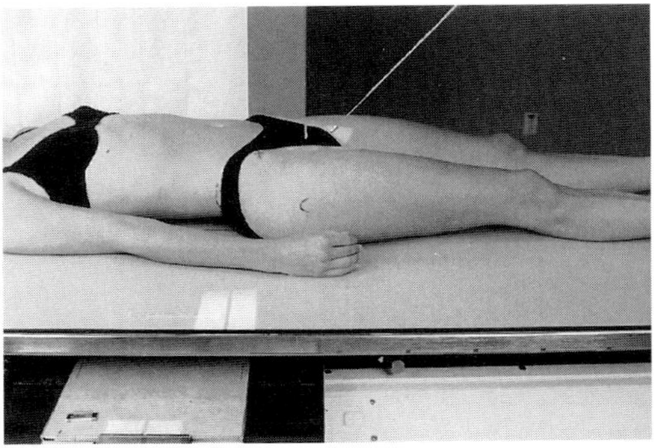

AP axial, CR 40° cephalad (female)

Position
- Supine, patient centered to centerline.
- No rotation of pelvis (ASIS' the same distance from table top).
- Center cassette to projected CR. Gondal shielding may not be possible without obscuring essential anatomy.

Central Ray
- CR: Male, 20–30° cephalad; Female, 30–45° cephalad.
- CR 1 1/2– 2" (4–5 cm) inferior to symphysis pubis.

SID: 40–48" (102–122 cm)

Collimation: Four sides to area of interest.

Respiration: Suspend during exposure.

mrad — without shields

S	89	G	89 M
ML	24		22 F

Technique: kVp (85±5) ________

(Increase total exposure 6-7 kVp from AP pelvis due to axial projection.)

	cm	kVp	mA	Time	mAs	SID	Film–Screen	Grid	F.S.
Model	17	86			7	44"	Kodak 400	12:1	S
Room									
S									
M									
L									

Bontrager Textbook, 3rd ed., p. 237

Sacroiliac Joints
AP Axial

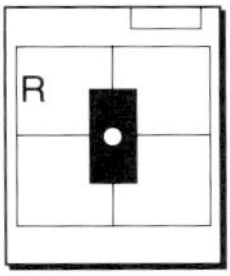

- 10 x 12" L.W. (24 x 30 cm)
- Grid

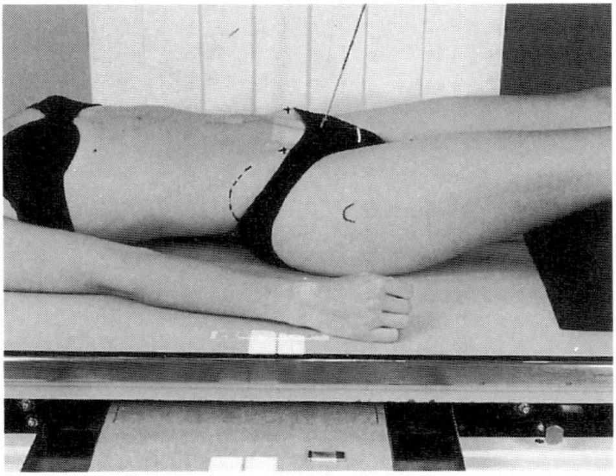
AP axial S–I joints (CR 30–35° cephalad)

Position
- Supine, center patient to centerline.
- No rotation of pelvis (ASIS' the same distance from table top).
- Center cassette to projected CR. **Shield gonads** for males.

Central Ray
- CR 30° (males) and 35° (females) cephalad, to midway between level of ASIS's and symphysis pubis.

SID: 40–48" (102–122 cm)

Collimation: Four sides to area of interest.

Respiration: Suspend during exposure.

mrad (without shields)

S	106	G 9 M
ML	30	26 F

Technique: kVp (85±5) _______

(Increase total exposure 5-6 kVp from AP pelvis due to axial projection.)

	cm	kVp	mA	Time	mAs	SID	Film–Screen	Grid	F.S.
Model	17	85			9	44"	Kodak 400	12:1	S
Room									
S									
M									
L									

Bontrager Textbook, 3rd ed., p. 239

Sacroiliac Joints

Posterior Obliques (Bilateral)

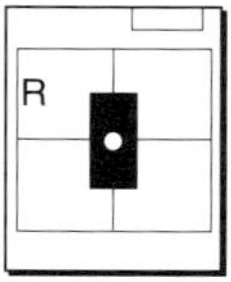

- 10 x 12" L.W. (24 x 30 cm)
- Grid

Two films – bilateral for comparison

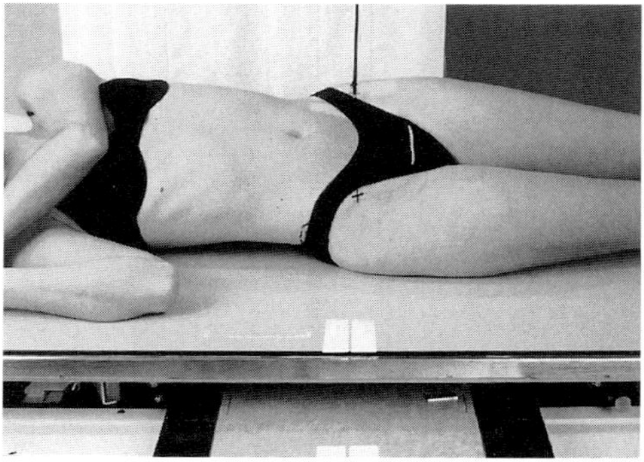

25–30° RPO for up-side (left) joint

Position

- Patient in 25–30° posterior oblique with side of interest elevated (use support to maintain this position).
- Align elevated SI joint to CR and to centerline, (about 1" or 2.5 cm medial to upside ASIS).
- Center cassette to CR. **Shield gonads** for males.

Central Ray: CR ⊥, to 1" (2.5 cm) medial to elevated ASIS.

SID: 40–48" (102–122 cm)

Collimation: Four sides to area of interest.

Respiration: Suspend during exposure.

Note: May also be taken in 25-30° anterior obliques demonstrating side down (joint closest to film).

Technique: kVp (80±5) ______

mrad (without shields)

S 106	G 67 M
ML 30	12 F

	cm	kVp	mA	Time	mAs	SID	Film–Screen	Grid	F.S.
Model	17	80			12	40"	Kodak 400	12:1	S
Room									
S									
M									
L									

Bontrager Textbook, 3rd ed., p. 240

Pediatric AP and Lateral Hips

Warning: Do not attempt "frog-leg" lat. with possible hip pathology unless so indicated by a physician after reviewing AP pelvis radiograph.

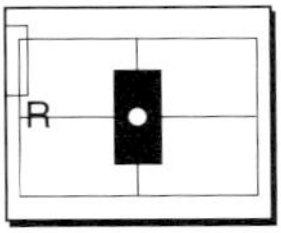

- Film C.W.
- Size determined by patient size
- Grid > 9 or 10 cm
  Screen < 9 or 10 cm

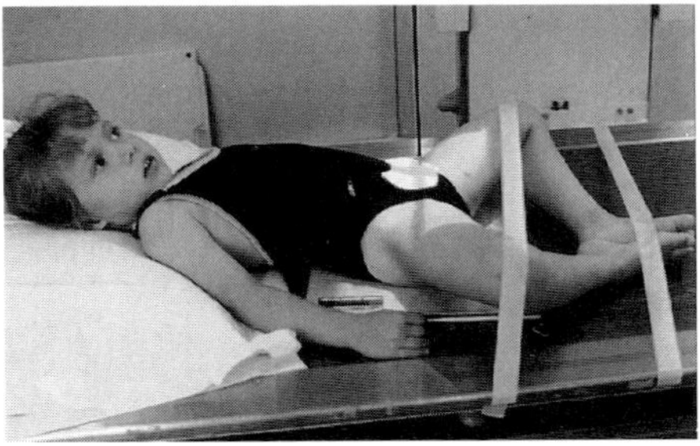

"Frog-leg" lateral hips

Position (AP and lateral)

- Supine, pelvis centered to CR and to cassette, use **gonadal shields on both male and female**. (Use appropriate size ovarian shield for female ensuring it does not cover hip areas).
- Immobilize arms and upper body with sandbags, tapes, or compression band as needed.

AP: Extend legs and internally rotate 15°.

Frog-leg Lateral: Flex knees and hips, place feet together and abduct both legs, secure with tape and sandbags.

Central Ray: CR ⊥, centered to level of hips.

SID: 40–48" (102–122 cm)

Collimation: To pelvic margins.

Respiration: Full inspiration if crying.

mrad (without shields)

S 58	G 58 M
ML 28	21 F

Technique: kVp: screen (65±5) _____, or grid (75±5) _____

	cm	kVp	mA	Time	mAs	SID	Film–Screen	Grid	F.S.
Model	10	66			12	40"	Kodak 100	–	S
Room									
S									
M									
L									

Bontrager Textbook, 3rd ed., p. 564

Hip or Pelvis

Position:

Central Ray:

SID:

Collimation:

Respiration:

Technique:

	Room	cm	kVp	mA	Time	mAs	SID	Film–Screen	Grid	F.S.
S										
M										
L										

Bontrager Textbook, 3rd ed.,

Chapter 7

Vertebral Column

Cervical Spine

Thoracic Spine

Lumbar Spine

Sacrum

Coccyx

Other

Topographical Landmarks

Landmarks which can be used to locate specific vertebrae are demonstrated in frontal and lateral views.[1] Positioning for demonstrating specific vertebrae requires an understanding of certain palpable landmarks. These begin at the upper or proximal vertebral column with **"A"** identifying the **mastoid tip** landmark as being at the level of **C1**. The distal vertebral column ends at the level of the **greater trochanter "L"** as the level of the **distal coccyx.**

Certain of these landmarks are also used for positioning for the pelvis and hips, and for various abdominal procedures as described in other chapters. (See following page for landmarks.)

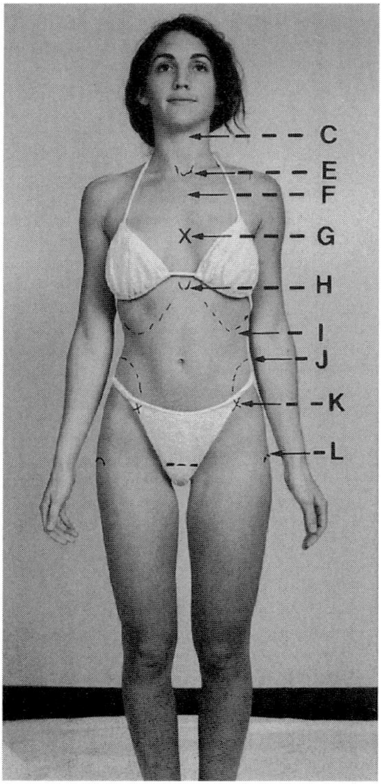

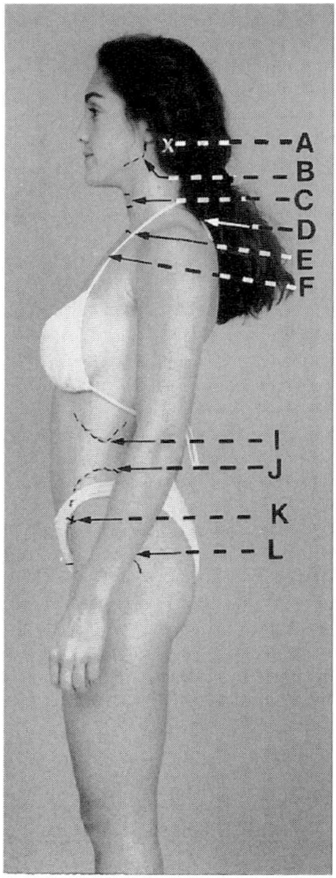

Topographical landmarks continued

Vertebral Column	Landmarks	Approximate levels
Cervical Spine	**A**. Mastoid tip (≈1" or 2.5 cm inferior to EAM.)	C 1
	B. Angle of mandible	C 2 or C 2–3 interspace
	C. Thyroid cartilage	C 4–5
	D. Vertebra prominens	C 7–T 1
Thoracic Spine	**E**. Jugular notch	T 2–3
	F. Sternal angle	T 4–5
	G. Midway between sternal angle & xiphoid process	T 7
	H. Xiphoid process	T 10
Lumbar Spine	**I**. Inferior costal margin	L 2–3
	J. Iliac crest	L 4–5 interspace
Sacrum	**K**. Anterior superior iliac spine (ASIS)	S 2
Coccyx	**L**. Greater trochanter (≈1" above symphysis pubis)	Distal coccyx

Intervertebral Foramina and Zygapophyseal Joints

Certain lateral and oblique projections best demonstrate these important foramina and joints of the spine as follows:[2]

	Zygapophyseal Joints	**Intervertebral Foramina**
Cervical Spine	Lateral position	45° posterior oblique (side away from film)
Thoracic Spine	70° posterior oblique (side away from film)	Lateral position
Lumbar Spine	45° posterior oblique (side closest to film)	Lateral position

AP for C1–2 (Atlas and Axis)

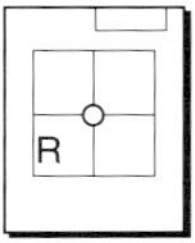

• 8 x 10" L.W. (20 x 24 cm)
• Grid

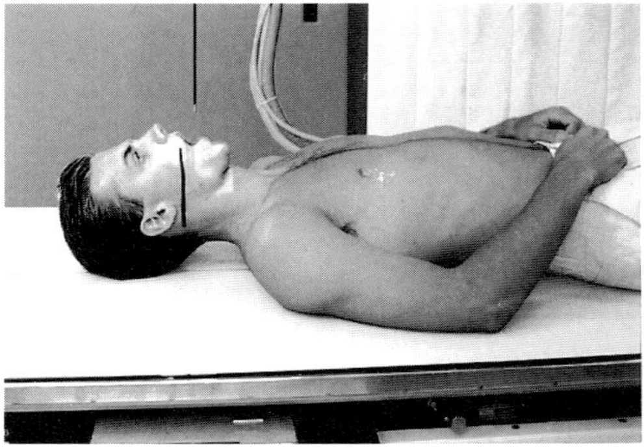

AP open mouth for C1-2

Position

- Supine, patient centered to CR and centerline.
- Adjust head without opening mouth – biting surface of upper incisors (junction of lips) aligned with base of skull (mastoid tips).
- Center cassette to CR.
- As a last step before making exposure – open mouth wide without moving head (make final check for head alignment).

Central Ray

- CR ⊥ through mid portion of open mouth (to C1–2).

SID: 40–48" (102–122 cm)

Collimation: Close collimation to C1-2 region.

Respiration: Suspend during exposure.

Technique: kVp (75±5) _____ mrad

S 131	G .<01 M
ML 32	NDC F

	cm	kVp	mA	Time	mAs	SID	Film–Screen	Grid	F.S.
Model Room	18	75			15	44"	Kodak 400	12:1	S

Bontrager Textbook, 3rd ed., p. 288

AP for Dens (Odontoid Process)
Fuchs Method (and Judd Method)[3,4]

Warning: Do not attempt on possible cervical trauma.

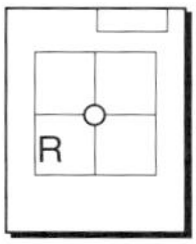

- 8 x 10" L.W. (20 x 24 cm)
- Grid

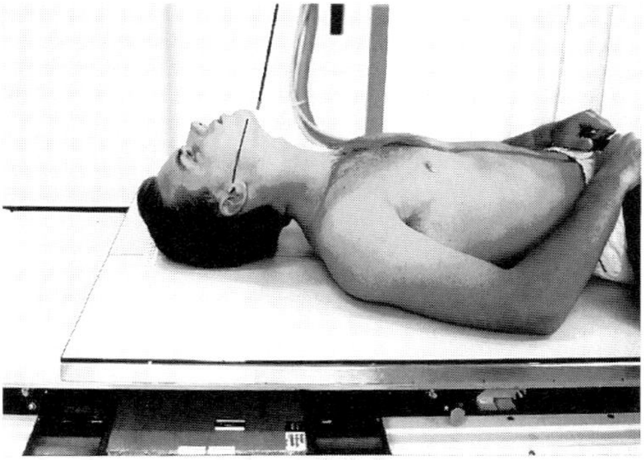

AP Fuchs for dens (within foramen magnum outline)

Position

- Supine or erect, MSP aligned to centerline, no rotation.
- Elevate chin until MML is near ⊥ to film (MML parallel to CR). (May require some cephalic CR angle if chin cannot be elevated sufficiently. This is similar to reverse Waters, except for CR.)

Note: May also be taken PA (Judd method) with chin against table top, with same CR alignment (Waters position).

- Center cassette to exiting CR.

Central Ray: CR ⊥, inferior to tip of mandible.

SID: 40–48" (102–122 cm)

Collimation: Close collimation to C1-2 region.

Respiration: Suspend during exposure.

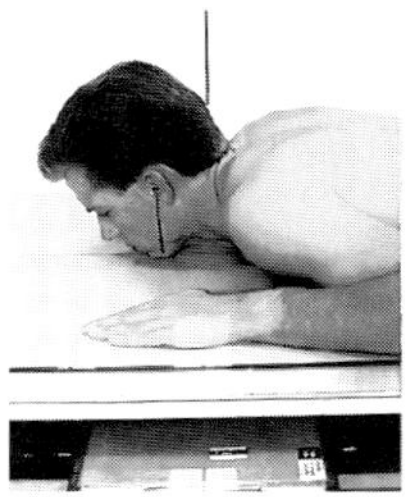

PA Judd method (reduces thyroid dose)

Technique: kVp (75±5) _____

	cm	kVp	mA	Time	mAs	SID	Film–Screen	Grid	F.S.
Model Room	11	75			15	44"	Kodak 400	12:1	S
S									
M									
L									

(AP) mrad

S 134	Thyroid
ML 18	89

(PA) mrad

S 134	Thyroid
ML 18	4

AP Cervical Spine

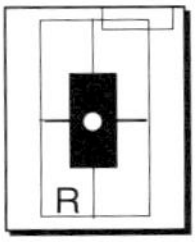

- 8 x 10" L.W. (20 x 24 cm)
- Grid

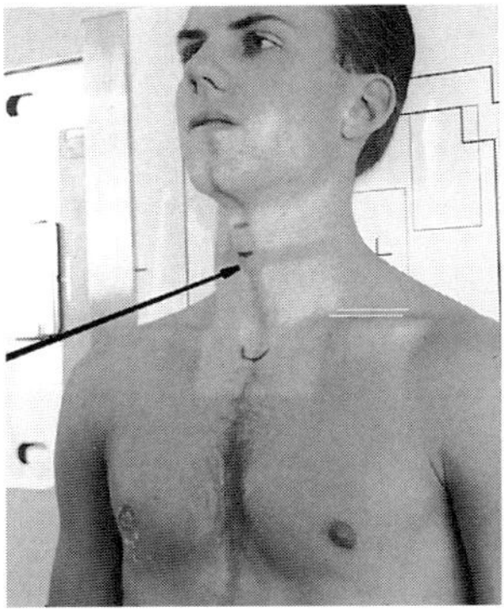

Erect

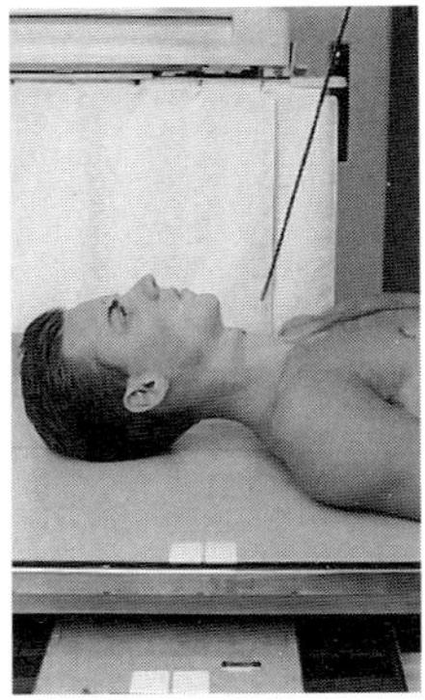

Supine

(CR 15—20° cephalad)

Position

- Supine or erect, center midsagittal plane to CR (and to centerline of cassette).
- Raise chin slightly as needed so the CR angle superimposes the mentum of the mandible over the base of the skull (to prevent mandible from superimposing more than C1-2).
- Center cassette to projected CR.

Central Ray: CR 15–20° cephalad, to enter at C–5 (inferior border of thyroid cartilage).

SID: 40–60" (102–152 cm)

Collimation: On four sides to C spine region.

Respiration: Suspend during exposure.

Technique: kVp (75±5) _____

mrad

S	74	Thyroid
ML	33	56

	cm	kVp	mA	Time	mAs	SID	Film–Screen	Grid	F.S.
Model	11	75			10	44"	Kodak 400	12:1	S
Room									

Bontrager Textbook, 3rd ed., p. 287

Obliques, Cervical Spine

Right and left obliques taken for comparison on two films (as either posterior or anterior obliques).

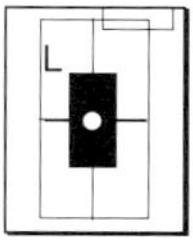

- 8 x 10" L.W. (20 x 24 cm)
- Grid (screen optional for small patient)

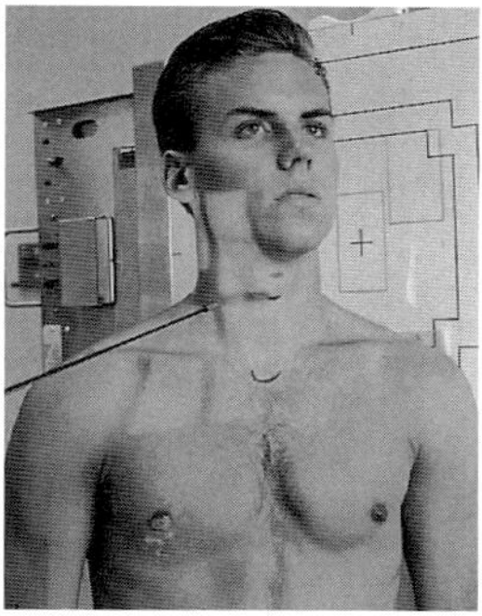

45° LPO
- CR 15° cephalad

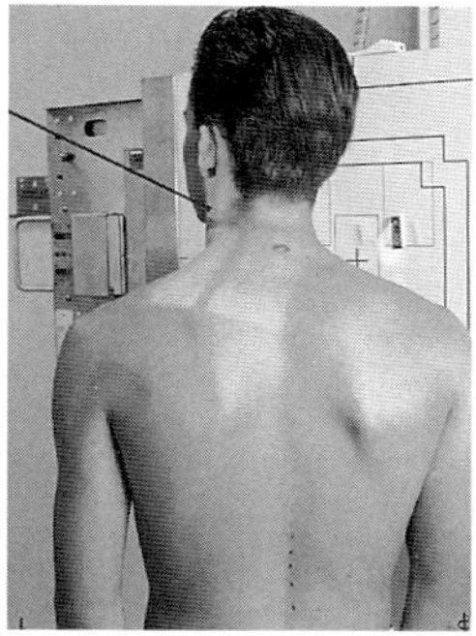

Optional 45° RAO
- CR 15° caudad

Position

- Erect preferred (sitting or standing), entire torso and head turned 45° to film, C spine aligned to CR (and centerline of cassette).
- Raise chin slightly, looking straight ahead (or turn head slightly toward film to prevent superimposing C1 by mandible).
- Center cassette to projected CR.

Central Ray (Posterior Obliques): CR 15-20° cephalad, to enter at C5. (Caudal angle required for anterior obliques.)

SID: 40–60" (102–152 cm) (60" may be preferred due to OFD.)

Collimation: On four sides to C spine region.

Respiration: Suspend during exposure.

Technique: kVp (75±5) _____

mrad

S	92	Thyroid* 7
ML	42	

(ant. obli.)

	cm	kVp	mA	Time	mAs	SID	Film–Screen	Grid	F.S.
Model Room	11	75			20	60"	Kodak 400	12:1	S
S									
M									
L									

Bontrager Textbook, 3rd Ed., p. 290

*Posterior oblique thyroid dose is similar to AP C spine, ≈ 56 mrad.

Lateral Cervical Spine

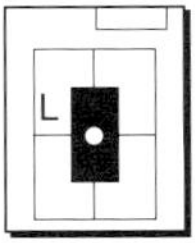

- 8 x 10" L.W. (20 x 24 cm)
- Grid (screen optional for small patient)

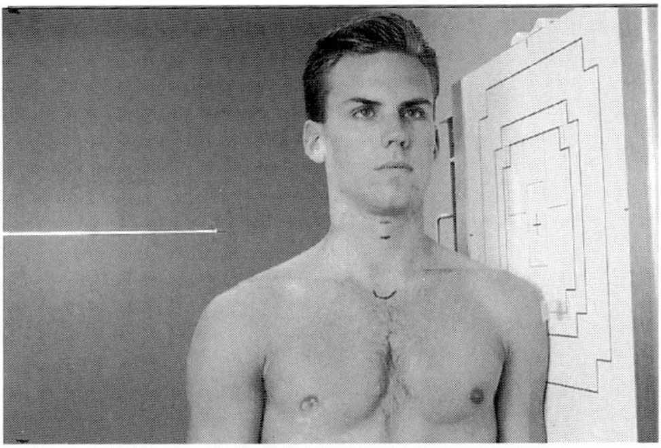

Erect lateral, 72"(183 cm) SID

Position

- Erect (sitting or standing) in lateral position, C spine aligned and centered to CR (and centerline of cassette).
- Top of cassette ≈1-2" (3-5 cm) above level of EAM.
- Raise chin slightly (to remove mandible angles from spine).
- Relax and depress both shoulders evenly (weights in each hand may be necessary to visualize C7).

(**Note:** See following pages for swimmer's lateral if C7 is still not visualized)

Central Ray: CR ⊥, to level of C4 (upper thyroid cartilage).

SID: 60–72" (152–183 cm). (Longer SID provides for better visualization of C7 due to less divergent rays.)

Collimation: On four sides to C spine region.

Respiration: Expose on complete expiration.

Technique: kVp (75±5) _____

mrad		
	S 78	Thyroid 6
	ML 37	

	cm	kVp	mA	Time	mAs	SID	Film–Screen	Grid	F.S.
Model	11	75			28	72"	Kodak 400	12:1	S
Room									
S									
M									
L									

Bontrager Textbook, 3rd ed., p. 289

Lateral Cervicothoracic Spine

Swimmer's (Twining Method) C7-T1 Region

See following page for alternate ways of visualizing C7-T1.

Pawlow method: Lateral recumbent (not shown).

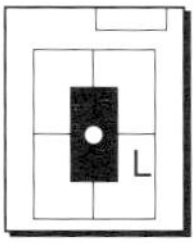

- 8 x 10" L.W. (20 x 24 cm)
- Grid

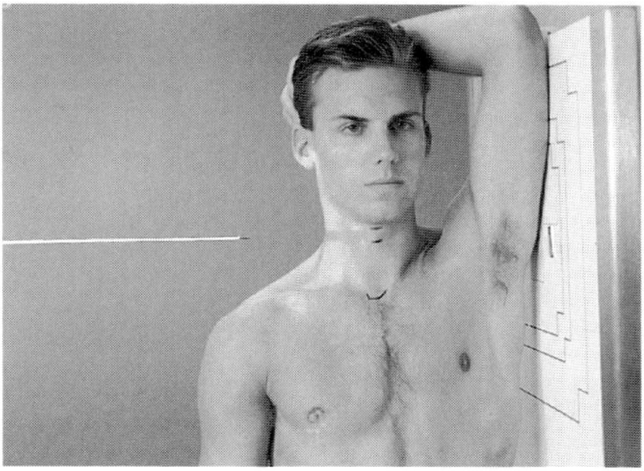

Swimmer's lateral, C7-T1

Position

- Erect preferred, align C spine to CR (and centerline of cassette).
- Elevate arm and shoulder closest to film and rotate this shoulder slightly anteriorly or posteriorly.
- Opposite arm down, relax and depress shoulder, with slight opposite rotation (from other shoulder) to separate humeral heads from vertebra. May also be taken in lateral recumbent position with one arm and shoulder down and one up - Pawlow method.

Central Ray: CR ⊥, centered to T1 (vertebra prominens).

SID: 40–60" (102–152 cm)

Collimation: Collimate closely to area of interest.

Respiration: Expose on full expiration.

Technique: kVp (80-±5) _____

mrad

S 474	G <.01 M
ML 82	NDC F

	cm	kVp	mA	Time	mAs	SID	Film–Screen	Grid	F.S.
Model Room	24	80			120	72"	Kodak 400	12:1	S
S									
M									
L									

Bontrager Textbook, 3rd ed., p. 291

Alternate Methods of Visualizing C7-T1
(Modified Swimmer's & Shoulders Forward Laterals)

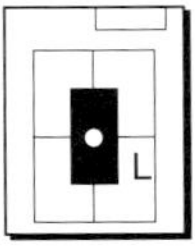

- 8 x 10" L.W. (20 x 24 cm)
- Grid

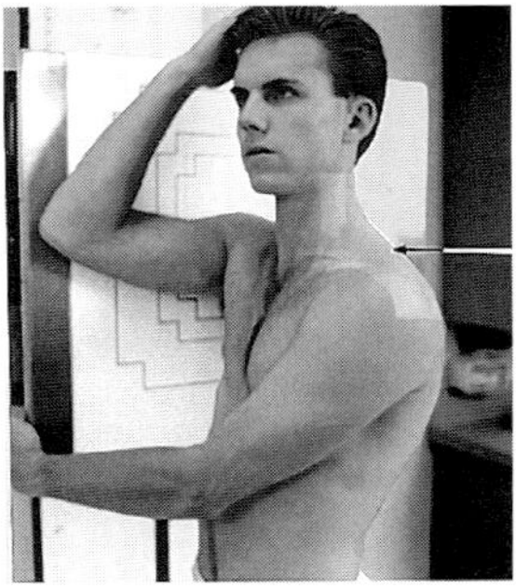

A. Modified Swimmer's[1]

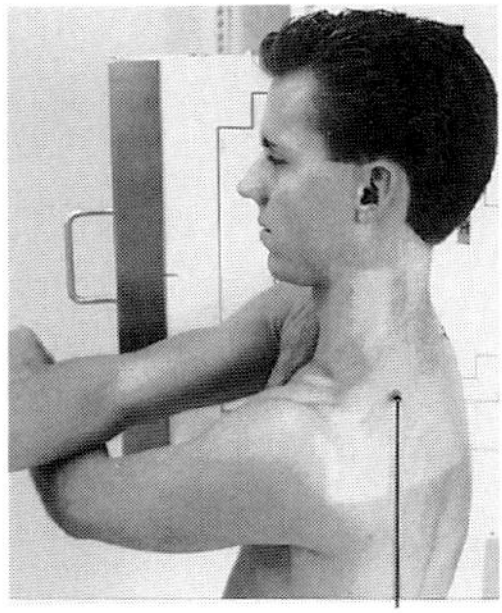

B. Shoulders forward lateral[2]

Position

- Erect (sitting or standing); may also be done cross table supine.
- Align C spine to CR (and to center of cassette), patient in true lateral position.

Method A[1]: Elevate arm closest to film and rest on head. Place opposite arm across the front pulling this shoulder anteriorly as far as possible while maintaining a lateral position.

Method B[2]: Have patient reach out in front and down pulling both shoulders anteriorly and downward as far as possible. (Works best for "rounded" shoulders.)

Central Ray: CR ⊥, centered to C7-T1.

SID: 40–60" (102–152 cm)

Collimation: To area of interest.

Respiration: Expose on full expiration.

Technique: kVp (80±5) _____

mrad

S 474	G <.01 M
ML 82	NDC F

	cm	kVp	mA	Time	mAs	SID	Film–Screen	Grid	F.S.
A. **Model** Room	24	80			120	72"	Kodak 400	12:1	S

[1] Described by Karen Brown, RT(R) [2] Described by Guy A.Copeman, RT(R)(T)

Lateral Cervical Spine
Hyperflexion – Hyperextension

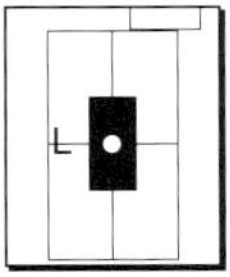

Warning: Do **NOT** attempt on possible trauma patients.

- 10 x 12" L.W. (24 x 30 cm)
- Grid or screen

Position

- Erect preferred (sitting or standing) in lateral position, C spine aligned to CR (and centerline of cassette).
- Relax and depress shoulders as much as possible.

First film: Depress chin to touch chest if possible.

Second film: Elevate chin as far as is comfortable. (Ensure that entire C spine is included on both films.)

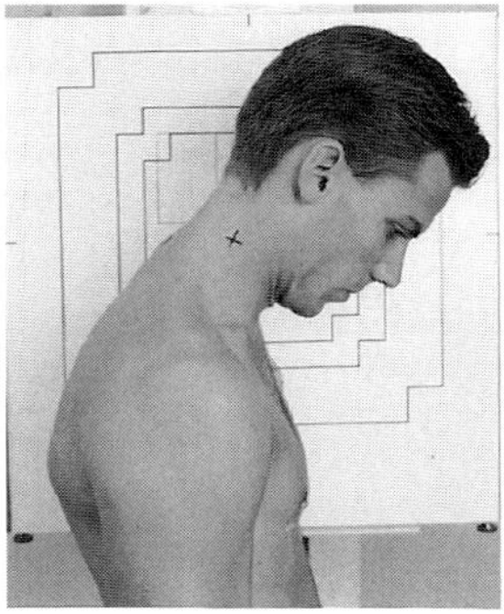

Hyperflexion

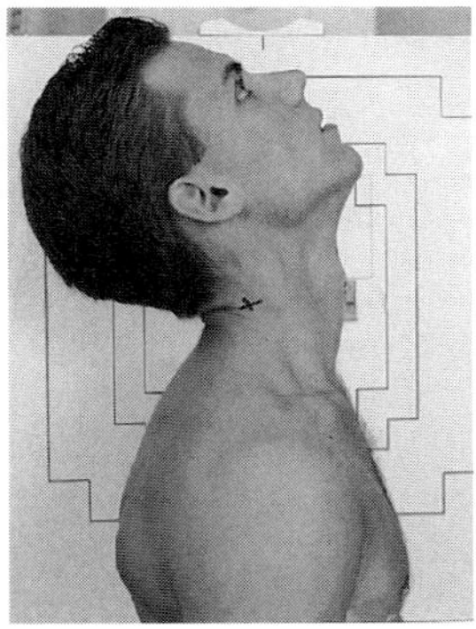

Hyperextension

Central Ray

- CR ⊥, to C-4 (level of upper border of thyroid cartilage).

SID: 60–72" (152–183 cm)

Collimation: To C spine area.

Respiration: Expose on total expiration.

Technique: kVp (75±5) _____

mrad per projection

S 78	ML 37	Thyroid 6

	cm	kVp	mA	Time	mAs	SID	Film–Screen	Grid	F.S.
Model	11	75			28	72"	Kodak 400	12:1	S
Room									
S									
M									
L									

Cervical Spine - Trauma Series

Warning: Do not remove cervical collar unless so indicated by the physician after viewing cross table lateral.

- 10 x 12" (24 x 30 cm) L.W.
- Screen or optional grid
- SID - 72" (183 cm) if possible
- CR ⊥, to C-4 (upper thyroid cartilage) (top of cassette ≈1–2" or 3–5 cm above EAM)
- Depress shoulders

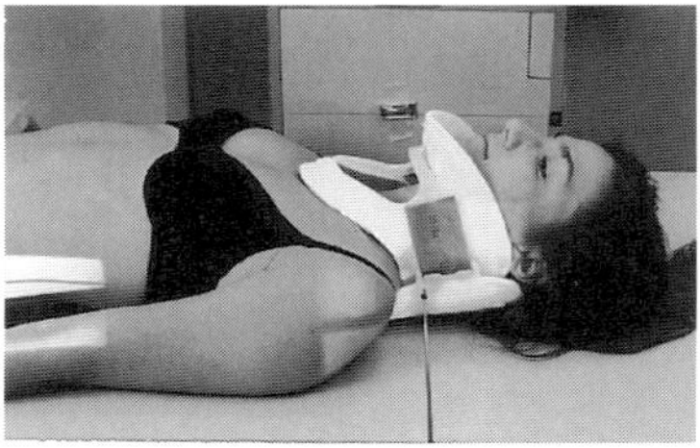

Cross table lateral

- 10 x 12" (24 x 30 cm) L.W.
- Grid – stationary or Bucky
- SID – 40-48" (102–122 cm)
- CR 15–20° cephalad, to enter at C5 (lower thyroid cartilage).

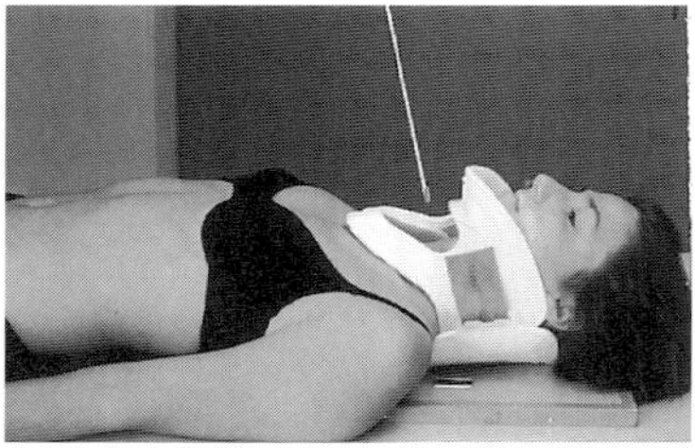

AP

- 10 x 12" L.W. (24 x 30 cm)
- Screen (or grid C.W.)
- SID - 40–48" (102–122 cm)
- CR 45° medially (and 15° cephalad if grid allows).
- CR to enter at level of C5.

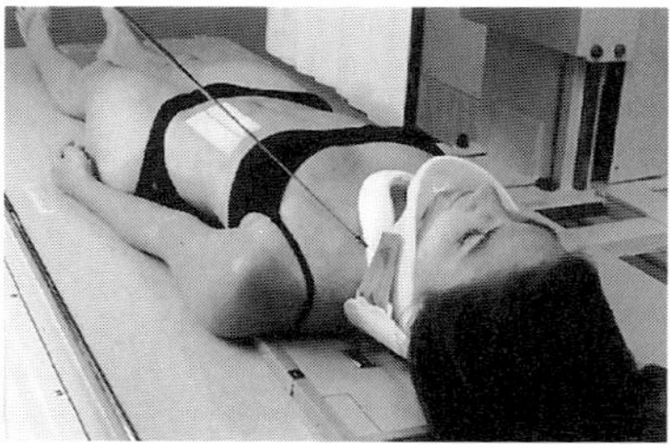

Oblique (both R and L obliques)

Optional Projection:

(If needed to visualize C7.)

- 10 x 12" (24 x 30 cm) L.W.
- Grid
- Elevate shoulder and arm nearest film, depress opposite shoulder
- SID – 40–48" (102–122 cm)
- CR ⊥ film, centered to T1.

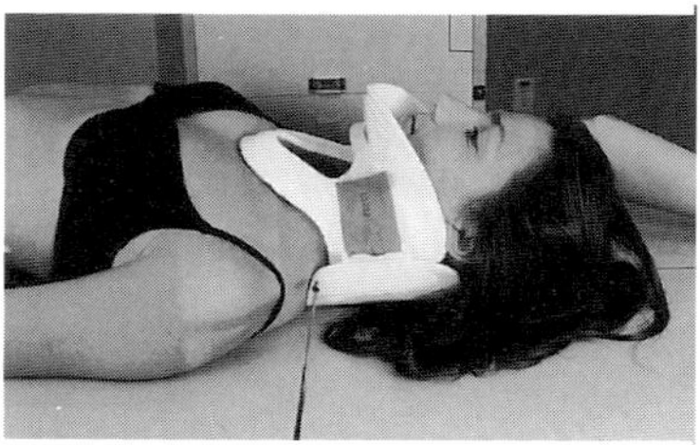

Swimmer's lateral

7 Cervical Spine

AP Thoracic Spine

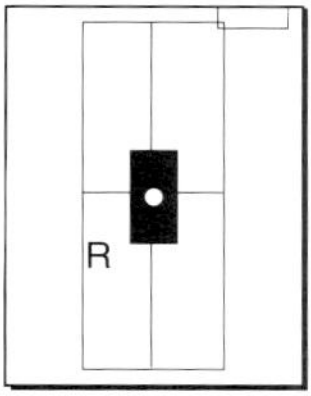

- 14 x 17" L.W. (35 x 43 cm)
- Grid
- Feet at cathode end (anode-heel effect)
- Wedge compensation filter optional

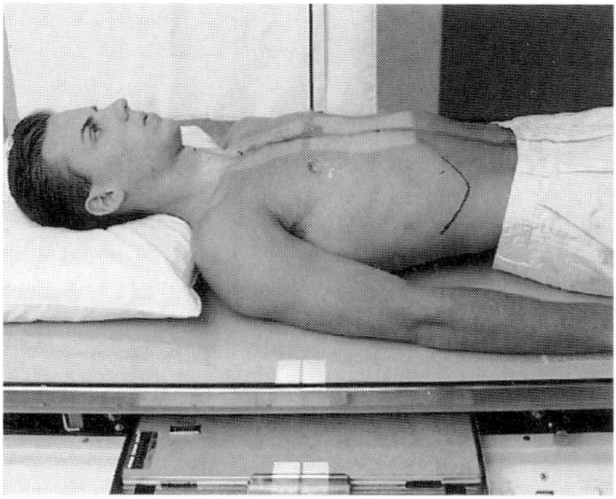

AP thoracic spine

Position

- Supine, spine aligned and centered to centerline, flex hips and knees to reduce lordotic curvature.
- Top of cassette 1 1/2" (3 cm) above shoulder.
- Ensure no rotation of thorax or pelvis. Shield gonads.

Central Ray: CR ⊥, to center of cassette (at level of T7 as for an AP chest, 3–4" or 8–10 cm below jugular notch).

SID: 40–48" (102–122 cm)

Collimation: Long narrow collimation field to T spine region.

Respiration: Expose on expiration for more uniform density.

mrad		
	S 124	Thyroid
	ML 21	8

Technique: kVp (80±5) ____ or (90±5 for greater latitude) ___

	cm	kVp	mA	Time	mAs	SID	Film–Screen	Grid	F.S.
Model Room	23	80			12	44"	Kodak 400	12:1	S
S									
M									
L									
InSight									

Bontrager Textbook, 3rd ed., p. 284

Lateral Thoracic Spine

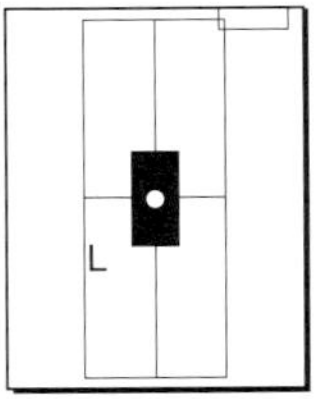

- 14 x 17" L.W. (35 x 43 cm)
- Grid
- Lead blocker posterior to patient

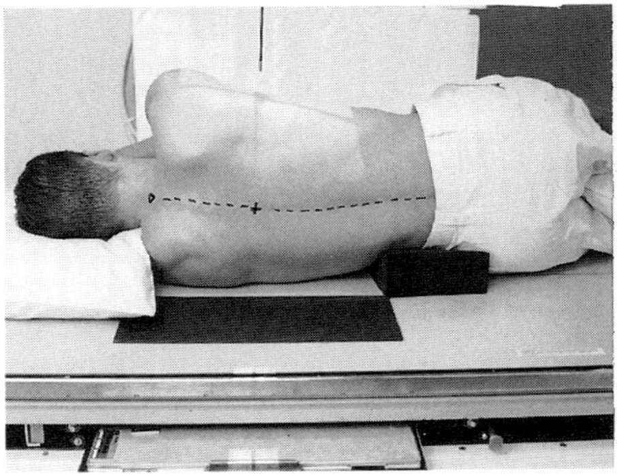

Lateral thoracic spine

Position

- Recumbent, support under head, lateral with hips and knees flexed, arms raised and elbows flexed. Shield gonads.
- Align and center midaxillary plane to centerline.
- Top of cassette 1 1/2" (3 cm) above shoulders; no rotation.
- Supports should be placed under lower back as needed to straighten and align spine near parallel to table top. (A slight natural curvature corresponding to divergent rays is helpful.)

Central Ray: CR ⊥ to thoracic spine, to center of cassette (T7).

SID: 40–48" (102–122 cm)

Collimation: Long narrow collimation field to T spine region.

Respiration: Breathing technique; or expose on expiration.

mrad		
	S 951	G<0.01M
	ML 67	0.2 F

Technique: kVp (80±5) ____ (breathing technique preferred)

	cm	kVp	mA	Time	mAs	SID	Film–Screen	Grid	F.S.
Model Room	33	80			70	44"	Kodak 400	12:1	S or L
S									
M									
L									
InSight									

Bontrager Textbook, 3rd ed., p. 285

Oblique Thoracic Spine

Both obliques generally taken on separate films for comparison. May also take as anterior obliques.

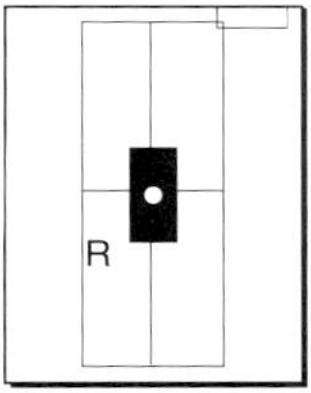

• 14 x 17" L.W. (35 x 43 cm)
• Grid

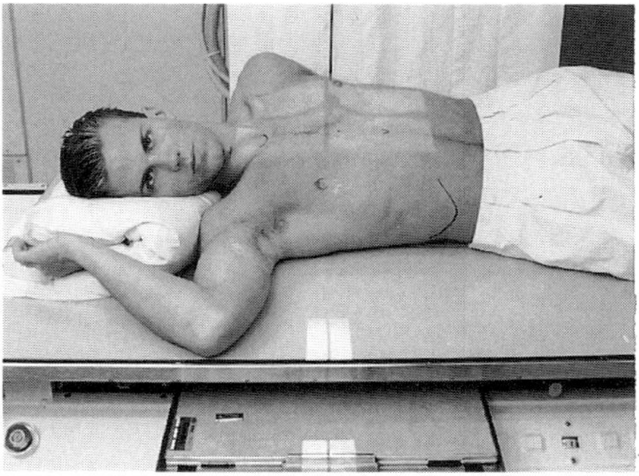

70° RPO (20° from lateral)

Position

- Recumbent, rotated posteriorly 20° from lateral. (Use some type of angle indicator.)
- Align and center spine to centerline, place arm away from film behind back and arm closest to film up in front of head.
- Top of cassette ≈1 1/2" (3 cm) above shoulders.

Central Ray: CR ⊥, to center of cassette (T7).

SID: 40–48" (102–122 cm)

Collimation: Long narrow collimation field to T spine region.

Respiration: Expose on expiration.

mrad

S 343	G<0.01M
ML 26	0.1 F

Technique: kVp (80±5) ____

	cm	kVp	mA	Time	mAs	SID	Film–Screen	Grid	F.S.
Model Room	32	80			26	44"	Kodak 400	12:1	S
S									
M									
L									
InSight									

Bontrager Textbook, 3rd ed., p. 286

AP (PA) Lumbar Spine

Note: May be taken PA for better opening of intervertebral spaces by divergent rays.

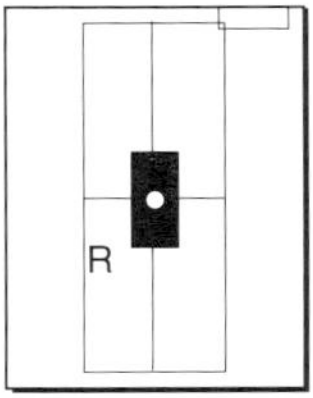

- 11 x 14" L.W. (30 x 35 cm) or 14 x 17" (35 x 43 cm)
- Grid

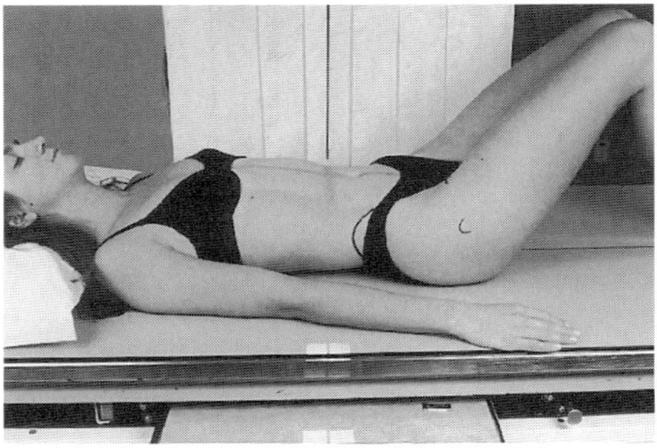

AP lumbar, hips and knees flexed

Position (AP)

- Supine, spine aligned to centerline
- Flex hips and knees (to reduce lordotic curvature).
- No rotation (ASIS' same distance from table).
- Center cassette to CR.

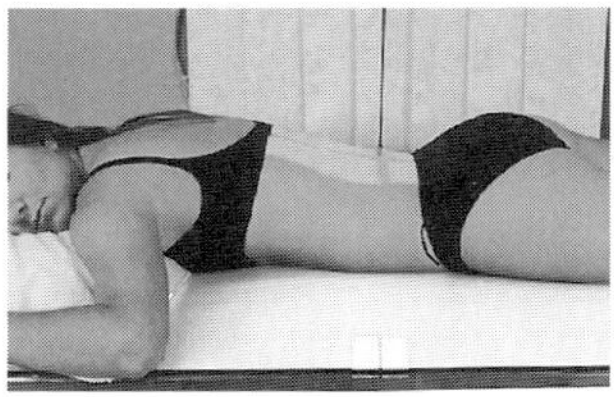

Alternate PA

Central Ray: CR ⊥, to ≈1" (2.5 cm) above iliac crest (L3); or center at crest for 14 x 17 film.

SID: 40–48" (102–122 cm)

Collimation: Long narrow collimation field to L spine region.

Respiration: Expose at end of expiration.

Technique: kVp (80±5) _____

(AP) mrad: S 133 | G 0.5 M | ML 36 | 12 F

(PA) mrad: S 133 | G<0.01 M | ML 36 | 12 F

	cm	kVp	mA	Time	mAs	SID	Film–Screen	Grid	F.S.
Model	17	80			15	44"	Kodak 400	12:1	S or L
Room									

Bontrager Textbook, 3rd ed., p. 261

Lateral Lumbar Spine

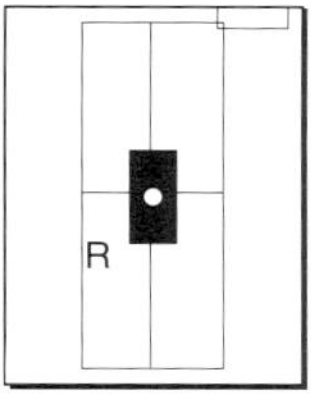

- 11 x 14 or 14 x 17" L.W. (30 x 35 or 35 x 43 cm)
- Grid
- Feet at cathode end
- Lead blocker posterior to patient

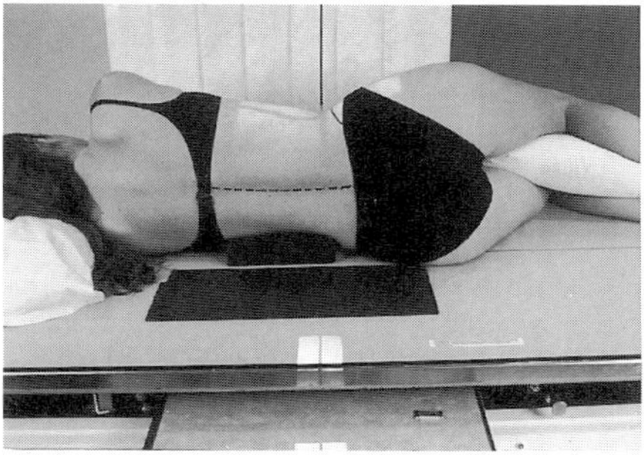

Lateral L spine – CR ⊥ to spine

Position

- Recumbent in true lateral position, flex hips and knees, align and center midaxillary plane to centerline.
- Place support under waist as needed to place entire spine parallel to table top (see note). Provide support between knees.
- Center cassette to CR.

Central Ray: CR ⊥ to spine. CR to level of ≈1" (2.5 cm) above iliac crest (L3); or at iliac crest for 14 x 17" film.

SID: 40–48" (102–122 cm)

Collimation: Long narrow collimation field to L spine region.

Respiration: Expose at end of expiration.

Note: Patient with wide pelvis and narrow thorax may require a 3–5° caudal CR. Also, elevating upper arm (side away from film) above head may straighten spine without the use of support under waist.

mrad

S 746	G 1.0 M
ML 105	28 F

Technique: kVp (90±5) _____

	cm	kVp	mA	Time	mAs	SID	Film–Screen	Grid	F.S.
Model Room	27	90			50	44"	Kodak 400	12:1	L
S									
M									
L									

Bontrager Textbook, 3rd ed., p. 263

Lateral L5-S1, Lumbar Spine

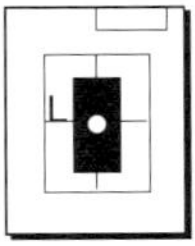

- 8 x 10" L.W. (20 x 24 cm)
- Grid
- Lead blocker posterior to patient

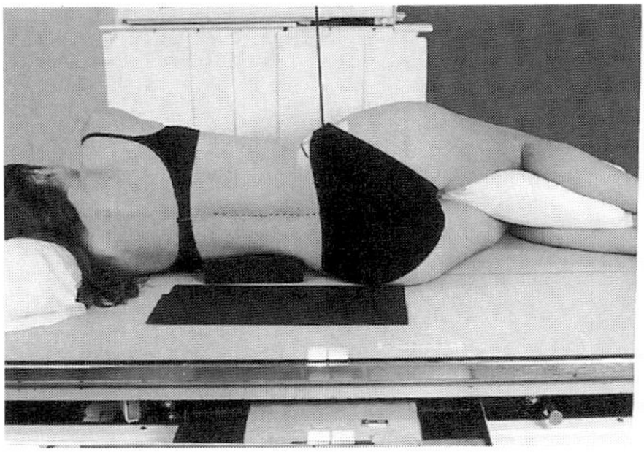

Lateral L5-S1 - CR 3–5° caudad

Position
- Recumbent in true lateral position, flex hips and knees, midaxillary plane aligned to centerline and CR.
- Place support under waist as needed to place spine parallel to table top. (Provide support between knees.)
- Center cassette to CR.

Central Ray
- CR ⊥, to film if entire spine is parallel to table; or 3–5 ° caudad if entire spine is not parallel (most often on females).
- CR centered to 1.5" (4 cm) distal to iliac crest and 1.5" (4 cm) anterior to spinous process of L5.

SID: 40–48" (102–122 cm)

Collimation: Collimate closely to area of interest.

Respiration: Suspend during exposure.

mrad

S 1016	G 0.5 M
ML 111	24 F

Technique: kVp (100±5) _____(+8–10 kVp from lateral L spine)

	cm	kVp	mA	Time	mAs	SID	Film–Screen	Grid	F.S.
Model	31	100			50	44"	Kodak 400	12:1	L
Room									

Bontrager Textbook, 3rd ed., p. 264

Obliques, Lumbar Spine

Both obliques on two films generally taken for comparison (as either ant. or post. obli.'s)

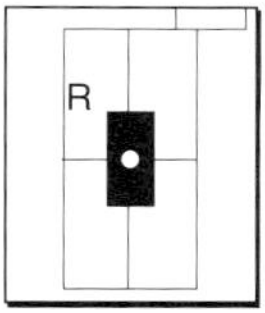

• 11 x 14" L.W. (30 x 35 cm)
• Grid

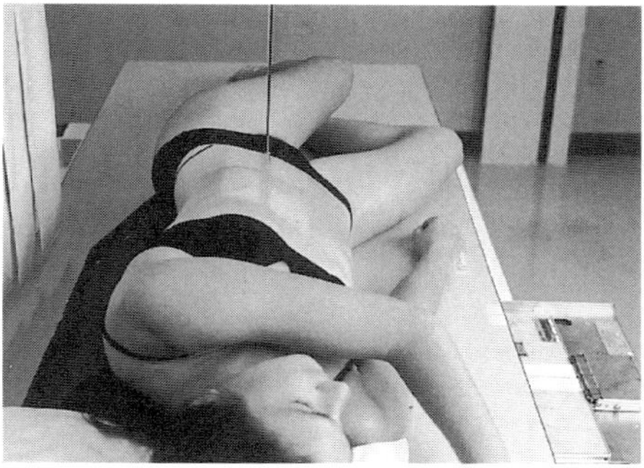

45° RPO (right zygapophyseal joints)

Position

- Semi-supine, 45° right & left posterior obliques. (Use support angle blocks under pelvis and shoulders to maintain position.)
- Align and center spine to CR and centerline.
- Center cassette to CR.

Central Ray

- CR ⊥, to body of L3 (1 1/2–2" or 4–5 cm above iliac crest and 2" or 5 cm lateral from midline of patient's anterior abdomen).

SID: 40–48" (102–122 cm)

Collimation: To area of interest.

Respiration: Suspend during exposure.

Note: 50° obli. is best for L1–2 zygapophyseal joints, and 30° for L5-S1.[5]

Technique: kVp (85±5) _____

mrad

S 168	G .5 M
ML 36	21 F

	cm	kVp	mA	Time	mAs	SID	Film–Screen	Grid	F.S.
Model	21	85			15	44"	Kodak 400	12:1	S
Room									
S									
M									
L									

Bontrager Textbook, 3rd ed., p. 262

Scoliosis Series
PA or AP Ferguson Method

PA reduces dose to radiation sensitive areas (breasts and thyroid).

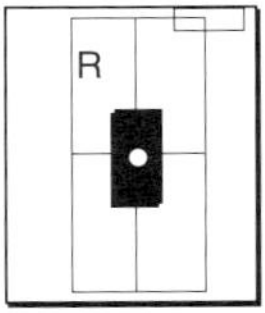

- 14 x 17" L.W. (35 x 43 cm)
- Grid

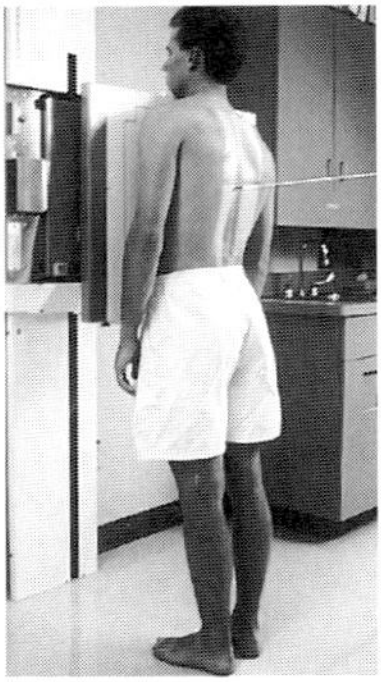

PA without block

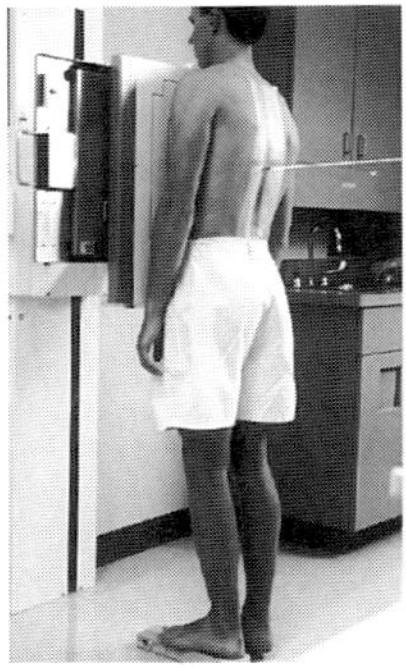

PA with block under foot on convex side of curve

Position

First Film: Erect, standing or seated, spine aligned and centered to centerline, arms at side, no rotation of pelvis or thorax.

- Center of cassette at level of L2–L3 (1–2" or 2.5–5 cm above crest) to include L5 and iliac crests on lower margin of film.

Second Film: Place 2–3"(5–7 cm) block under foot (or buttock if seated) on convex side of curvature. (Identifies primary deforming curves from compensatory curve.)

Shielding: Use gonad shields (and breast shields on young females).

Central Ray: CR ⊥, to center of cassette.

SID: 40–72" (102–180 cm) longer SID is recommended.

Collimation: Long and narrow to vertebral column region.

Respiration: Expose on full expiration.

mrad, 2 proj's

S 294	G <0.1 M
ML 62	28 F

Technique: kVp (80-100) _____ (higher kVp reduces dose and increases exposure latitude)

	cm	kVp	mA	Time	mAs	SID	Film–Screen	Grid	F.S.
Model Room	23	90			25	60"	Kodak 400	12:1	L

Bontrager Textbook, 3rd ed., p. 268

Lumbar Spine

AP (PA) Right and Left Bending

Note: May be taken erect PA to reduce ovarian and breast dose.

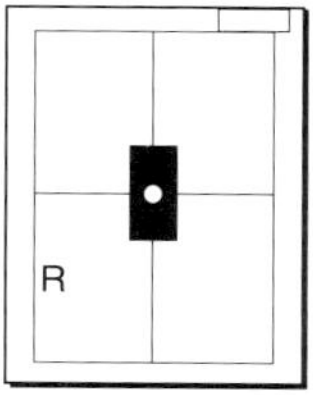

- 14 x 17" L.W.
  (35 x 43 cm)
- Grid

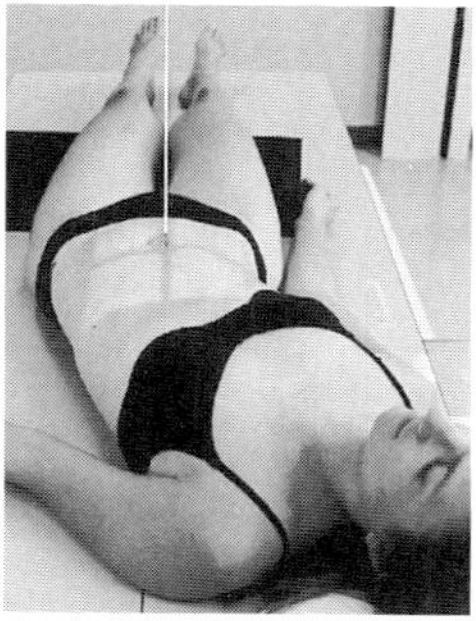

AP, right bending

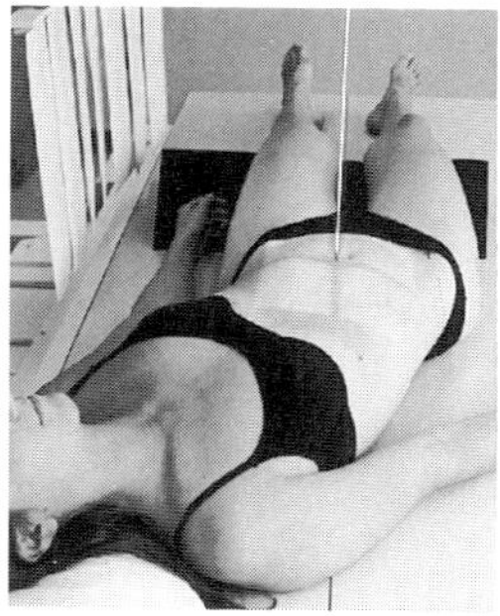

AP, left bending

Position

- Supine or erect,
  spine centered to CR and centerline of table.
- Bend laterally as far as possible (right then left) without tilting pelvis (pelvis remains stationary and acts as a fulcrum).
- Ensure no rotation of pelvis and upper torso.
- Center cassette to CR.

Central Ray: CR ⊥, to L2-3 level (2" [5 cm] superior to iliac crest). (Higher centering if thoracic spine is area of interest.)

SID: 40–48" (102–122 cm)

Collimation: Include vertebral column of interest.

Respiration: Expose at end of expiration.

mrad, two projections

S 272	G 1.4 M
ML 69	60 F

Technique: kVp (80±5) _____

	cm	kVp	mA	Time	mAs	SID	Film–Screen	Grid	F.S.
Model Room	17	80			15	44"	Kodak 400	12:1	S or L
S									
M									
L									

Bontrager Textbook, 3rd ed., p. 269

Lumbar Spine
Lateral Flexion and Extension

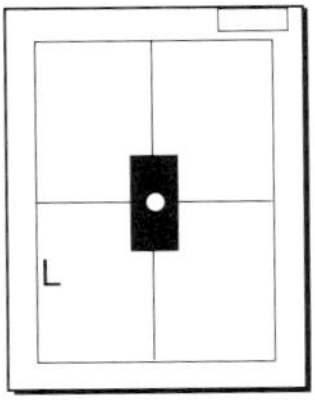

- 14 x 17" L.W. (35 x 43 cm)
- Grid
- Lead blocker posterior to patient

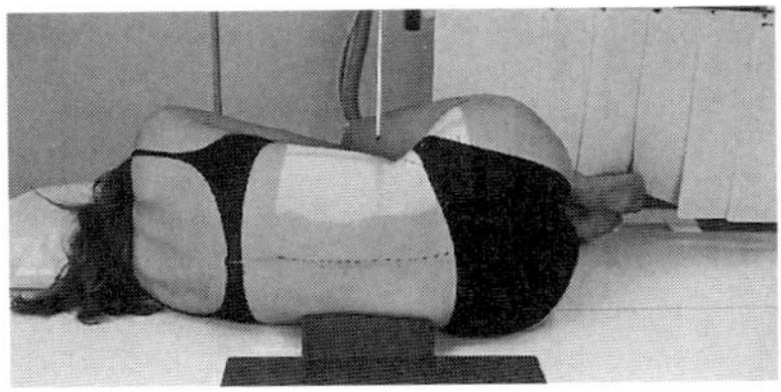

Hyperflexion lateral

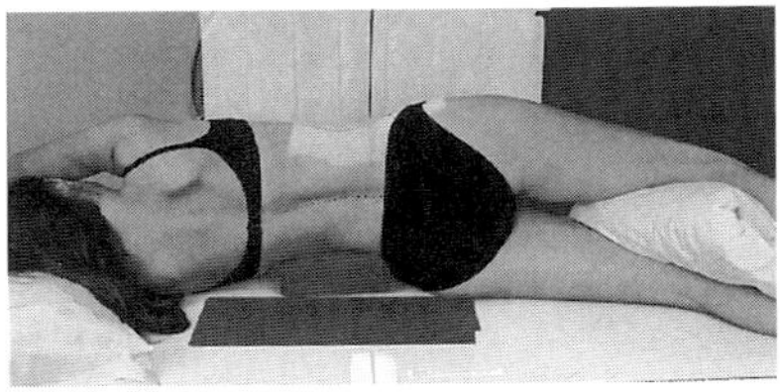

Hyperextension lateral

Position

- Recumbent or erect, spine centered to table.
- Support under waist to align spine parallel to table top.
- Hyperflex forward as far as possible, then hyperextend back as far as possible for second film; maintain true lateral position.
- Center cassette to CR.

Central Ray

- CR⊥, to level of L3 (1–1 1/2" or 2 1/2 –4 cm above iliac crest).

SID: 40–48" (102–122 cm)

Collimation: On four sides to near borders of film.

Respiration: Expose at end of expiration.

mrad, two projections

S 1516	G 1.2 M
ML 200	58 F

Technique: kVp (90±5) _____

	cm	kVp	mA	Time	mAs	SID	Film–Screen	Grid	F.S.
Model	27	90			50	44"	Kodak 400	12:1	L
Room									

Bontrager Textbook, 3rd ed., p. 270

AP Sacrum

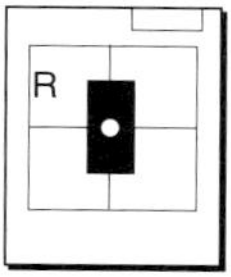

- 10 x 12" L.W. (24 x 30 cm)
- Grid

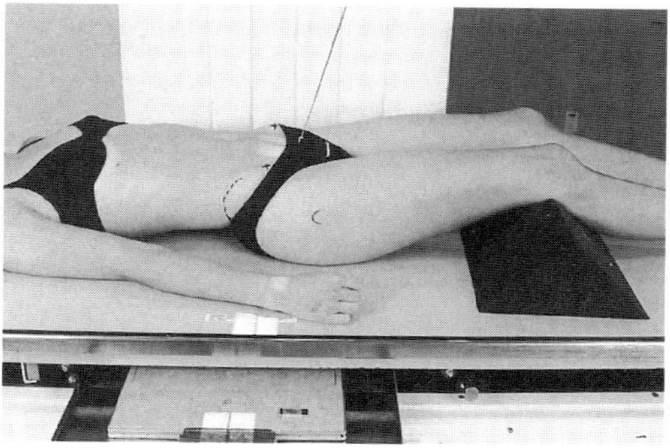

AP sacrum, CR 15° cephalad

Position

- Supine, spine centered to CR and centerline.
- No rotation of pelvis (both ASIS' same distance from table).
- Center cassette to projected CR. (**Shield gonads for males**.)

Central Ray

- CR 15° cephalad, at midpoint between level of ASIS and symphysis pubis.

SID: 40–48" (102–122 cm)

Collimation: On four sides to area of sacrum.

Respiration: Suspend during exposure.

mrad		
	S 132	G 12 M
	ML 37	26 F

Technique: kVp (80±5) _____ (or 92±5 and reduce mAs by half to decrease patient exposure) _____

	cm	kVp	mA	Time	mAs	SID	Film–Screen	Grid	F.S.
Model	17	80			15	44"	Kodak 400	12:1	S
Room									
S									
M									
L									

Lateral Sacrum

Note: Lateral sacrum and lateral coccyx may be taken as one projection if both sacrum and coccyx are being examined (reduces patient exposure).

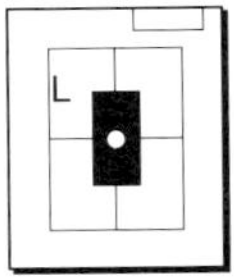

- 10 x 12" L.W. (24 x 30 cm)
- Grid
- Lead blocker posterior to patient

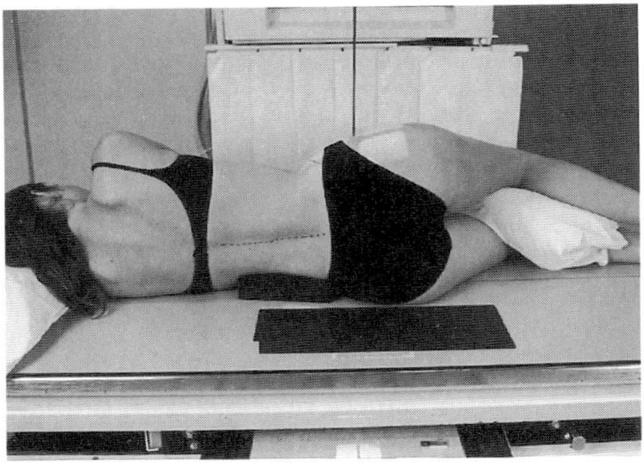

Lateral sacrum

Position

- Lateral recumbent, hips and knees flexed, true lateral position.
- Center sacrum to CR and centerline. (Align patient and cassette to correctly centered CR.)

Central Ray

- CR ⊥, to level of ASIS, 1 1/2–2" (4–5 cm) anterior to posterior surface of sacrum.

SID: 40–48" (102–122 cm)

Collimation: On four sides to area of sacrum.

Respiration: Suspend during exposure.

Technique: kVp (90±5) _____

mrad

S 908	G 89 M
ML 92	89 F

	cm	kVp	mA	Time	mAs	SID	Film–Screen	Grid	F.S.
Model	31	90			55	44"	Kodak 400	12:1	L
Room									

Bontrager Textbook, 3rd ed., p. 260

AP Coccyx

Note: May be done PA with 10° cephalic angle if patient cannot sustain weight on the coccyx area in a supine position.

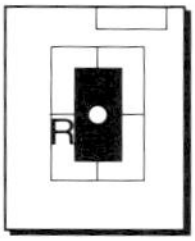

- 8 x 10" L.W. (20 x 24 cm)
- Grid

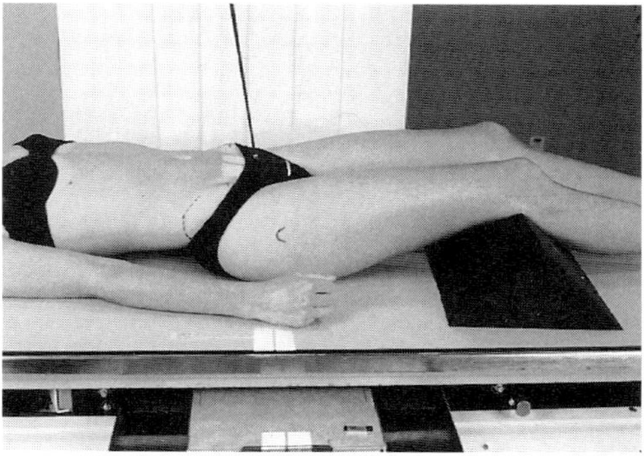

AP coccyx, CR 10° caudad

Position

- Supine, support under knees, gonad shield for males.
- Align and center midsagittal plane to centerline, no rotation.
- Center cassette to level of projected CR.

Central Ray

- CR 10° caudad, centered midway between level of ASIS' and symphysis pubis.

SID: 40–48" (102–122 cm)

Collimation: Close collimation to area of coccyx.

Respiration: Suspend during exposure.

(AP) mrad

S 112	G 10 M
ML 24	22 F

Technique: kVp (75±5) _____

(PA) mrad

S 112	G <.01 M
ML 30	22 F

	cm	kVp	mA	Time	mAs	SID	Film–Screen	Grid	F.S.
Model	17	75			15	44"	Kodak 400	12:1	S
Room									
S									
M									
L									

Lateral Coccyx

Note: Lateral sacrum and lateral coccyx are commonly taken with one projection if both sacrum and coccyx are being examined (reduces patient exposure).

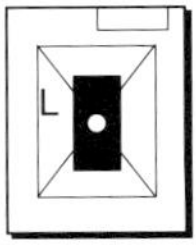

- 8 x 10" L.W. (20 x 24 cm)
- Grid
- Lead blocker posterior to patient

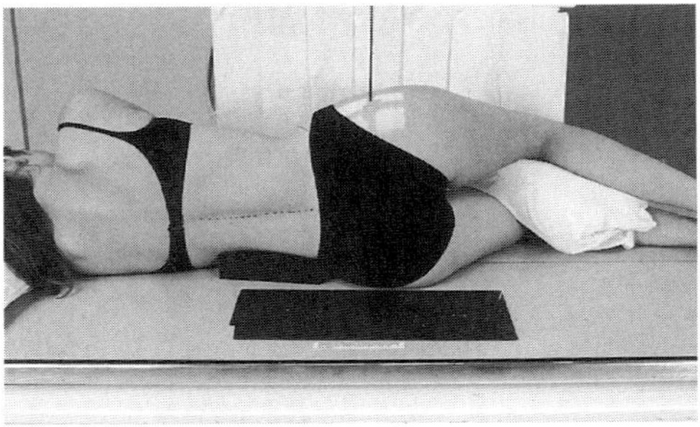

Lateral coccyx

Position

- Lateral recumbent, with hips and knees flexed 90°, true lateral position.
- Center coccyx to CR and centerline of table (remember the coccyx is located superficially between buttocks slightly superior to level of greater trochanter).
- Center cassette to CR.

Central Ray: CR ⊥, to 2" (5 cm) inferior to level of ASIS and ≈1" (2.5 cm) anterior to posterior sacral surface.

SID: 40–48" (102–122 cm)

Collimation: To area of distal sacrum and coccyx.

Respiration: Suspend during exposure.

mrad		
	S 1003	G 78 M
	ML 83	78 F

Technique: kVp (75±5) _____ (requires less kVp than lat. sacrum)

	cm	kVp	mA	Time	mAs	SID	Film–Screen	Grid	F.S.
Model	31	80			80	44"	Kodak 400	12:1	L
Room									

Bontrager Textbook, 3rd ed., p. 258

Vertebral Column

Position:

Central Ray:

SID:

Collimation:

Respiration:

Technique:

	Room	cm	kVp	mA	Time	mAs	SID	Film–Screen	Grid	F.S.
S										
M										
L										

Vertebral Column

Position:

Central Ray:

SID:

Collimation:

Respiration:

Technique:

Room	cm	kVp	mA	Time	mAs	SID	Film–Screen	Grid	F.S.

Chapter 8

Skull

Cranial landmarks and positioning lines used in skull and facial bones positioning.[1,2]

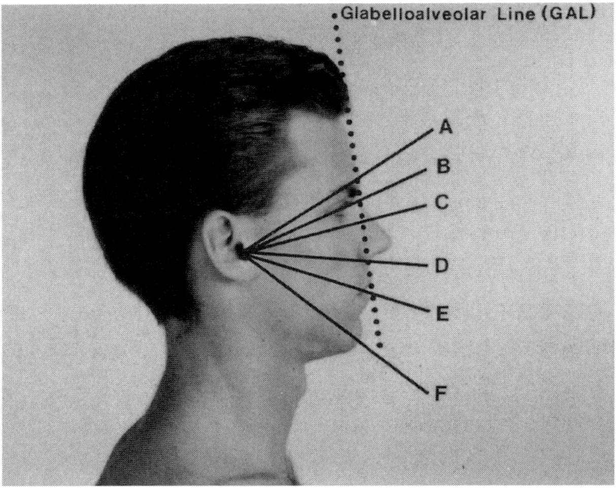

Positioning Lines

A. Glabellomeatal line
B. Orbitomeatal line **(OML)**
C. Infraorbitomeatal line (**IOML**) (Reid's base line, or "base line," base of cranium)
D. Acanthomeatal line **(AML)**
E. Lips-Meatal Line **(LML)** (used for modified Waters)
F. Mentomeatal line **(MML)** (used for Waters)

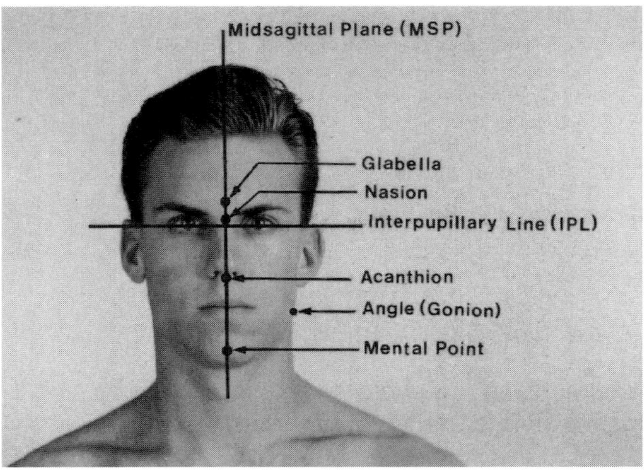

AP (PA) Axial Skull
AP Towne (or PA Haas method)

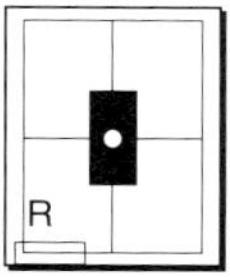

- 10 x 12" L.W. (24 x 30 cm)
- Grid

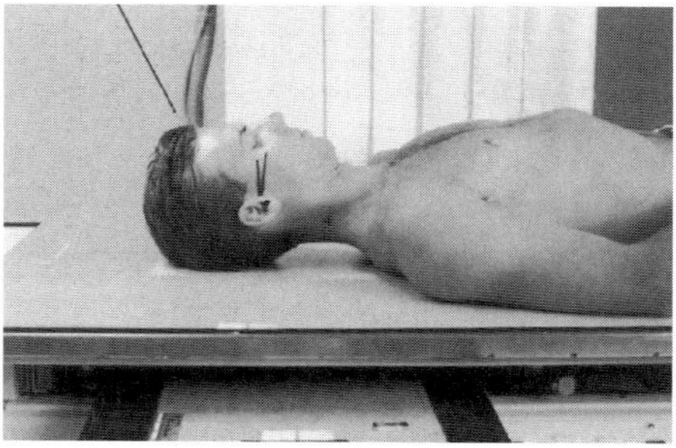

AP Towne – CR 30° caudad to OML

Position

- Seated erect, or supine, midsagittal plane aligned to CR and centerline, perpendicular to film – no rotation or tilt.
- Depress chin to bring OML or IOML perpendicular to film. (Place support under head if needed.)
- Center cassette to projecting CR.

Central Ray: CR 30° caudal to OML; or 37° caudal to IOML.

- CR to ≈2.5" or 6 cm above glabella (through ≈1" or 2.5 cm superior to level of EAM's).

SID: 40–48" (102–122 cm)

Collimation: On four sides to skull margins.

Respiration: Suspend during exposure.

Note: PA Haas is an alternate to AP Towne. Adjust head to bring OML ⊥ to film.

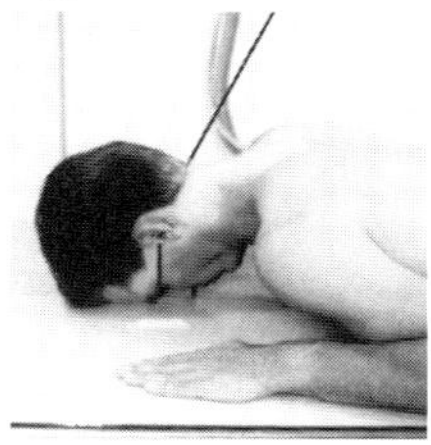

PA Haas method, OML ⊥ - CR 25° cephalad, through level of EAM's

Technique: kVp (80±5) ______

	cm	kVp	mA	Time	mAs	SID	Film–Screen	Grid	F.S.
Model Room	21	80			20	44"	Kodak 400	12:1	S
S									
M									
L									

(AP) mrad		
	S 179	Thyroid
	ML 45	52

Bontrager Textbook, 3rd ed., p.328

Lateral Skull

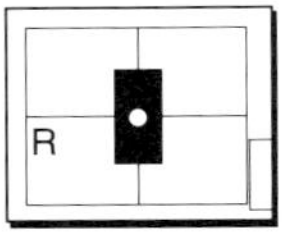

• 10 x 12" C.W. (24 x 30 cm)
• Grid

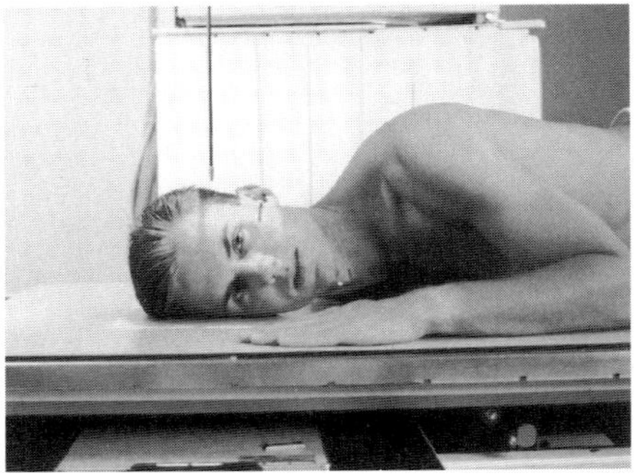

Lateral skull

Position

• Seated erect, or semiprone on table.
• No rotation or tilt, midsagittal plane parallel to film, and IPL perpendicular to film.
• Adjust chin to place IOML parallel to upper and lower cassette edges.
• Center cassette to CR.

Central Ray

• CR ⊥ to film, ≈ 2" (5 cm) superior to EAM.

SID: 40–48" (102–122 cm)

Collimation: On four sides to skull margins.

Respiration: Suspend during exposure.

Technique: kVp (80±5) ______

mrad		Thyroid
S	68	9
ML	20	

	cm	kVp	mA	Time	mAs	SID	Film–Screen	Grid	F.S.
Model Room	15	80			8	44"	Kodak 400	12:1	S
S									
M									
L									

Bontrager Textbook, 3rd ed., p. 329

PA (0° & 15 or 23°) Caldwell Skull

Note: Some departmental routines include a 0° PA to better demonstrate the frontal bone in addition to the 15 or 23° PA Caldwell.

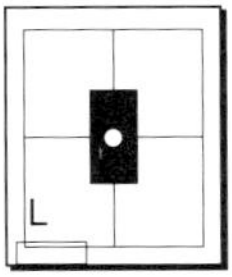

- 10 x 12" L.W. (24 x 30 cm)
- Grid

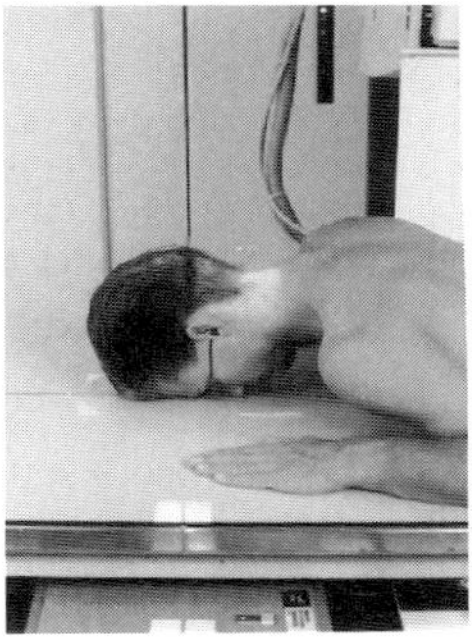

PA – 0°

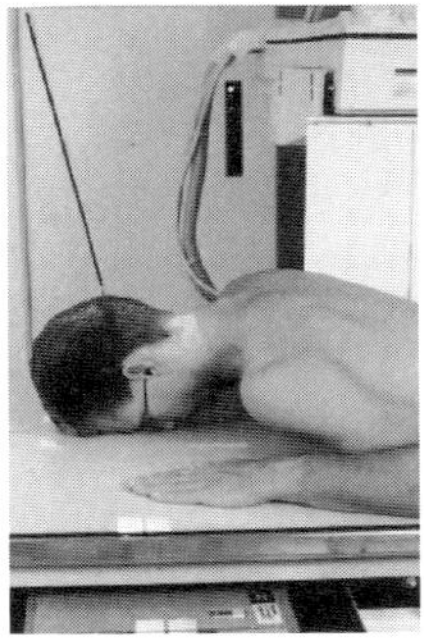

PA – 15° Caldwell

Position

- Seated erect, or prone on table, head aligned to CR and centerline of cassette.
- With forehead and nose resting on table top, adjust head to place OML perpendicular to film.
- No rotation or tilt, midsagittal plane perpendicular to film.
- Center cassette to projected CR.

Central Ray: PA – CR ⊥ to film, centered to exit at glabella.

- PA Caldwell – CR 15° caudad to OML, centered to exit at nasion (some prefer 23° caudad).

SID: 40–48" (102–122 cm)

Collimation: On four sides to skull margins.

Respiration: Suspend during exposure.

per projection

mrad		
	S 177	Thyroid
	ML 33	5

Technique: kVp (80±5) ______

	cm	kVp	mA	Time	mAs	SID	Film–Screen	Grid	F.S.
Model	21	80			18	44"	Kodak 400	12:1	S
Room									
S									
M									
L									

Bontrager Textbook, 3rd ed., p. 330, 331

Submentovertex (SMV) Skull

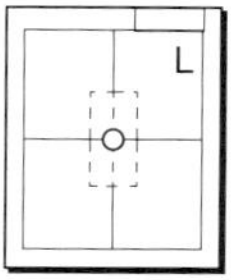

- 10 x 12" L.W. (24 x 30 cm)
- Grid
- AEC optional

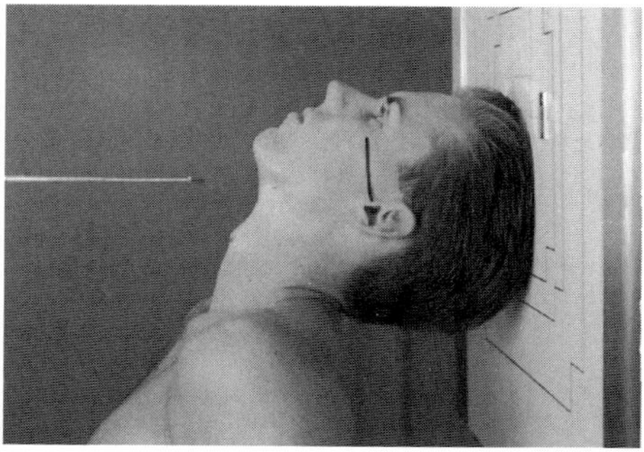

SMV – CR ⊥ to IOML

Position

- Seated erect, or supine with head extended over end of table resting top of head against grid cassette (may tilt table up slightly as shown).
- Adjust cassette and head to place IOML parallel to film.
- Ensure no rotation or tilt.
- Center cassette to CR.

Central Ray: CR angled to be ⊥ to IOML, centered to midpoint between angles of mandible.

Note: If patient cannot extend head this far, adjust CR as needed to remain perpendicular to IOML.

SID: 40–48" (102–122 cm)

Collimation: On four sides to skull margins.

Respiration: Suspend during exposure.

Technique: kVp (80±5) ______

mrad		
	S 288	G NDC M
	ML 58	NDC F

	cm	kVp	mA	Time	mAs	SID	Film–Screen	Grid	F.S.
Model Room	21	80			30	44"	Kodak 400	12:1	S
S									
M									
L									

Bontrager Textbook, 3rd ed., p. 332

Lateral Trauma Skull

Warning: Do **NOT** elevate or move patient's head before cervical spine injuries have been ruled out.

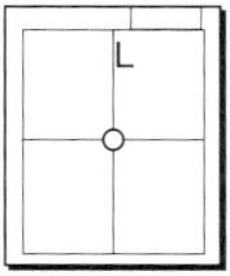

- 10 x 12" vertical (24 x 30 cm)
- Grid

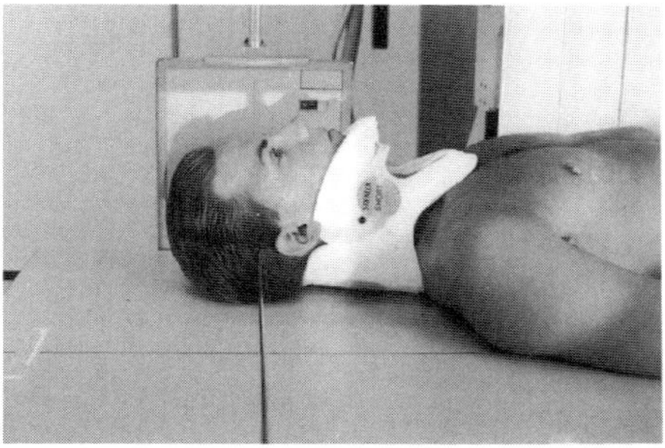

Lateral, with possible spinal injury

Position

- Supine, without removing cervical collar if present.
- With possible spinal injury, move patient to back edge of table and place cassette about 1" (2.5 cm) below table top and posterior skull (move floating table top forward).
- Center cassette to cross table CR (to include entire skull).
- Ensure no rotation or tilt.

Central Ray: CR cross table, ⊥ to film, centered to ≈2" (5 cm) superior to EAM.

SID: 40–48" (102–122 cm)

Collimation: On four sides to skull margins.

Respiration: Take as is for trauma patient.

Technique: kVp (75±5) ______

mrad		
	S 59	G NDC M
	ML 17	NDC F

	cm	kVp	mA	Time	mAs	SID	Film–Screen	Grid	F.S.
Model Room	15	75			8	40"	Kodak 400	6:1	S
S									
M									
L									

Bontrager Textbook, 3rd ed., p. 333

AP Trauma Skull Series

Warning: With possible spine or severe head injuries, take all projections AP without moving head or without removing cervical collar if present.

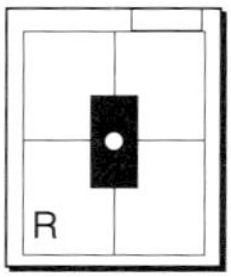

- 10 x 12" L.W. (24 x 30 cm)
- Grid (Bucky)

Position

- Patient carefully moved onto x–ray table in supine position.
- All projections taken as is without moving head.

SID: 40–48" (102–122 cm)

Collimation: On four sides to skull margins.

Respiration: Suspend during exposure, or take "as is".

CR Angle and Centering:

- As indicated under each photo.
- Cassette centered to projected CR.

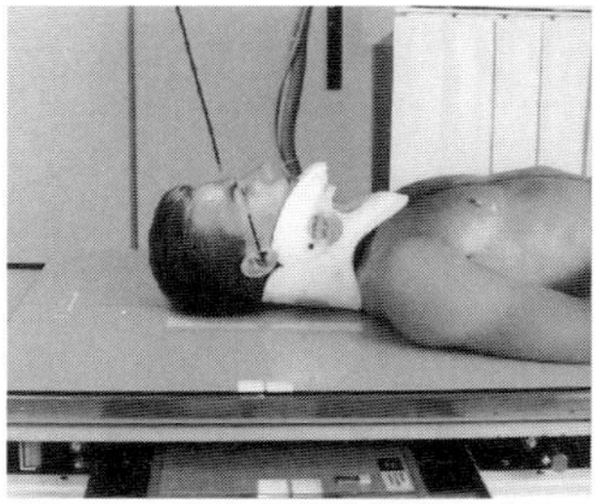

AP, 0° to OML
CR – parallel to OML
– centered to glabella

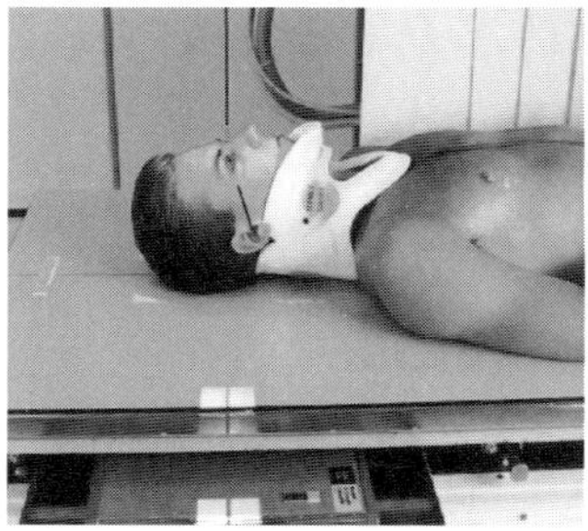

AP Reverse Caldwell
CR – 15° cephalad to OML
– centered to nasion

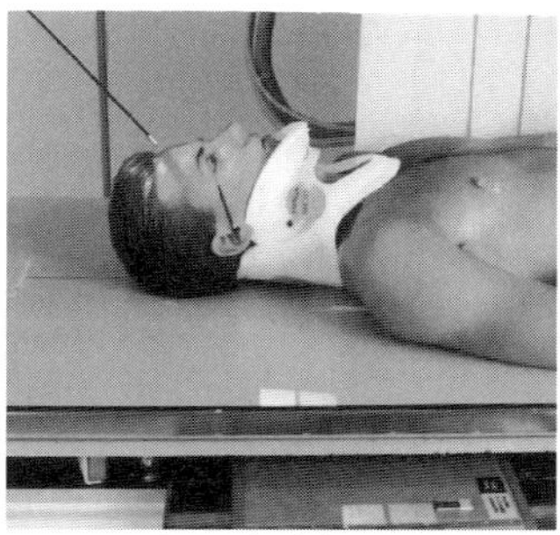

AP semiaxial Towne
CR – 30° caudad to OML
– centered to midpoint between EAM's

Bontrager Textbook, 3rd ed., p. 334

Facial Bones – Lateral

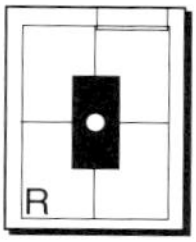

- 8 x 10" L.W. (20 x 24 cm)
- Grid

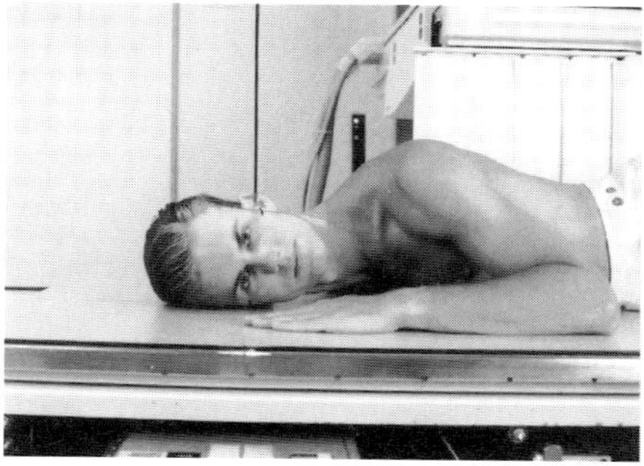

Lateral facial bones

Position

- Seated erect, or semi-prone on table.
- No rotation or tilt, midsagittal plane parallel to film, IPL perpendicular to film.
- Adjust chin to place IOML parallel to top and bottom edge of cassette.
- Center cassette to CR.

Central Ray

- CR ⊥ to film, centered to midway between EAM and outer canthus.

SID: 40–48" (102–122 cm)

Collimation: On four sides to area of facial bones.

Respiration: Suspend during exposure.

Technique: kVp (75±5) _____

mrad		
S	49	G NDC M
ML	13	NDC F

	cm	kVp	mA	Time	mAs	SID	Film–Screen	Grid	F.S.
Model Room	15	70			8	44"	Kodak 400	12:1	S
S									
M									
L									

Bontrager Textbook, 3rd ed., p. 358

Facial Bones - Parietoacanthial
(Waters & Modified Waters)

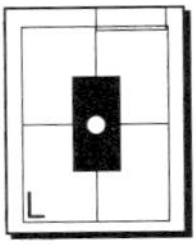

- 10 x 12" L.W. (24 x 30 cm) or 8 x 10" L.W. (20 x 24 cm)
- Grid

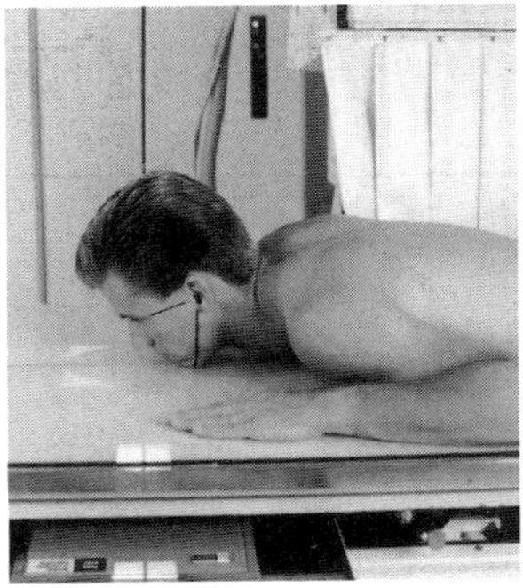

PA Waters, OML 37° - CR and MML ⊥

Position

Waters:
- Seated erect or prone on table.
- Extend head resting on chin, place MML ⊥ to film, which places the OML 37° to film.
- Center cassette to CR.

Modified Waters: OML is 55° to the plane of the film; or line from junction of lips to EAM (LML) is ⊥ (18-20° from MML).

Central Ray: CR ⊥ to film, to exit at acanthion (both projections).

SID: 40–48" (102–122 cm)

Collimation: To skull margins.

Respiration: Suspend during exposure.

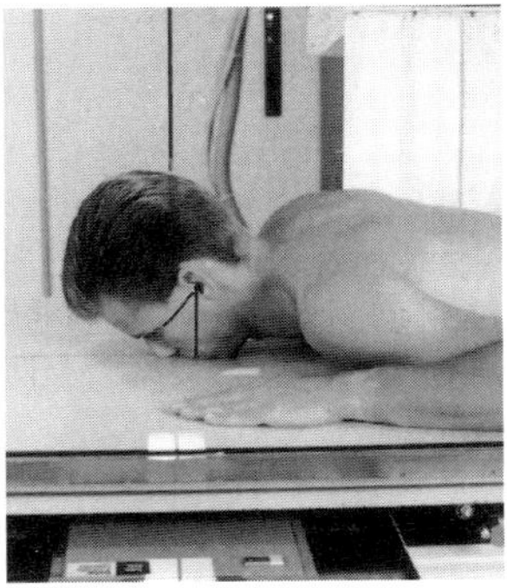

PA modified Waters, OML 55° - CR and LML ⊥

Technique: kVp (80±5) _____

mrad per projection		
S	189	G NDC M
ML	29	NDC F

	cm	kVp	mA	Time	mAs	SID	Film–Screen	Grid	F.S.
Model Room	24	80			18	44"	Kodak 400	12:1	S
S									
M									
L									

Bontrager Textbook, 3rd ed., p. 334

Facial Bones - PA (Caldwell)

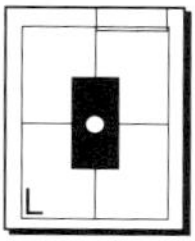

- 10 x 12" L.W. (24 x 30 cm)
  or
  8 x 10" L.W. (20 x 24 cm)
- Grid

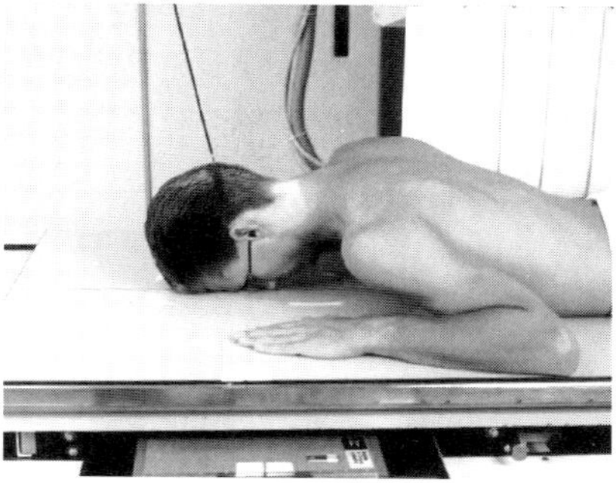

PA - 15° Caldwell (OML ⊥)
- CR to exit at nasion

Position

- Seated erect or prone on table, MSP aligned to CR and to centerline of cassette.
- With forehead and nose resting on table top, adjust head to place OML perpendicular to film. Ensure no rotation or tilt.
- Center cassette to projected CR (to nasion).

Central Ray

- CR 15° caudal to OML, centered to exit at nasion.

  Note: A 30° CR angle is required to project lower orbits below petrous ridges if this is an area of interest.

SID: 40–48" (102–122 cm)

Collimation: On four sides to skull (facial bones) margins.

Respiration: Suspend during exposure.

Technique: kVp (75±5) _____

mrad

S 118	G NDC M
ML 22	NDC F

	cm	kVp	mA	Time	mAs	SID	Film–Screen	Grid	F.S.
Model Room		75			18	44"	Kodak 400	12:1	S
S									
M									
L									

Bontrager Textbook, 3rd ed., p. 361

Facial Bones - Trauma Series

Warning: With possible spine or severe head injuries, take all projections AP without moving head or without removing cervical collar if present.

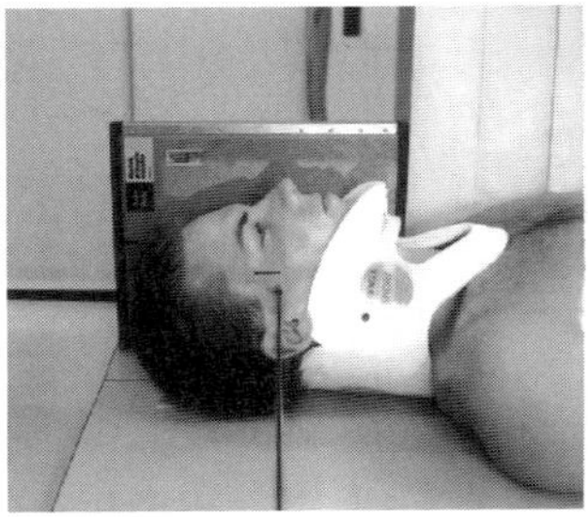

Trauma cross table lateral
- CR to midway between outer canthus and EAM

Lateral (cross table)

- 8 x 10" (20 x 24 cm) L.W.
- Grid, placed on edge against lateral cranium.
- Ensure no rotation or tilt, MSP parallel to film.
- CR horizontal, to midway between outer canthus and EAM.

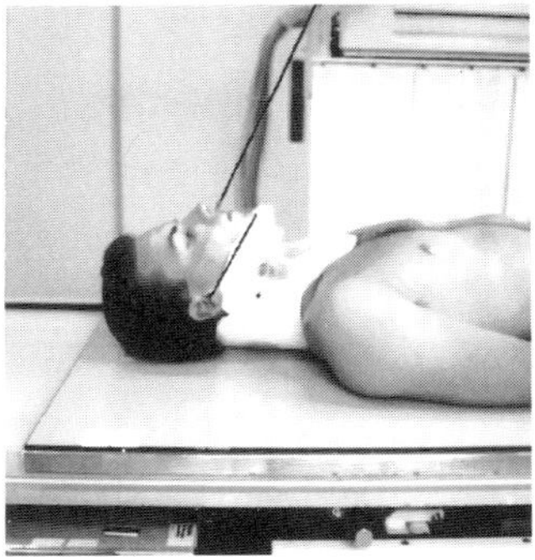

Trauma reverse Waters
- CR parallel to MML, to acanthion

Reverse Waters

- 8 x 10" (20 x 24 cm) L.W.
- Grid (Bucky), AEC - center field
- MSP aligned to CR and centerline of table and/or film.
- Ensure no rotation or tilt.
- CR parallel to MML.
- CR centered to acanthion. (CR angled cephalad as needed unless head can be tilted back if cervical injury has been ruled out)

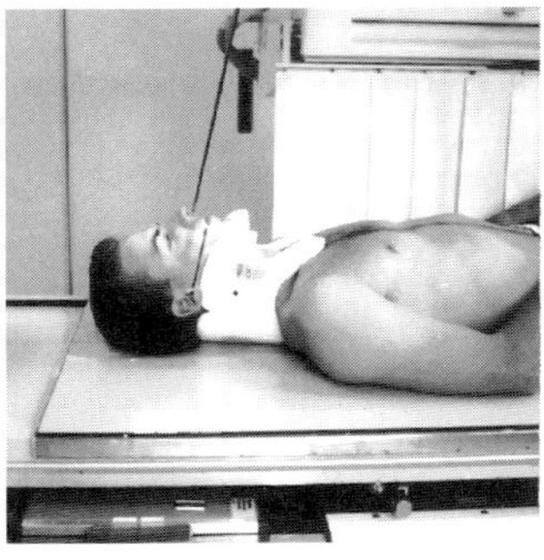

Trauma reverse modified Waters
- CR parallel to LML, to acanthion

Reverse Modified Waters

Same as reverse Waters except--
- CR parallel to junction of lips - meatal line (LML), which is 18-20° from MML.
- CR centered to acanthion.

Bontrager Textbook, 3rd ed., pp. 362-364

Optic Foramina – Parieto-orbital
(Rhese Oblique Method)

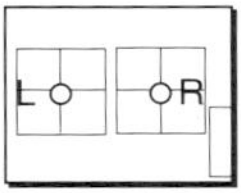

- 8 x 10" C.W. (20 x 24 cm)
- Grid

R and L sides taken for comparison.

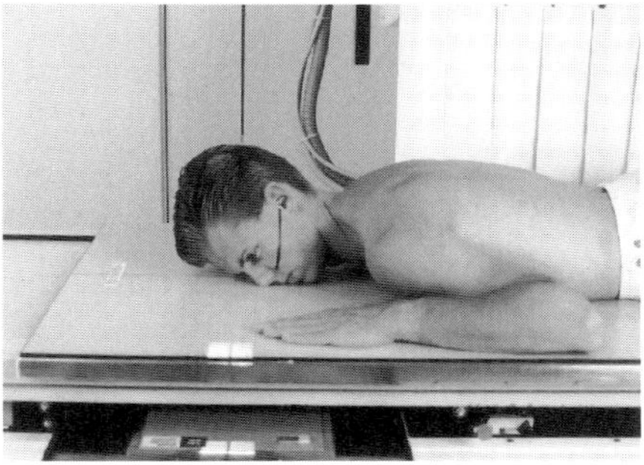

Rhese oblique (right side)
- AML and CR ⊥
- 53° rotation of head from lateral

Position
- Seated erect, or prone on table.
- As a starting reference, adjust the head so the nose, cheek, and chin are touching the table top.
- Adjust the head so the AML is perpendicular to the film, and the midsagittal plane is 53° to the film (use angle indicator).
- Center cassette to CR (to down-side orbit).

Central Ray
- CR ⊥ to film, to center of down-side orbit.

SID: 40–48" (102–122 cm)

Collimation: Closely collimate to 3–4" (8–10 cm) square.

Respiration: Suspend during exposure.

Technique: kVp (80±5) _____

mrad

S	171	G NDC M
ML	30	NDC F

	cm	kVp	mA	Time	mAs	SID	Film–Screen	Grid	F.S.
Model	21	80			18	44"	Kodak 400	12:1	S
Room									
S									
M									
L									

Bontrager Textbook, 3rd ed., p. 374

Zygomatic Arches - Bilateral
Submentovertex (SMV) Projection

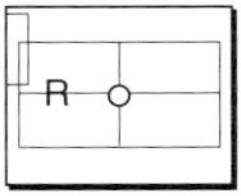

- 8 x 10" C.W. (20 x 24 cm)
- TT or grid

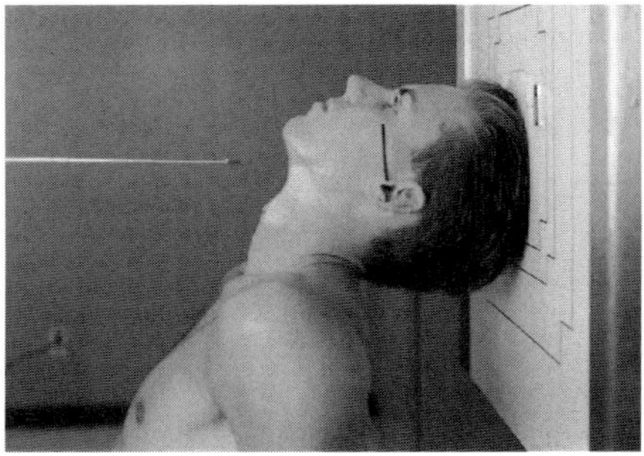

SMV, bilateral zygomatic arches, erect - CR ⊥ to IOML (non-grid may be preferred—not shown)

Position

- Seated erect, or supine with head extended over end of table resting top of head against grid cassette (may tilt table up slightly).
- Adjust cassette and head to place IOML parallel to film.
- Ensure no rotation or tilt.
- Center cassette to CR.

Central Ray: CR angled as needed to be ⊥ to IOML, centered to midway between zygomatic arches (≈ 1.5" or 4 cm inferior to mandibular symphysis).

SID: 40–48" (102–122 cm)

Collimation: To include area of zygomatic arches.

Respiration: Suspend during exposure.

mrad

S	35	G NDC M
ML	6	NDC F

Technique: kVp (65±5) _____ (near soft tissue technique)

	cm	kVp	mA	Time	mAs	SID	Film–Screen	Grid	F.S.
Model Room	20	65			6	44"	Kodak 100	–	S
S									
M									
L									

Bontrager Textbook, 3rd ed., p. 369

Zygomatic Arches - Tangential
(Oblique Axial Projection)

R and L sides generally taken for comparison.

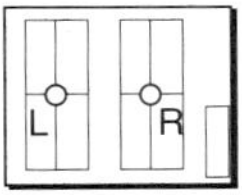

- 8 x 10" C.W. (20 x 24 cm)
- TT or grid

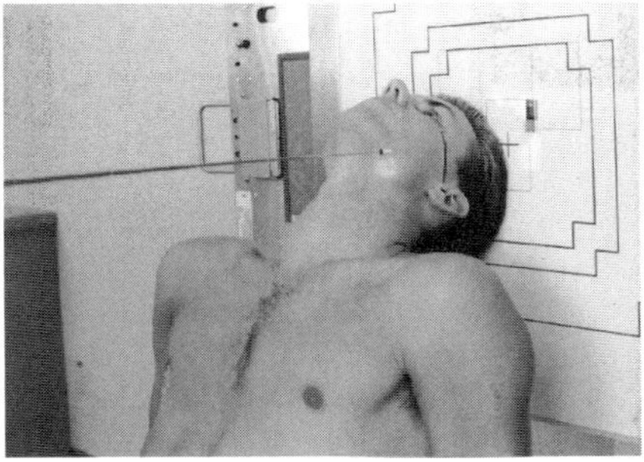

Tangential of left zygomatic arch
(non-grid may be preferred–not shown)

Position

- Position as for a SMV skull with the IOML parallel to the film.
- Rotate the head ≈15° toward side being examined.
- Tilt the midsagittal plane with the chin towards the side of interest about 15° or as needed to free the zygomatic arch from superimposition by mandible or parietal bone.
- Center cassette to CR.

Central Ray: CR angled if needed to be ⊥ to IOML, centered to mid zygomatic arch.

SID: 40–48" (102–122 cm)

Collimation: Collimate closely to area of interest.

Respiration: Suspend during exposure.

Technique: kVp (65±5) _____

mrad

S	44	G NDC M
ML	8	NDC F

	cm	kVp	mA	Time	mAs	SID	Film–Screen	Grid	F.S.
Model	20	65			6	44"	Kodak 100	–	S
Room									
S									
M									
L									

Bontrager Textbook, 3rd ed., p. 372

Zygomatic Arches - AP Axial
(Modified Towne)

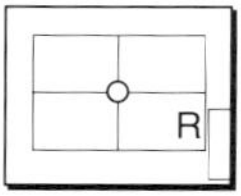

- 8 x 10" C.W. (20 x 24 cm)
- Grid

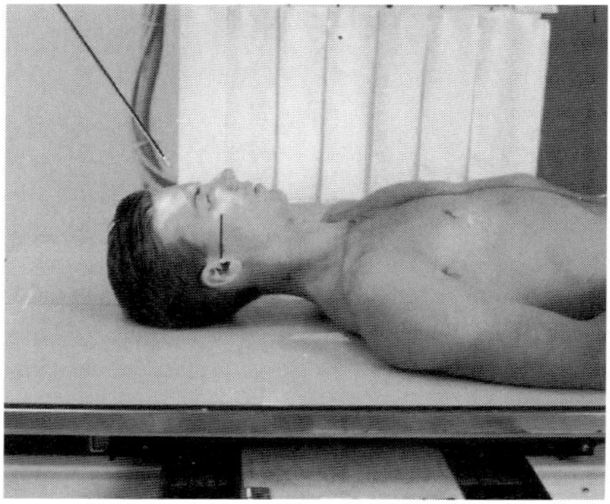

AP axial – CR 37° to IOML

Position

- Seated erect, or supine on table, midsagittal plane aligned to midline of table or cassette – ensure no rotation or tilt.
- Depress chin to bring either the OML or the IOML perpendicular to film.
- Center cassette to projected CR.

Central Ray

- CR 30° caudal to OML; or 37° to IOML.
- CR slightly superior to glabella to pass through level of mid arches.

SID: 40–48" (102–122 cm)

Collimation: On four sides to area of bilateral arches.

Respiration: Suspend during exposure.

Technique: kVp (70±5) _____

mrad

S	193	G NDC M
ML	49	NDC F

	cm	kVp	mA	Time	mAs	SID	Film–Screen	Grid	F.S.
Model Room	17	70			30	44"	Kodak 400	12:1	S
S									
M									
L									

Bontrager Textbook, 3rd ed., p. 371

Nasal Bones - Lateral

R and L laterals generally taken for comparison.

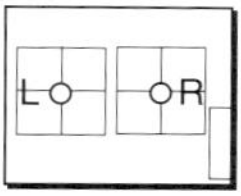

- 8 x 10" C.W. (20 x 24 cm)
- TT – detail screens

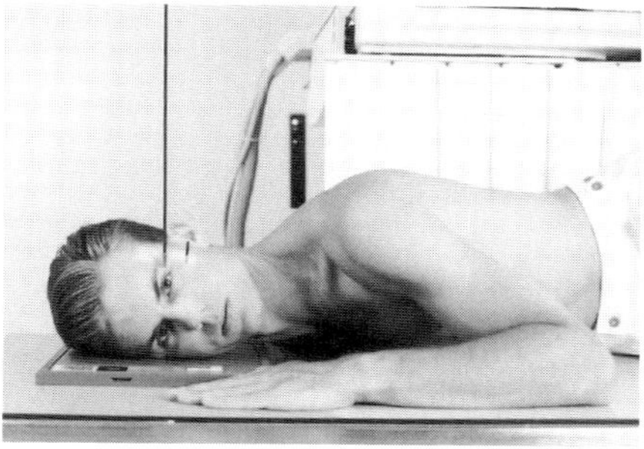

Right lateral – nasal bones

Position

- Seated erect, or semiprone on table.
- Center nasal bones to half of cassette and to CR.
- Adjust head to bring IOML parallel to top and bottom edge of cassette.
- Ensure a true lateral, IPL perpendicular to film, and midsagittal plane parallel to film.

Central Ray

- CR ⊥ to film, centered to ≈3/4" (2 cm) inferior to nasion.

SID: 40–48" (102–122 cm)

Collimation: Closely collimate to ≈4" (10 cm) square.

Respiration: Suspend during exposure.

Technique: kVp (55±5) _____

mrad

S	8	G NDC M
ML	8	NDC F

	cm	kVp	mA	Time	mAs	SID	Film–Screen	Grid	F.S.
Model Room	2	55			3	40"	Kodak 100	–	S
S									
M									
L									

Bontrager Textbook, 3rd ed., p. 365

Nasal Bones

Superoinferior Axial

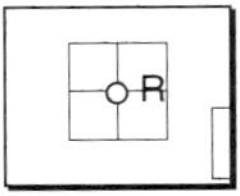

- 8 x 10" C.W. (20 x 24 cm)
- TT (detail screens)

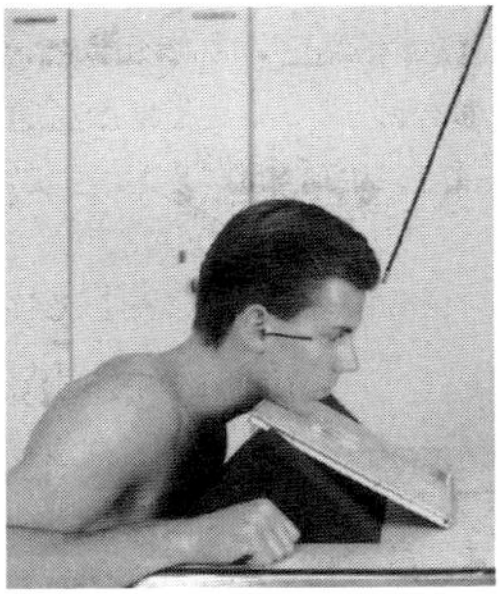

Erect

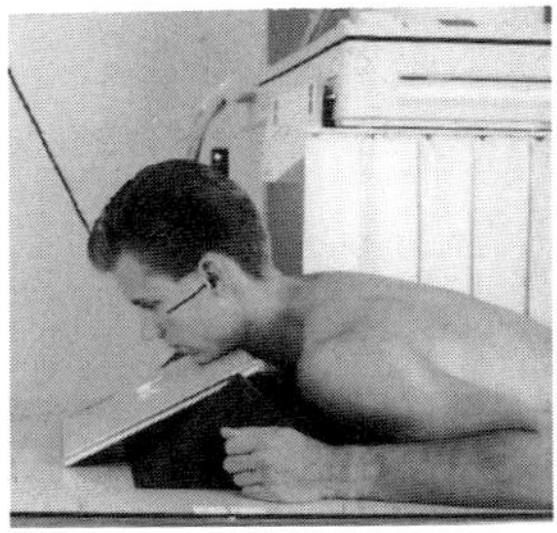

Prone

Position

- Seated erect at end of table, or prone on table.
- If prone, place supports under chest and under cassette.
- Rest extended chin on cassette which should be perpendicular to GAL (glabelloalveolar line) and to CR.

Central Ray

- CR directed along GAL, ⊥ to film.

SID: 40–48" (102–122 cm)

Collimation: Closely collimate to ≈4" (10 cm) square.

Respiration: Suspend during exposure.

Technique: kVp (55±5) _____

mrad		
S	27	G NDC M
ML	27	NDC F

	cm	kVp	mA	Time	mAs	SID	Film–Screen	Grid	F.S.
Model		60			6	40"	Kodak 100	–	S
Room									
S									
M									
L									

Bontrager Textbook, 3rd ed., p. 368

Mandible - PA

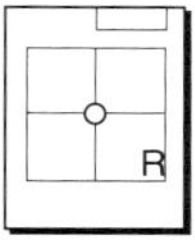

- 8 x 10" L.W. (20 x 24 cm)
- Grid

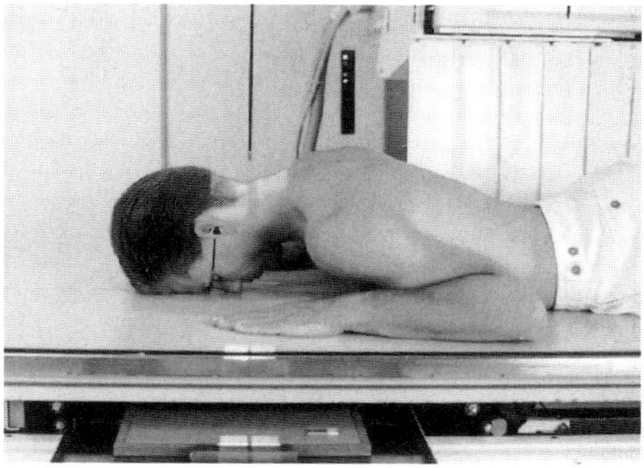

PA mandible – CR and OML ⊥ to film

Position

- Seated erect, or prone on table, head aligned to centerline.
- With forehead and nose resting on table top, adjust head to place OML ⊥ to film.
- No rotation or tilt, midsagittal plane ⊥ to film.
- Center cassette to CR (level of junction of lips).

Central Ray: CR ⊥ to film, to exit at level of lips.

Note: A CR angle of 20-25° cephalad best demonstrates proximal rami and condyles.

SID: 40–48" (102–122 cm)

Collimation: Collimate to area of mandible (square area).

Respiration: Suspend during exposure.

Technique: kVp (75±5) _____

mrad		
S	91	G NDC M
ML	24	NDC F

	cm	kVp	mA	Time	mAs	SID	Film–Screen	Grid	F.S.
Model Room	17	75			12	44"	Kodak 400	12:1	S
S									
M									
L									

Bontrager Textbook, 3rd ed., p. 361

Mandible - Axiolateral Obliques

R and L sides generally taken for comparison unless contraindicated.

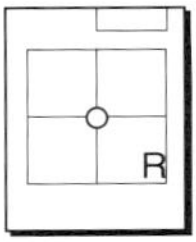

- 8 x 10" L.W. (20 x 24 cm)
- Grid - lengthwise

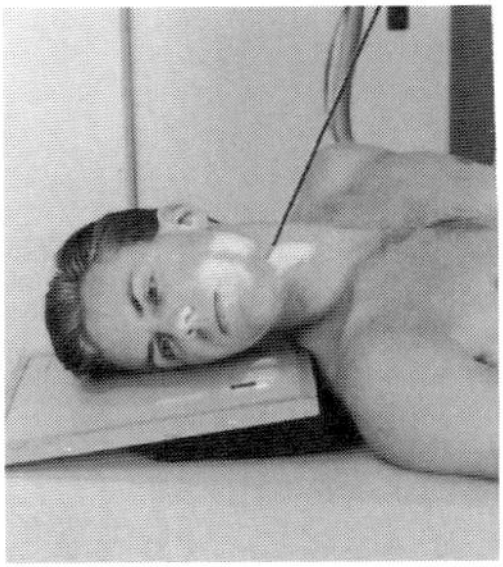
Semi-supine

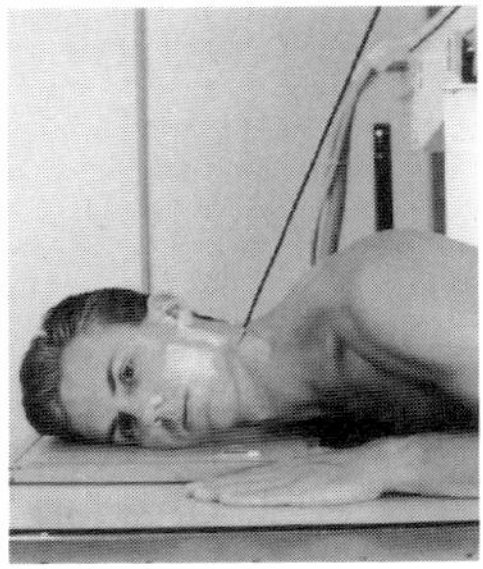
Semi-prone

CR 25-30° cephalad
10-15° rotation for general survey (as shown above)
– 0° rotation for ramus
– 30° rotation for body (most common)
– 45° rotation for mentum

Position

- Seated erect, semi-prone or semi-supine with support under shoulder and hip.
- Extend chin, with side of interest against cassette.
- Adjust head so IPL is perpendicular to film, no tilt.
- Rotate head toward film as determined by area of interest.

Central Ray: CR 25–30° cephalad to IPL, centered to down-side mid mandible (≈2" or 5 cm below up-side angle).

SID: 40–48" (102–122 cm)

Collimation: To area of mandible (square area).

Respiration: Suspend during exposure.

Technique: kVp (75±5) _____

mrad

S	35	G NDC M
ML	12	NDC F

	cm	kVp	mA	Time	mAs	SID	Film–Screen	Grid	F.S.
Model	13	75			5	40"	Kodak 400	6:1	S
Room									
S									
M									
L									

Bontrager Textbook, 3rd ed., p. 376

Mandible -Trauma Axiolateral Obli's
(cross table)

For trauma or inebriated patients unable to cooperate.

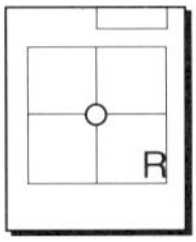

- 8 x 10" L.W. (20 x 24 cm)
- Grid lengthwise

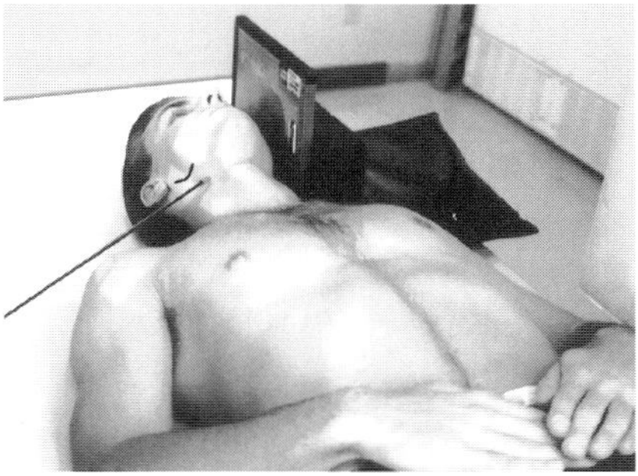

Cross table axiolateral[3] - CR 30° cephalad

Position

- Supine, no rotation of head, MSP ⊥ to TT.
- Cassette on edge next to face, parallel to MSP with lower edge of cassette ≈1" (2.5 cm) below lower border of mandible.
- Depress shoulders and elevate or extend chin if possible.

Note: May rotate head toward film slightly (10-15°) to better visualize body or mentum of mandible if this is area of interest.

Central Ray: CR cross table, 30° cephalad (from lateral or IPL) angled down (posteriorly) slightly if needed to clear shoulder.

- CR centered to ≈2" (5 cm) distal to angle of mandible on side away from film.

SID: 40–48" (102–122 cm)

Collimation: To area of mandible (square area).

Respiration: Suspend during exposure.

Technique: kVp (75±5) _____

mrad		
S	35	G NDC M
ML	12	NDC F

	cm	kVp	mA	Time	mAs	SID	Film–Screen	Grid	F.S.
Model Room	13	75			5	40"	Kodak 400	6:1	S
S									
M									
L									

[3]Clark's Positioning in Radiography, 11th ed., p. 243

AP Axial Mandible
(and Temperomandibular Joints)

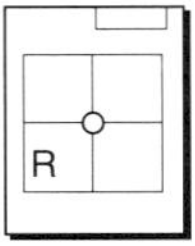

- 10 x 12" L.W. (24 x 30 cm)
- Grid

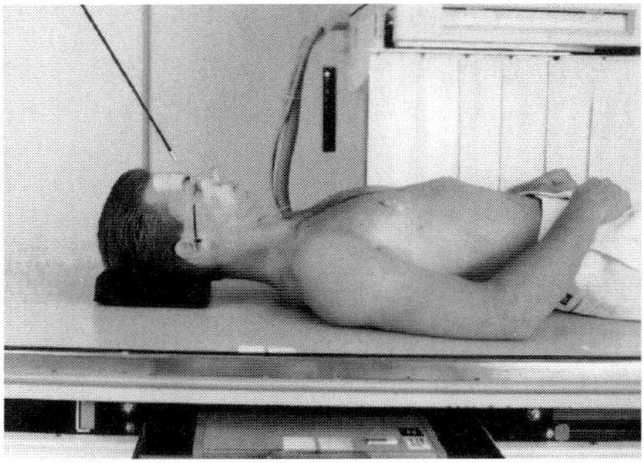

AP axial, CR 35–40° to OML
(CR centered for mandible)

Position
- Seated erect, or supine on table, midsagittal plane centered to midline of table – ensure no rotation or tilt.
- Depress chin to bring OML perpendicular to film if possible (or bring IOML perpendicular and add 7° to CR angle).
- Center cassette to projected CR.

Central Ray: CR 35–40° caudad to OML (42–47° to IOML).
- CR centered to glabella for mandible.

Note: CR centered ≈ 2" (5 cm) above glabella if TMJ's are of primary interest.

SID: 40–48" (102–122 cm)

Collimation: To include from TMJ's to body of mandible.

Respiration: Suspend during exposure.

Technique: kVp (80±5) _____

mrad

S	177	G NDC M
ML	32	NDC F

	cm	kVp	mA	Time	mAs	SID	Film–Screen	Grid	F.S.
Model	21	80			16	44"	Kodak 400	12:1	S
Room									
S									
M									
L									

Temperomandibular Joints

Axiolateral Oblique (Law Method)

R & L sides for comparison in both open & closed mouth positions.

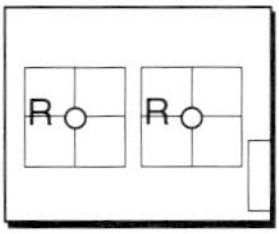

- 10 x 12" C.W. (24 x 30 cm)
- Grid

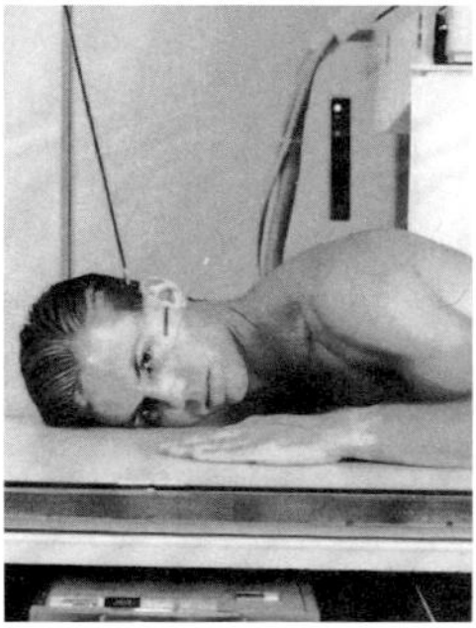

Closed mouth

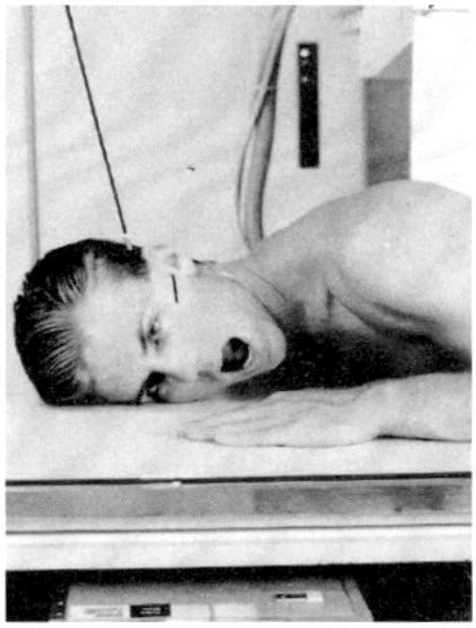

Open mouth

– 15° oblique (from lateral) and 15° CR (caudad)

Position

- Seated erect, or semiprone on table, affected side down.
- Adjust chin to place IOML parallel to top edge of cassette.
- Anterior head (midsagittal plane) rotated 15° toward film, no tilt, IPL remains perpendicular to film.
- Portion of cassette being exposed centered to projected CR.
- Second exposure in same position except with mouth fully open.

Central Ray: CR 15° caudad, center to exit through down-side TMJ (to enter ≈1" or 2.5 cm superior to up-side EAM).

SID: 40–48" (102–122 cm)

Collimation: Collimate to 3–4" (8–10 cm) square.

Respiration: Suspend during exposure.

Technique: kVp (75±5) _____

mrad, per projection

S	101	G NDC M
ML	30	NDC F

	cm	kVp	mA	Time	mAs	SID	Film–Screen	Grid	F.S.
Model Room	15	75			14	44"	Kodak 400	12:1	S
S									
M									
L									

Bontrager Textbook, 3rd ed., p. 383

Temperomandibular Joints
Axiolateral (Schuller Method)

R & L sides for comparison in both open & closed mouth positions.

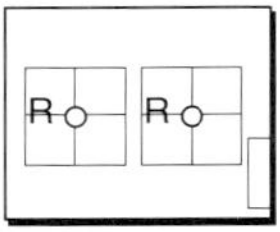

• 10 x 12" C.W. (24 x 30 cm)
• Grid

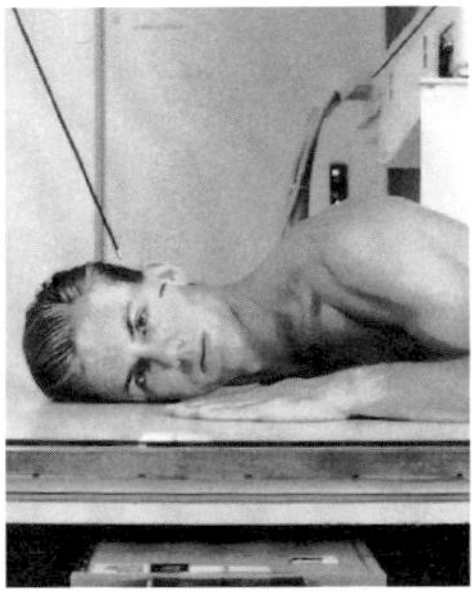
closed mouth

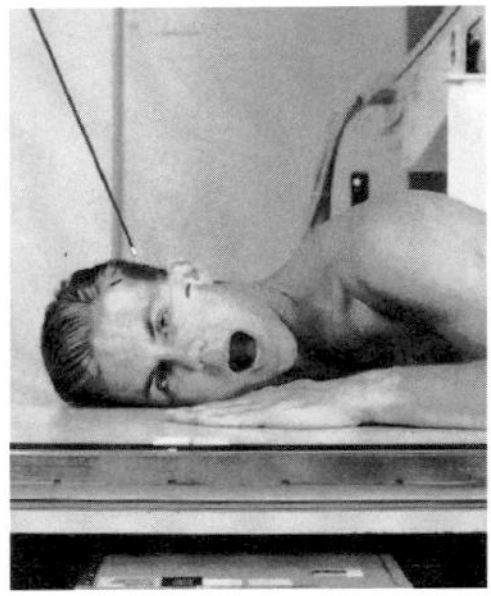
open mouth

– 0° rotation and CR 25-30° caudad

Position

- Seated erect, or semiprone, affected side down.
- Adjust chin to place IOML parallel to top and bottom edges of cassette, true lateral, no rotation or tilt.
- Portion of cassette being exposed centered to projected CR.
- Second exposure in same position except with mouth fully open.

Central Ray: CR 25–30° caudad, center to exit through down-side TMJ (to enter ≈2" or 5 cm superior and 1" or 2.5 cm anterior to up-side EAM).

SID: 40–48" (102–122 cm)

Collimation: Collimate to 3–4" (8–10 cm) square.

Respiration: Suspend during exposure.

Technique: kVp (80±5) _____

mrad — per projection

S 101	G NDC M
ML 30	NDC F

	cm	kVp	mA	Time	mAs	SID	Film–Screen	Grid	F.S.
Model Room	15	75			14	44"	Kodak 400	12:1	S
S									
M									
L									

Bontrager Textbook, 3rd ed., p. 384

Lateral Paranasal Sinuses

Requires an **erect position with horizontal CR** to demonstrate air-fluid levels.

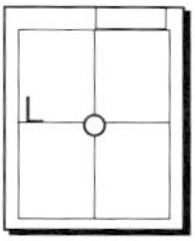

- 8 x 10" L.W. (20 x 24 cm)
- Grid

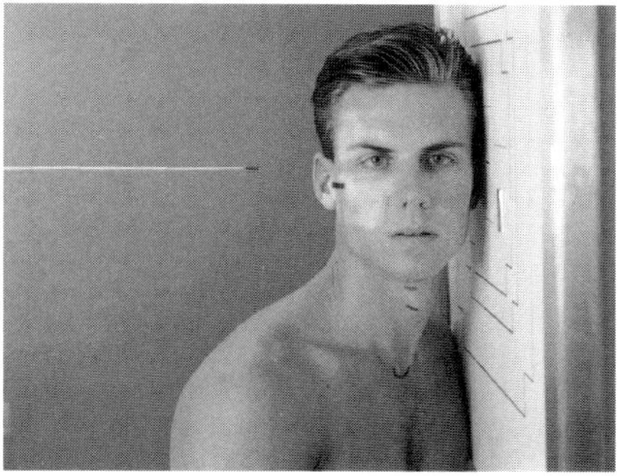

Erect lateral

Position

- Erect, seated facing film, turn head into lateral position.
- Adjust height of cassette to center film to level of EAM.
- Raise chin to bring IOML parallel to floor.
- No rotation, midsagittal plane parallel and IPL ⊥ to film.
- Center cassette to CR.

Central Ray

- CR horizontal, to midpoint between EAM and outer canthus.

SID: 40–48" (102–122 cm)

Collimation: Collimate on four sides to area of sinuses.

Respiration: Suspend during exposure.

Technique: kVp (75±5) _____

mrad

S	31	G NDC M
ML	8	NDC F

	cm	kVp	mA	Time	mAs	SID	Film–Screen	Grid	F.S.
Model Room	15	70			5	44"	Kodak 400	12:1	S
S									
M									
L									

Bontrager Textbook, 3rd ed., p. 400

PA Paranasal Sinuses
(Caldwell Method)

Requires an **erect position with horizontal CR** to demonstrate air-fluid levels.

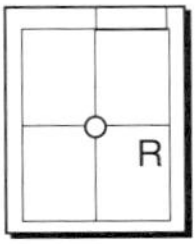

- 8 x 10" L.W. (20 x 24 cm)
- Grid

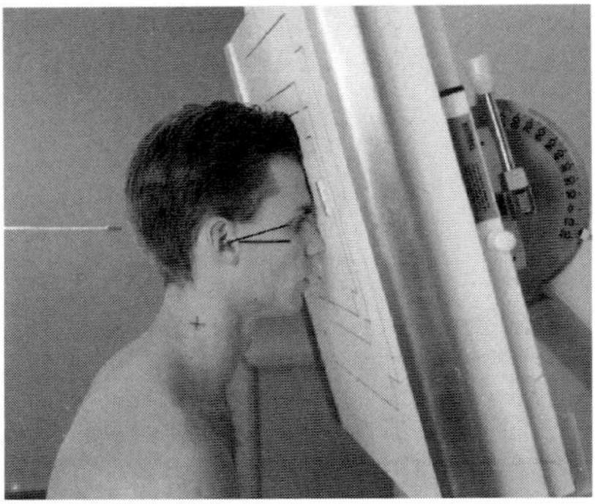

PA Caldwell
(If film holder can be tilted)

Position

PA Caldwell

- Seated erect, facing film, tilt top of film 15° toward patient.
- Adjust head so OML is ⊥ to film, no rotation.
- Film centered to CR (nasion).

Modified PA Caldwell

- Tilt head back to bring OML 15° from horizontal.

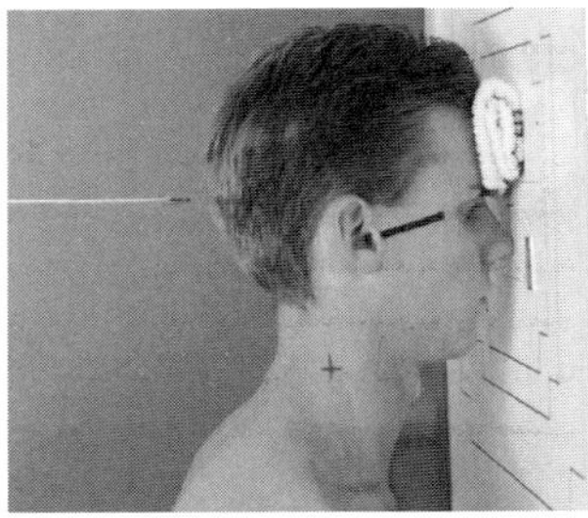

Modified PA Caldwell
(If film holder cannot be tilted)

Central Ray: CR horizontal, centered to exit at nasion.

SID: 40–48" (102–122 cm)

Collimation: To area of sinuses.

Respiration: Suspend during exposure.

Technique: kVp (75±5) _____

mrad

S	202	G NDC M
ML	35	NDC F

	cm	kVp	mA	Time	mAs	SID	Film–Screen	Grid	F.S.
Model Room	21	75			24	44"	Kodak 400	12:1	S
S									
M									
L									

Bontrager Textbook, 3rd ed., p. 401

Paranasal Sinuses

(Waters Method) Parietoacanthial

Requires an **erect position with horizontal CR** to demonstrate air-fluid levels.

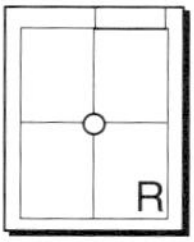

- 8 x 10" L.W. (20 x 24 cm)
- Grid

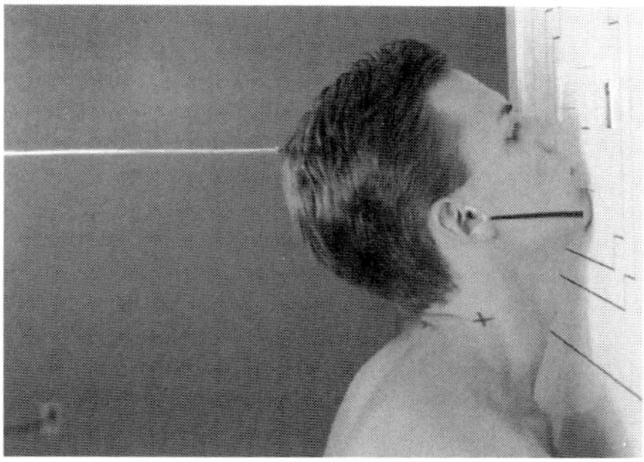

PA Erect Waters, MML ⊥ and CR horizontal

Position

- Seated erect, chin extended and touching film holder.
- Adjust height of cassette to center film to acanthion.
- Adjust MML perpendicular to film (OML is 37° to film).
- No rotation, midsagittal plane perpendicular to film holder.
- Center cassette to CR.

Optional Open-mouth Position: Patient opens mouth wide to better visualize sphenoid sinuses through the open mouth.

Central Ray

- CR horizontal and ⊥ to film, to exit at acanthion.

SID: 40–48" (102–122 cm)

Collimation: Collimate on four sides to area of sinuses.

Respiration: Suspend during exposure.

Technique: kVp (75±5) _____

mrad

S 253	G NDC M
ML 35	NDC F

	cm	kVp	mA	Time	mAs	SID	Film–Screen	Grid	F.S.
Model Room	24	75			28	44"	Kodak 400	12:1	S
S									
M									
L									

Bontrager Textbook, 3rd ed., pp. 402 and 404

Paranasal Sinuses
Submentovertex (SMV)

Requires an **erect position with horizontal CR** to demonstrate air-fluid levels.

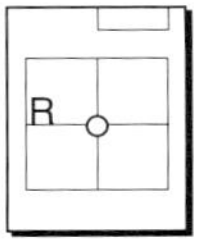

- 8 x 10" L.W. (20 x 24 cm)
- Grid

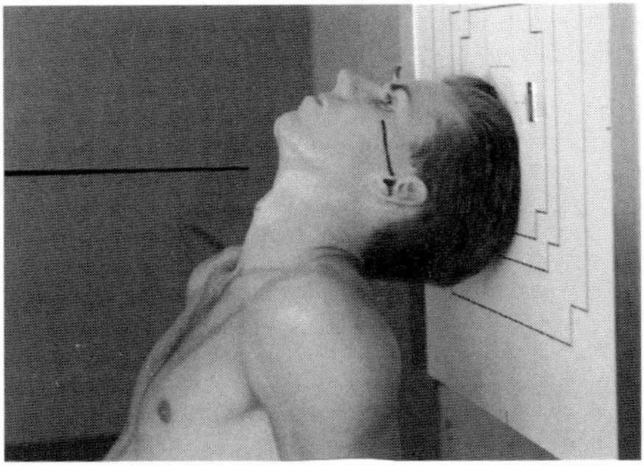

SMV sinuses
- CR ⊥ to IOML and film

Position

- Seated erect, leaning back in chair and extending head to rest top of head against film holder.
- Adjust head to place IOML as near parallel to plane of film as possible; ensure no rotation or tilt.
- Center cassette to CR.

Central Ray: CR horizontal and ⊥ to IOML, centered to midpoint between angles of mandible.

SID: 40–48" (102–122 cm)

Collimation: On four sides to area of sinuses.

Respiration: Suspend during exposure.

Technique: kVp (75±5) _____

mrad

S 277	G NDC M
ML 53	NDC F

	cm	kVp	mA	Time	mAs	SID	Film–Screen	Grid	F.S.
Model Room	20	75			34	44"	Kodak 400	12:1	S
S									
M									
L									

Bontrager Textbook, 3rd ed., p. 403

Mastoids – Axiolateral Oblique
(Law Method)

R & L sides taken for comparison.

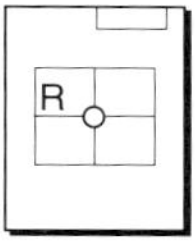

- 8 x 10" L.W. (20 x 24 cm)
- Grid

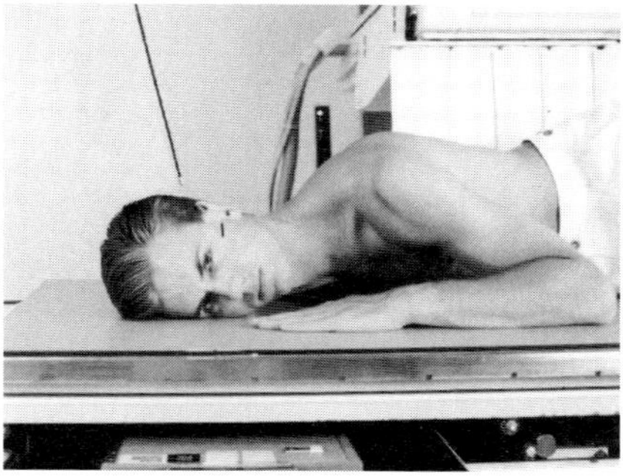

Axiolateral oblique – right side – 15° rotation and 15° CR (caudad)

Position

- Tape auricles of both ears forward.
- Erect or semiprone, side of interest down.
- IMOL parallel to top and bottom edge of film.
- Rotate anterior head (midsagittal plane) 15° toward film, no tilt, IPL remains perpendicular to film.
- Center cassette to projected CR.

Central Ray: CR 15° caudad, centered to ≈1 1/2" (4 cm) posterior and superior to up-side EAM (centers down-side mastoids to film).

SID: 40–48" (102–122 cm)

Collimation: On four sides to ≈ 4 x 5" (10 x 12 cm) field.

Respiration: Suspend during exposure.

Technique: kVp (75±5) _____

mrad

S	115	G NDC M
ML	35	NDC F

	cm	kVp	mA	Time	mAs	SID	Film–Screen	Grid	F.S.
Model Room	15	75			16	44"	Kodak 400	12:1	S
S									
M									
L									

Bontrager Textbook, 3rd ed., p. 405

Mastoids–Posterior Profile Obli.
(Stenvers Method)

R & L sides taken for comparison.

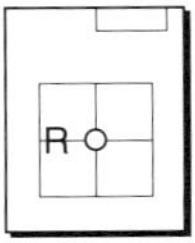

• 8 x 10" L.W. (20 x 24 cm)
• Grid

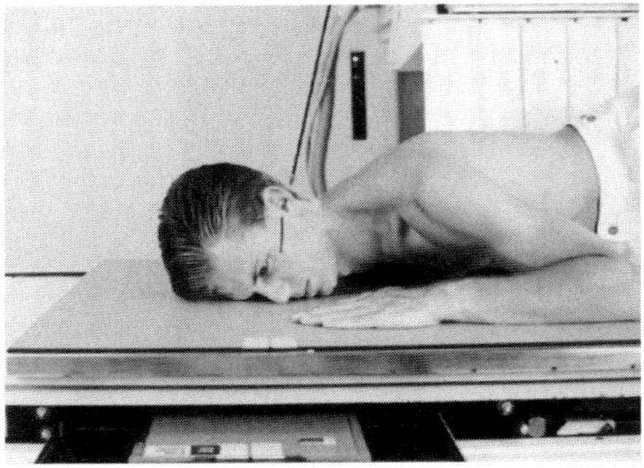

Posterior profile – right side
– 45° oblique and 12° CR (cephalad)

Position

• Erect or prone, rotate head 45°, begin by placing forehead, nose and cheek against table top.
• Adjust head as needed to bring IMOL perpendicular to table-top as viewed from the front.
• Center cassette to projected CR.

Central Ray: CR 12° cephalad, centered to ≈2" (5 cm) posterior and ≈1/2" (1 cm) inferior to up-side EAM.

SID: 40–48" (102–122 cm)

Collimation: On four sides to ≈ 4" (10 cm) square.

Respiration: Suspend during exposure.

Technique: kVp (75±5) _____

mrad

S	144	G NDC M
ML	43	NDC F

	cm	kVp	mA	Time	mAs	SID	Film–Screen	Grid	F.S.
Model Room	15	75			20	44"	Kodak 400	12:1	S
S									
M									
L									

Bontrager Textbook, 3rd ed., p. 406

Mastoids–Anterior Profile Obli.
(Arcelin Method – Reverse Stenvers)

R and L sides taken for comparison.

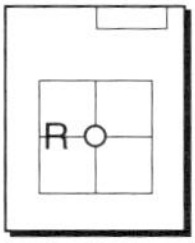

- 8 x 10" L.W. (20 x 24 cm)
- Grid

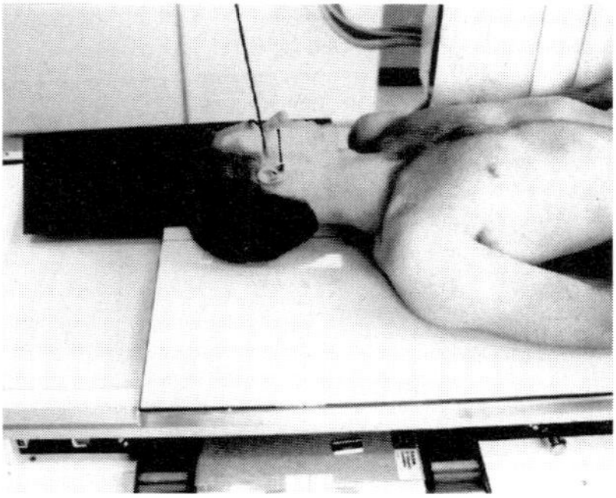

Anterior profile – right side (up side) – 45° oblique and CR 10° caudad

Position
- Supine, align upside mastoid area to centerline of table.
- Rotate head 45° away from side of interest.
- Adjust head as needed to bring IOML perpendicular to table top.
- Center cassette to projected CR.

Central Ray
- CR 10° caudad, centered to ≈ 1" (2.5 cm) anterior and ≈ 3/4" (2 cm) superior to up-side EAM.

SID: 40–48" (102–122 cm)

Collimation: On four sides to ≈ 4" (10 cm) square.

Respiration: Suspend during exposure.

Technique: kVp (75±5) _____

mrad

S	144	G NDC M
ML	42	NDC F

	cm	kVp	mA	Time	mAs	SID	Film–Screen	Grid	F.S.
Model Room	15	75			20	44"	Kodak 400	12:1	S
S									
M									
L									

Merrill's Atlas, 8th ed., p . 1-410

Mastoids – AP Axial
(Towne)

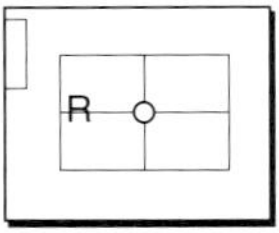

• 8 x 10" C.W. (20 x 24 cm)
• Grid

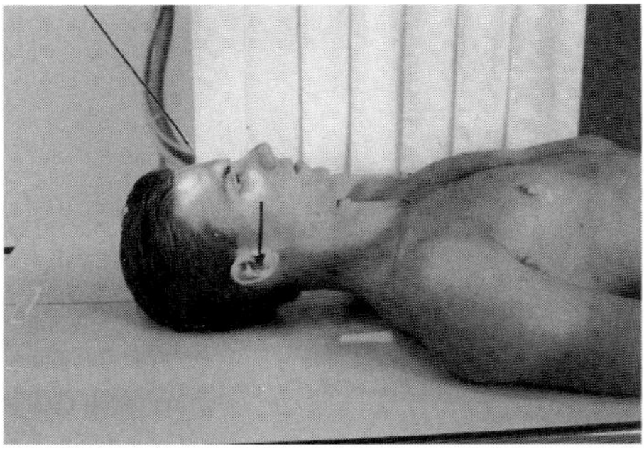
AP axial, IOML ⊥, CR 37° caudad

Position
• Seated erect, or supine on table, midsagittal plane centered to midline of cassette, no rotation or tilt.
• Depress chin to bring OML ⊥ to film, or if this is difficult for patient, place IOML ⊥ and increase CR to 37°.
• Center cassette to projected CR.

Central Ray: CR 30° caudad to OML, or 37° to IOML.
• CR to pass through skull midway between EAM's (enters ≈2" or 5 cm superior to glabella).

SID: 40–48" (102–122 cm)

Collimation: To include mastoid and temporal bone area.

Respiration: Suspend during exposure.

Technique: kVp (80±5) _____

mrad

S	255	G NDC M
ML	66	NDC F

	cm	kVp	mA	Time	mAs	SID	Film–Screen	Grid	F.S.
Model Room	17	80			26	44"	Kodak 400	12:1	S
S									
M									
L									

Bontrager Textbook, 3rd ed., p. 407

Mastoids – Axioposterior Obli.
(Mayer Method and Owen Modification)

R & L sides taken for comparison.

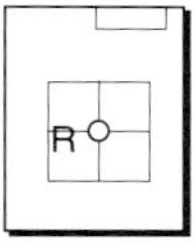

- 8 x 10" C.W. (20 x 24 cm)
- Grid

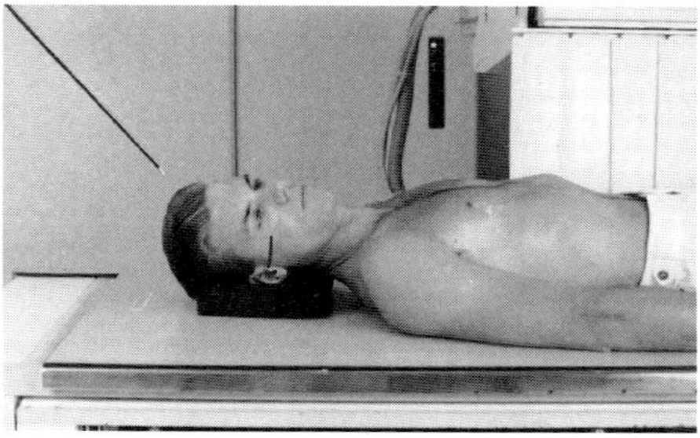

45° RPO (for right side)
– 45° CR (caudad)

Position
- Seated erect, or supine on table.
- Rotate head 45° (side of interest is down-side).
- Depress chin, IOML ⊥ to film (as viewed from front).
- Center cassette to projected CR.

Central Ray: CR 45° caudad, centered to exit through down-side EAM.

SID: 40–48" (102–122 cm)

Collimation: To ≈4" (10 cm) square field.

Alternate Owen modification: similar, with less obliquity and less CR angle.

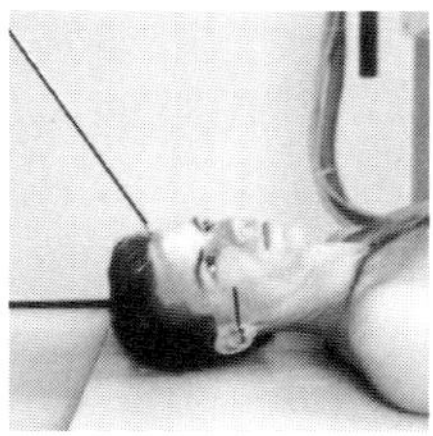

Owen modification
- 30–40° RPO
- 30–40° caudad

Respiration: Suspend during exposure.

Technique: kVp (80±5) _____

mrad

S	253	G NDC M
ML	64	NDC F

	cm	kVp	mA	Time	mAs	SID	Film–Screen	Grid	F.S.
Model	17	80			26	44"	Kodak 400	12:1	S
Room									
S									
M									
L									

Bontrager Textbook, 3rd ed., p. 408

Pediatric Skull – AP

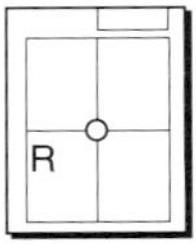

- 8 x 10" L.W. (20 x 24 cm) or 10 x 12" L.W. (24 x 30 cm)
- Grid

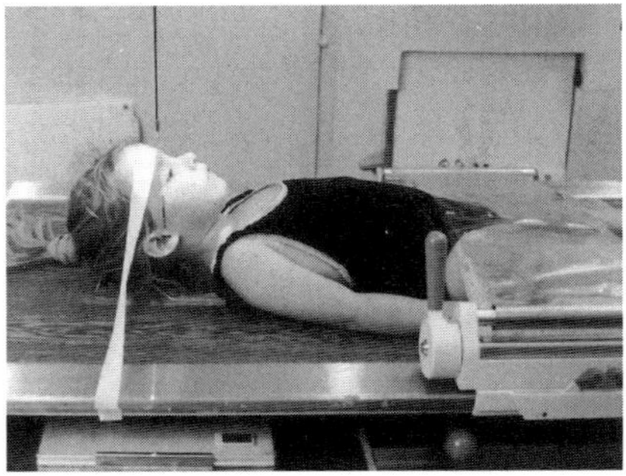

AP skull, CR 0°, OML ⊥

Position

- Patient supine, mummify or secure arms and legs with ace bandages and/or tape, sandbags or compression band.
- Immobilize head with head clamps or tape. (Tape should be twisted so adhesive side is not against skin.)
- Adjust chin as needed to place OML perpendicular to film; ensure no rotation.
- Center cassette to CR.

Central Ray: CR centered to glabella.
AP: CR 0° (perpendicular)
AP reverse Caldwell: CR 15° cephalad
AP axial Towne: CR 30° caudad

SID: 40–48" (102–122 cm)

Collimation: Four sides to skull margin.

Technique: kVp (65–70) _____

mrad		
S	127	G NDC M
ML	35	NDC F

	cm	kVp	mA	Time	mAs	SID	Film–Screen	Grid	F.S.
Model Room	16	70			20	44"	Kodak 400	12:1	S
S									
M									
L									

Bontrager Textbook, 3rd ed., p. 566

Pediatric Skull – Lateral

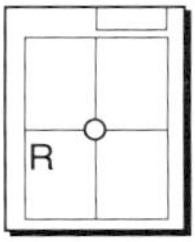

- 8 x 10" C.W. (20 x 24 cm) or 10 x 12" L.W. (24 x 30 cm)
- Grid

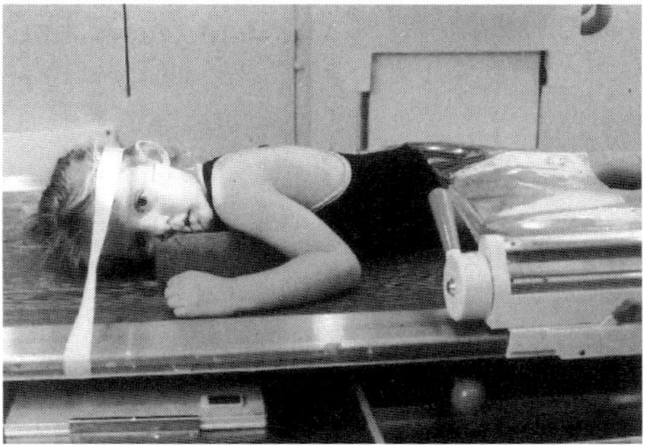

Lateral skull

Position

- Patient semi-prone, mummified or restrained as for AP skull.
- Turn head into true lateral position, place support under chin.
- Use sandbags, tape or compression band to maintain lateral position.
- Center cassette to CR (and to entire skull).

Note: May also be done as a cross table lateral if a board-type restraining device is used such as a "Tam-em Board".

Central Ray

- CR perpendicular, centered to mid skull (midway between glabella and occipital protuberance).

SID: 40–48" (102–122 cm)

Collimation: Four sides to skull margins.

Technique: kVp (65–70) _____

mrad			
	S	83	G NDC M
	ML	30	NDC F

	cm	kVp	mA	Time	mAs	SID	Film–Screen	Grid	F.S.
Model	13	70			14	44"	Kodak 400	12:1	S
Room									
S									
M									
L									

Bontrager Textbook, 3rd ed., p. 567

Skull

Position:

Central Ray:

SID:

Collimation:

Respiration:

Technique:

	Room	cm	kVp	mA	Time	mAs	SID	Film–Screen	Grid	F.S.
S										
M										
L										

Chapter 9

Abdomen and Common Contrast Media Procedures

Abdomen and Common Contrast Procedures

Prevention of Motion

Preventing motion, both voluntary and involuntary, is important in procedures involving the abdomen. **High kVp and mA** along with the **shortest exposure time possible** should be used on all radiographic procedures of the abdomen.

Breathing control can be achieved by asking the patient to hold their breath at the end of expiration, or by just asking the patient to stop breathing, to "hold their breath." To minimize involuntary motion from peristaltic activity, **allow one or two seconds after the patient is holding their breath before making exposure.**

Radiation Protection

Collimation

Accurate collimation is an important radiation protection practice in radiographic exams of the abdomen. For the average adult abdomen, lateral collimation borders should be to the abdominal lateral soft tissue margins. For adult full abdomen radiographs, top and bottom collimation borders should closely coincide with the film margins to not "cut off" essential anatomy and yet minimize patient exposure. (Remember the path of the divergent rays as they project onto the film.)

Gonadal Shielding

Male: Gonadal shields should be used on **all** males of reproductive age, with upper edge of shield placed at symphysis pubis.

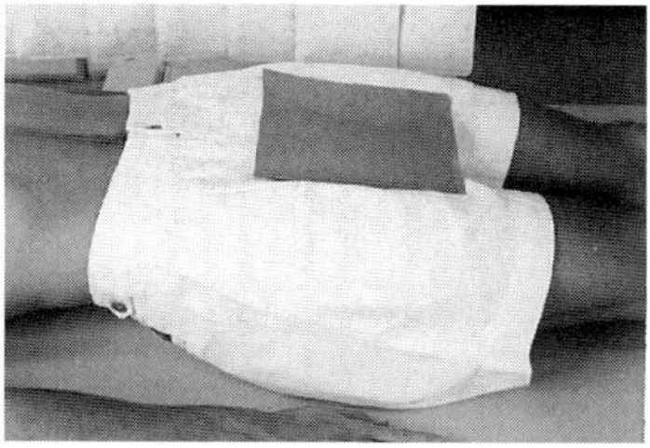

Male gonadal shield
(Top of shield at symphysis pubis)

Females: Ovarian gonadal shields placed correctly may be used for abdomen exams on females of reproductive age only **if** such shields do not cover essential anatomy for that exam as determined by a radiologist (shielding is especially important for children).

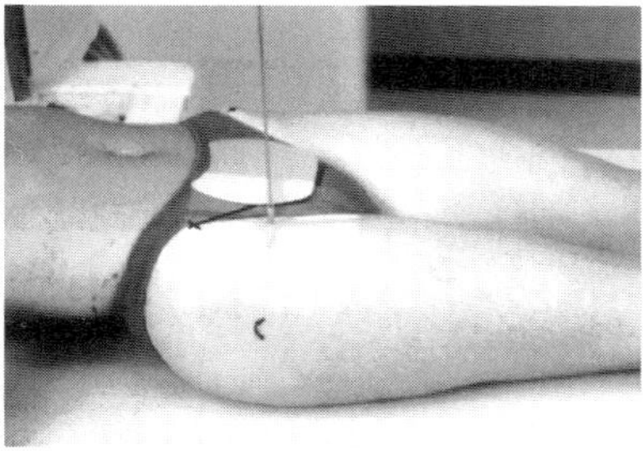

Female ovarian shield
(Top of shield at or slightly above the level of ASIS', lower border just above symphysis pubis)

Pregnancies

Generally no radiographic procedures exposing the pelvic region should be performed during pregnancy without special instruction from a radiologist, especially higher dose procedures such as any fluoroscopic exam of the abdominal or pelvic regions.

Topographical Positioning Landmarks[1,2]

Certain positioning landmarks are essential for positioning the general abdomen and specific organs within the abdomen since the borders of these organs and the upper and lower margins of the general abdomen itself are not visible from the exterior.

Abdominal borders and organ locations however, can be determined by certain landmarks which can be located by gentle palpation with the finger tips, being careful of painful or sensitive areas. (The patient should be informed of the purpose for this prior to beginning the palpation process.)

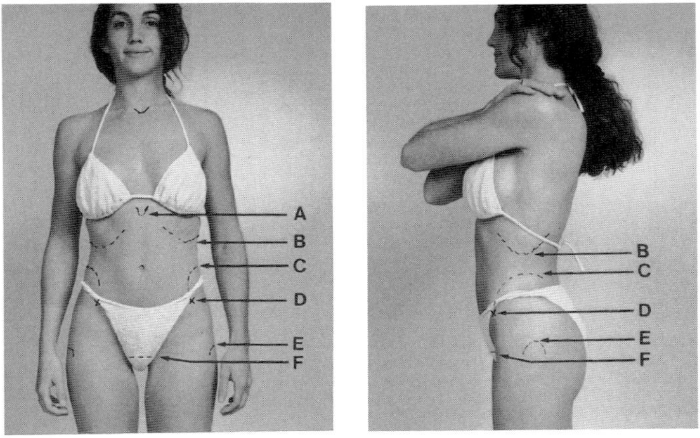

Positioning Landmarks

A. Xiphoid Process: (T9-10) Indicates the approximate level of the most superior, anterior portion of the diaphragm on expiration.

B. Inferior Costal (Rib) Margin: (L2-3) Used to determine the location of the gall bladder and/or other abdominal organs.

C. Iliac Crest: (L4-5) The uppermost curved border of the pelvis, which is the most commonly used abdominal landmark. This is the **approximate mid abdominal level.**

D. Anterior Superior Iliac Spine (ASIS): Easily palpated (on females) as the prominent anterior border of the iliac crest.

E. Greater Trochanter: More easily palpated on thin patients. Gentle but firm palpation is required to locate this landmark by feeling the movement of the trochanter while rotating the leg internally and externally. For most patients this level is just superior to the level of the symphysis pubis.

F. Symphysis Pubis: This is the **inferior margin of the abdomen.** Palpation of this area may be embarrassing for some patients, and with practice one can also determine this level by placing the iliac crest at the center of the film.

Body Habitus[3,4]

The four classes of body types within the general population are **hypersthenic, sthenic, hyposthenic** and **asthenic**. The hyposthenic and asthenic can be combined for purposes of organ locations because of general similarities as seen on these drawings. The location of certain organs within the abdomen such as the gallbladder, stomach, and large intestine change dramatically with the different body types. The gall bladder varies as much as 6" (15 cm) or more in location. Therefore each radiographer must learn to recognize these body types to be able to accurately position for procedures involving these organs.

Hypersthenic

Represents 5% of the most broad and very "stocky" population. The dome of the diaphragm is high with the ribs near horizontal. The upper abdomen is the widest part of the abdomen. The characteristic locations of abdominal organs are as follows:

Gall Bladder

High, transverse and to the right, well away from the midline.

- Level of T10-11 (≈1" or 2.5 cm caudal to xiphoid process)
- Approximately midway between midline and right lateral abdominal margin.

Stomach

High and more transverse in abdomen, in general is near midline of abdomen.

- Level of T9-12
- Center of stomach ≈1" (2.5 cm caudal to xiphoid process.

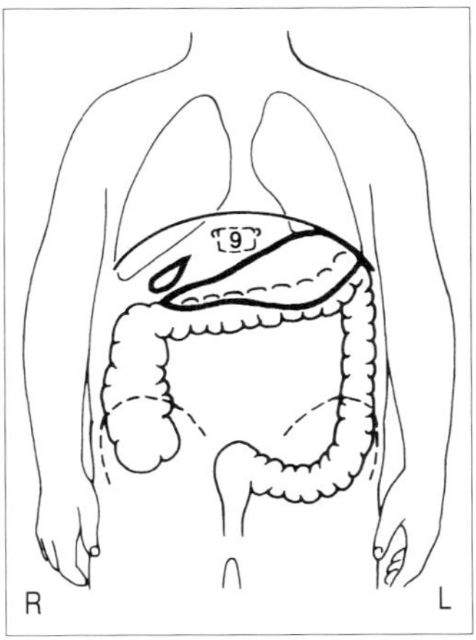

Hypersthenic (5%)

- Duodenal bulb at level of T11-12, to right of midline.

Large Intestine

Extends around periphery of abdominal cavity with transverse colon and left colic flexure located high in abdomen. (Requires 2 films placed crosswise to include entire large intestine.)

Sthenic

(Nearer average type.)

The sthenic (50%) are nearer the average non-slender and medium to slightly heavy set but not as broad in proportion to height as the hypersthenic.

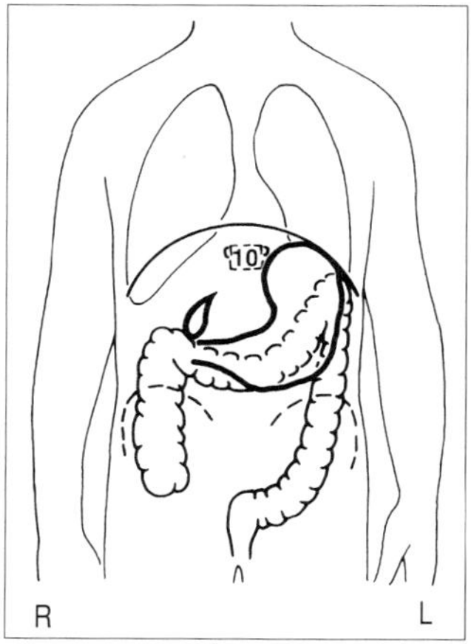

Sthenic (50%)

Gall Bladder

- Level of T12-L1, or approximately midway between xiphoid and lower rib margin.
- 2-3" (5-7 cm) caudal to xiphoid process and ≈2" (5 cm) to the right of the mid line.

Stomach

J-shaped and more vertical, and primarily to left of midline of abdomen.

- Level of T10 or 11 - L2.
- Approximately midway between midline and left lateral border of abdomen.
- Duodenal bulb at level of L1-2, near midline.

Large Intestine

Left colic flexure tends to be high in abdomen, with transverse colon lower to mid abdomen region.

These two types together represent about 45% of the more slender population with a long, narrow and shallow (anterior to posterior) thorax with ribs sloping more downward. The dome of the diaphragm is lower in the abdomen. The lower abdominal cavity is generally the widest part of the abdomen for the most asthenic type.

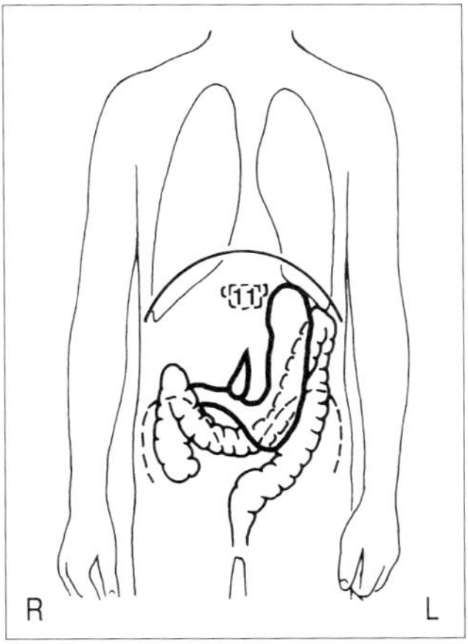

Hyposthenic (35%)/Asthenic (10%)

Gall Bladder

- Level of L3-4 (slightly above level of ilac crest).
- Near midline of abdomen (or only slightly to right).

Stomach

Elongated, vertical and low in abdomen.

- Level of T11 to L5 (extends from just below xiphoid tip to below level of ilac crest).
- Vertical portion is slightly to left of midline.
- Duodenal bulb is near midline at level of L3-4.

Large Intestine

Left colic flexure and transverse colon located lower in the abdomen.

Additional factors which affect abdominal organ location:

- Inspiration vs. expiration (primarily GB and upper stomach which move with diaphragm)
- Erect vs. recumbent position (all drop in erect position)
- Muscle tone due to age (older person's organs generally all drop farther in an erect position).
- Contents of organs (barium-filled drop more than air-filled).

Barium Distribution and Body Positions

The air-barium distribution within the stomach and large intestine changes with various body positions. By knowing these distribution patterns one can determine in which body position a radiograph was taken. Air always rises to the highest levels and the heavy barium settles to the lowest levels (air is black, barium is white).

Stomach

The fundus is located more posteriorly, therefore in the supine position it would be the lowest portion of the stomach and would be filled with barium.

In both the prone and erect positions the fundus would be filled with air as seen on the drawings below, with a straight air-barium line on the erect.

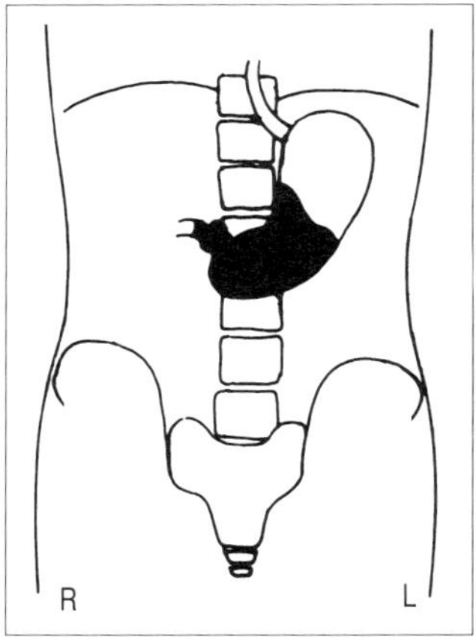

Supine (barium in fundus)

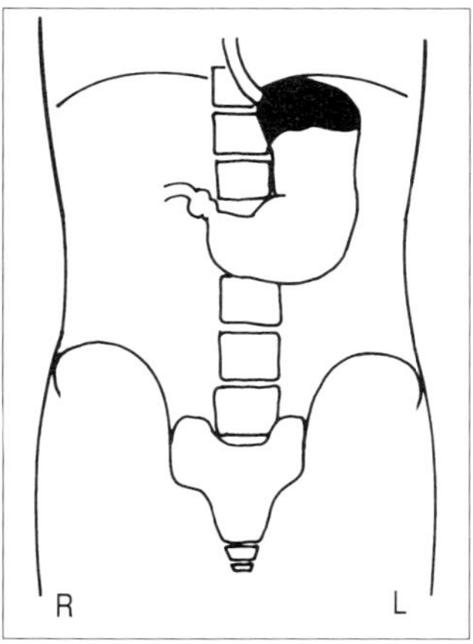

Prone
(Barium in body and pylorus)

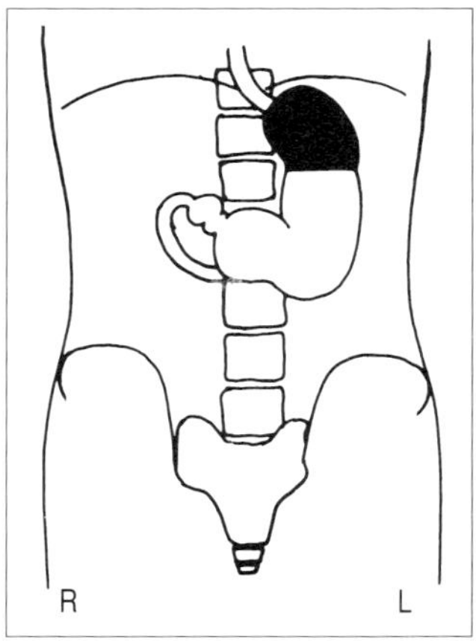

Erect
(Straight line barium-air level)

Barium = white   Air = black

Large Intestine

The ascending and descending portions are located more posteriorly and thus more of these parts would in general be filled with barium (white) in the **supine position,** and with air (black) in the **prone position.**

Note: This much separation of barium and air occurs generally only with double contrast barium-air studies.

Straight air-fluid levels would be seen in the **erect position**, and the air would rise to the highest position in each of the various sections of the large intestine as shown below.

Right and left decubitus projections (not shown on these drawings) would also demonstrate air-fluid levels with air again rising to highest portions.

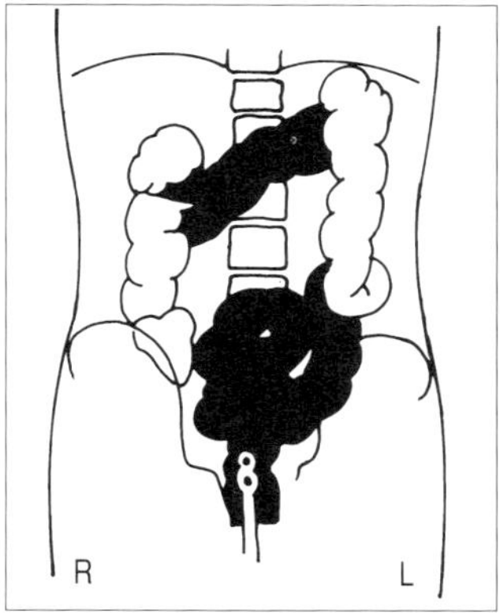

Supine

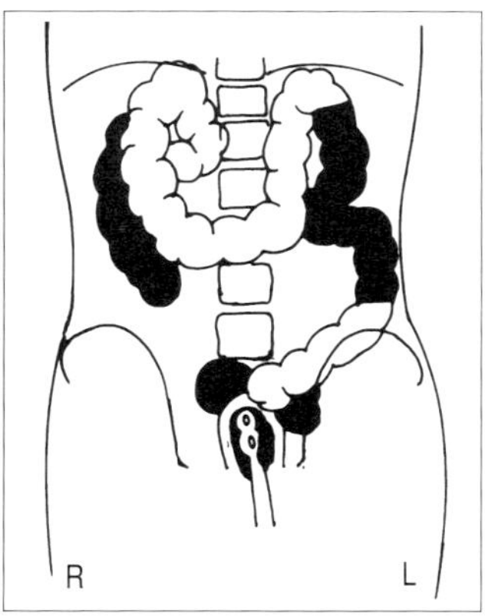

Prone

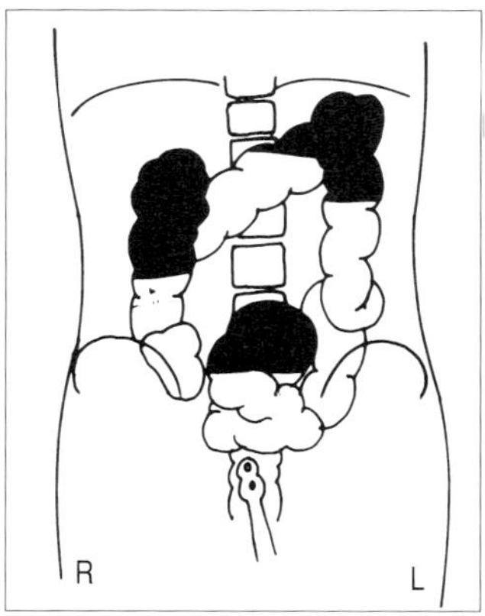

Erect

AP Abdomen (KUB)

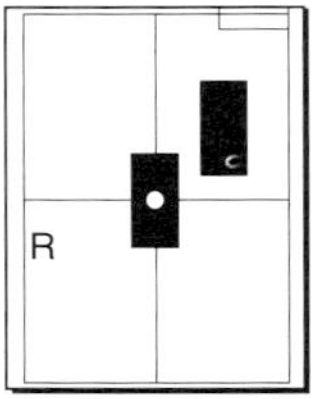

- 14 x 17" L.W. (35 x 43 cm)

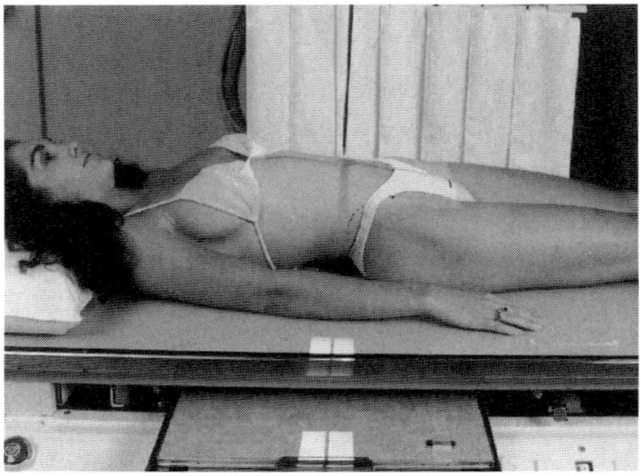

KUB abdomen

Position

- Supine, legs extended, arms at sides.
- Midsagittal plane aligned and centered to centerline.
- Ensure no rotation (ASIS' equal distance from table top).
- Center of cassette to level of iliac crests, ensuring that upper margin of symphysis pubis is included on lower film margin. (A large hypersthenic patient may require the film be placed crosswise with a second film centered higher.)

Central Ray

- CR ⊥, to center of cassette (level of iliac crests).

SID: 40–48" (102–122 cm)

Collimation: To abdomen and/or film borders.

Respiration: Expose at end of expiration.

Technique: kVp (80±5) _____

mrad

S	117	G	2 M
ML	27		26 F

	cm	kVp	mA	Time	mAs	SID	Film–Screen	Grid	F.S.
Model Room	17	75			15	44"	Kodak 400	12:1	S
S									
M									
L									

Bontrager Textbook, 3rd ed., p. 91

Erect AP Abdomen

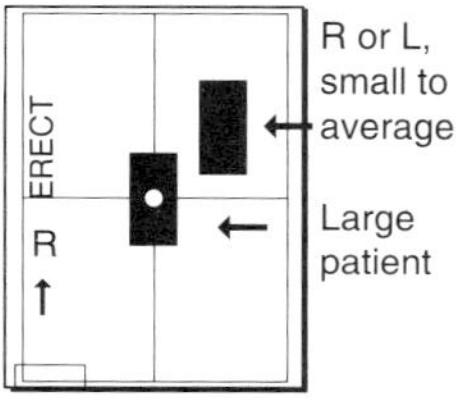

- 14 x 17" L.W. (35 x 43 cm)
- Grid
- Erect marker

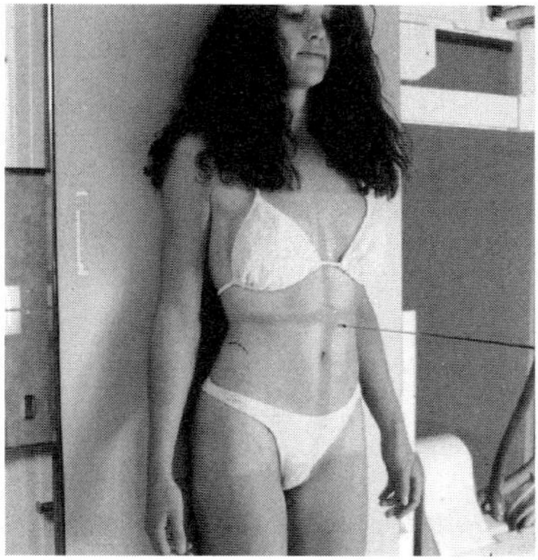
Erect AP (include diaphragm)

Position
- Erect, back against table, arms at sides.
- Midsagittal plane aligned and centered to centerline.
- Ensure no rotation.
- Center of cassette about 1-2" (3-5 cm) above iliac crest (top of film approximately at axilla to ensure that diaphragm is included).

Central Ray: CR horizontal, to center of cassette (1-2" or 3-5 cm above iliac crest).

SID: 40–48" (102–122 cm)

Collimation: To abdomen and/or film borders.

Respiration: Expose at end of expiration.

Technique: kVp (80±5) _____

mrad

S 139	G 3 M
ML 32	33 F

	cm	kVp	mA	Time	mAs	SID	Film–Screen	Grid	F.S.
Model Room	18	80			15	44"	Kodak 400	12:1	S
S									
M									
L									

Bontrager Textbook, 3rd ed., p. 94

Abdomen
Lateral Decubitus (AP)

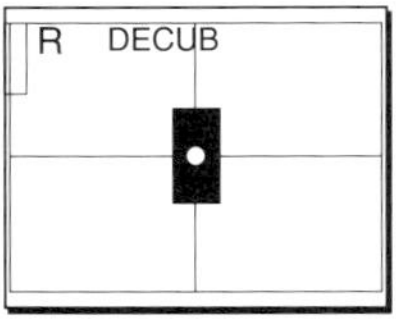

- 14 x 17" C.W. (35 x 43 cm)
- Grid
- Decub. marker

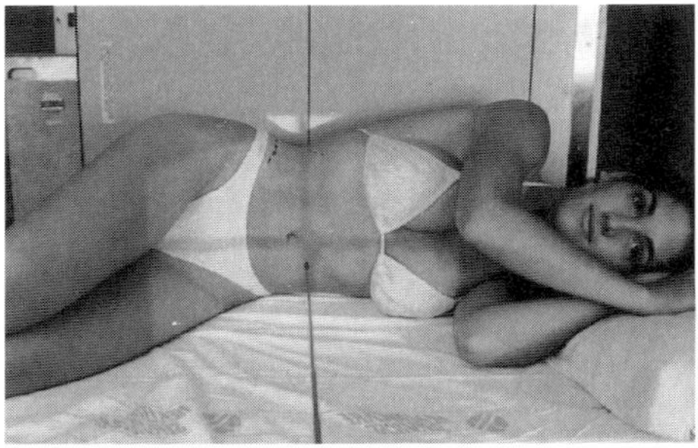

Left lateral decubitus (AP)

Position
- Lock wheels of stretcher.
- Patient on side, knees partially flexed, arms up near head.
- Adjust patient and stretcher so center of cassette and table (and CR) is 1–2" (3–5 cm) above level of iliac crest (to include diaphragm).
- Adjust height of cassette to ensure that "up-side" of abdomen is included on film for possible free air.

Central Ray
- CR horizontal, to center of cassette and table (1–2" or 3–5 cm above iliac crests).

SID: 40–48" (102–122 cm)

Collimation: Ensure that "up-side" is not cut off by collimation.

Respiration: Expose at end of expiration.

Technique: kVp (80±5) _____

mrad

S	126	G	2 M
ML	23		28 F

	cm	kVp	mA	Time	mAs	SID	Film–Screen	Grid	F.S.
Model Room	20	75			15	44"	Kodak 400	12:1	S
S									
M									
L									

Bontrager Textbook, 3rd ed., p. 93

Abdomen
Dorsal Decubitus (lateral)

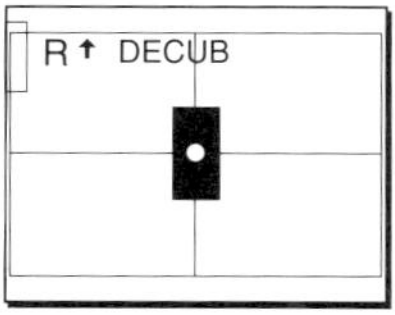

- 14 x 17" C.W. (35 x 43 cm)
- Grid
- Include decub marker

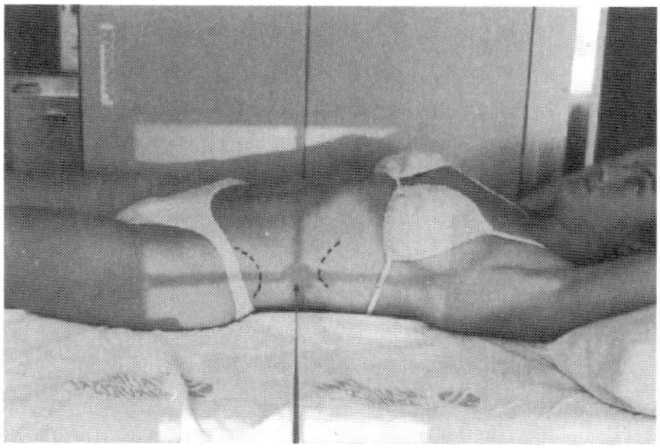

Dorsal decubitus (R lateral)

Position
- Patient supine, side against table, arms above head.
- Secure stretcher (lock wheels).
- Center of cassette and table (and CR) is 1– 2" (3–5 cm) above level of iliac crest (to include diaphragm).
- Adjust height of cassette to align midcoronal plane to centerline of cassette.

Central Ray
- CR horizontal, to center of cassette and table (1–2" or 3–5 cm above iliac crests at midcoronal plane).

SID: 40–48" (102–122 cm)

Collimation: To abdomen and/or film borders.

Respiration: Expose at end of expiration.

Technique: kVp (80±5) _____

mrad

S 279	G 1 M
ML 37	16 F

	cm	kVp	mA	Time	mAs	SID	Film–Screen	Grid	F.S.
Model Room	24	75			30	44"	Kodak 400	12:1	S
S									
M									
L									

Bontrager Textbook, 3rd ed., p.95

Abdomen

9

AP Pediatric Abdomen (KUB)

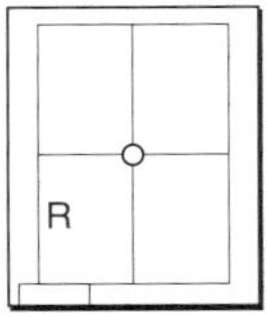

- 8 x 10", 10 x 12" or 11 x 14" L.W.
- Screen < 9–10 cm, Grid > 9–10 cm

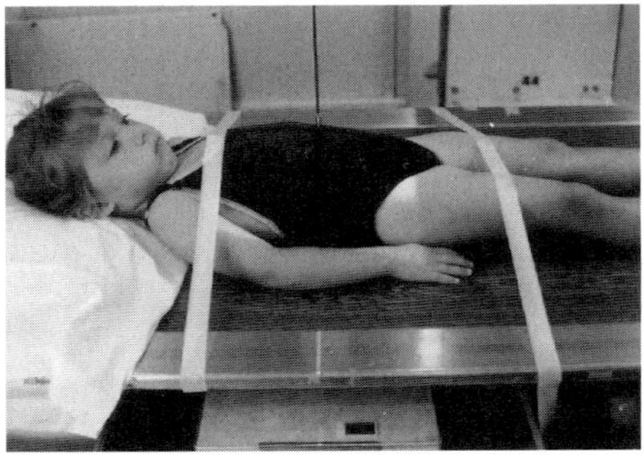

Child AP abdomen (KUB)

Position (Infant)
- Immobilize arms above head (use stockinette, ace bandage, tape or sandbags).
- Immobilize legs with ace bandage or tape and sandbags.
- Center cassette to CR.
- Shield gonads if possible.

Parental Assistance for infant: Use only if necessary. Supply with lead apron and gloves and have them hold arms above head with one hand and legs with other hand preventing rotation.

Central Ray
- Infants and young child: CR to 1" or 2.5 cm above umbilicus. Older child: CR to level of umbilicus.[5]

SID: 40–48" (102–122 cm)

Collimation: On four sides to abdominal borders.

Respiration: Expose on expiration or when abdomen has least movement. If crying, time exposures at full expiration.

Technique: kVp for screens (65±5) _____, or grid kVp (70±5) _____

	cm	kVp	mA	Time	mAs	SID	Film–Screen	Grid	F.S.
Model Room	11	66			10	44"	Kodak 400	12:1	S
S									
M									
L									

Bontrager Textbook, 3rd ed., p. 558

mrad

S 49	G 5 M
ML 20	20 F

AP Erect Pediatric Abdomen

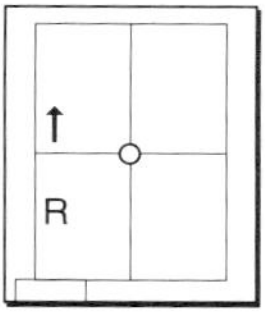

- 8 x 10", 10 x 12" or 11 x 14"
- Screen < 9–10 cm
  Grid > 9–10 cm

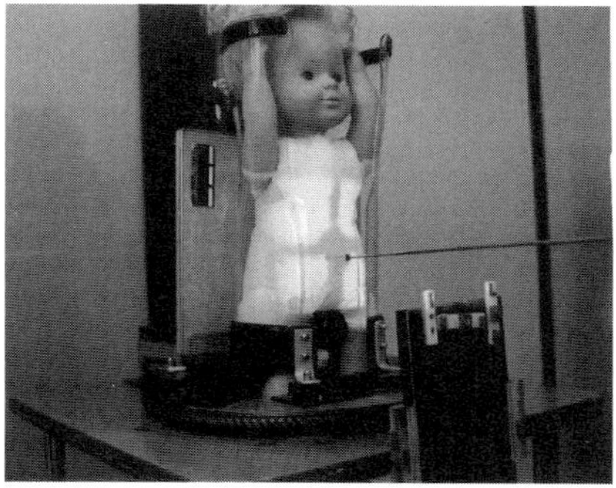

Utilizing Pigg-O-Stat

Position

- Patient seated, legs through openings.
- Arms above head, side body clamps firmly in place.
- Lead shield at level of symphysis pubis.
- Center cassette to CR

Parental Assistance: If necessary, have parent hold arms overhead with one hand, and with other hand hold legs to prevent rotation of pelvis or thorax (provide with lead apron and gloves).

Central Ray

- Infants and young child: CR to 1" (2.5 cm) above umbilicus. Older child: CR to level of umbilicus.[6]

SID: 40–48" (102–122 cm)

Collimation: On four sides to abdominal borders.

Respiration: Expose on expiration, or during least movement.

Technique: kVp for screens (65±5) _____, or grid kVp (70±5) _____

	cm	kVp	mA	Time	mAs	SID	Film–Screen	Grid	F.S.
Model Room	9	66			4	44"	Kodak 400	–	S
S									
M									
L									

Bontrager Textbook, 3rd ed., p. 559

mrad

S	16	G	2 M
ML	8		8 F

Abdomen

9

Esophagram – RAO

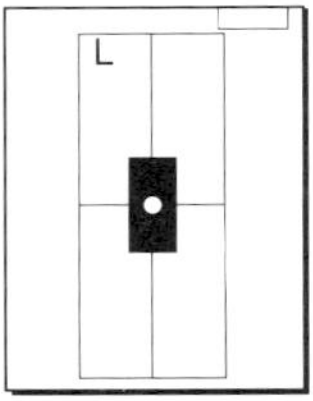

- 14 x 17" L.W. (35 x 43 cm)
- Grid

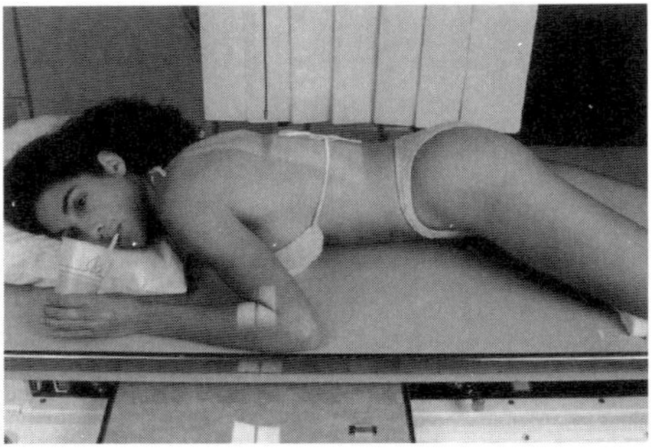

35–40° RAO for esophagus (barium swallow)

Position

- Recumbent or erect, recumbent preferred for better filling of esophagus.
- Rotate 35–40° from prone position onto right side, right arm down, left arm up, hold cup with left hand, straw in mouth.
- Center obliqued thorax to centerline.
- Top of cassette ≈2" (5 cm) above level of shoulder.

Central Ray: CR ⊥, to center of cassette (≈3" or 7 cm) distal to jugular notch (T6)).

SID: 40–48" (102–122 cm)

Collimation: To area of interest (≈5–6" [12–15 cm] wide).

Respiration: With thin barium, expose while swallowing (after 3 or 4 swallows). With thick barium, expose immediately after swallowing (while holding breath).

Technique: kVp (100–115) _____

mrad		
	S 60	G <0.01 M
	ML 14	0.1 F

	cm	kVp	mA	Time	mAs	SID	Film–Screen	Grid	F.S.
Model	22	110			3	44"	Kodak 400	12:1	L
Room									
S									
M									
L									

Bontrager Textbook, 3rd ed., p. 440

Esophagram – Lateral

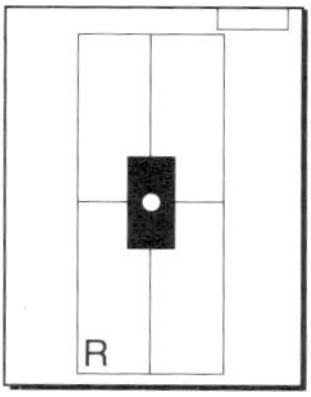

• 14 x 17" L.W. (35 x 43 cm)
• Grid

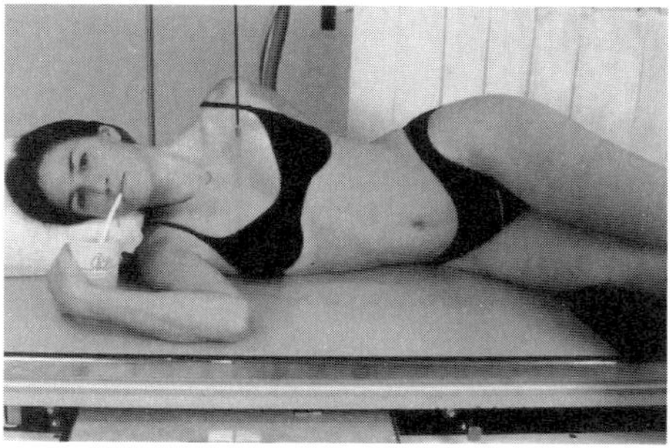

R lat. esophagram (barium swallow) in "swimmer's" position

Position

- Recumbent or erect, recumbent preferred.
- Right lateral position, right arm and shoulder up and forward (holding cup), left arm and shoulder down and back.
- Center midcoronal plane to centerline.
- Top of cassette ≈2" (5 cm) above top of shoulder.

Central Ray: CR ⊥, to center of film (≈3" (7 cm) distal to jugular notch (T6)).

SID: 40–48" (102–122 cm)

Collimation: To area of interest (5–6" [12–15 cm] wide).

Respiration: With thin barium expose while swallowing (after 3 or 4 swallows). With thick barium expose immediately after swallowing, while holding breath.

Technique: kVp (110–125) _____

mrad

S 87	G <0.01 M
ML 17	0.1 F

	cm	kVp	mA	Time	mAs	SID	Film–Screen	Grid	F.S.
Model Room	25	110			4	44"	Kodak 400	12:1	L
S									
M									
L									

Bontrager Textbook, 3rd ed., p.436

Esophagram – AP (PA)

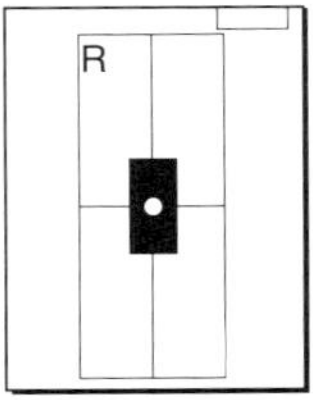

• 14 x 17" L.W.
(35 x 43 cm)
• Grid

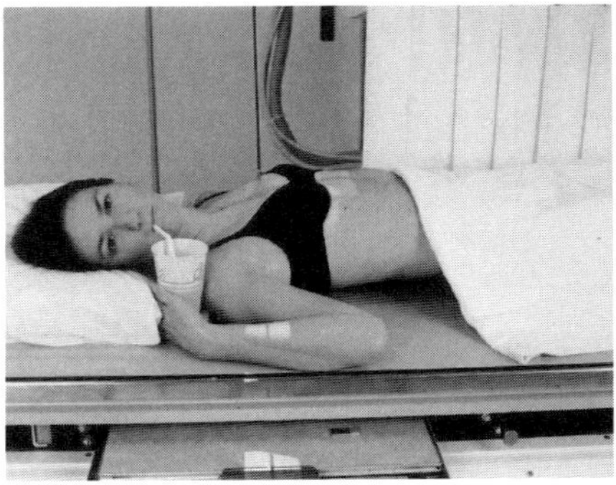

AP barium swallow

Position

• Supine or erect, supine preferred (may be taken PA if erect).
• Center patient to centerline.
• Top of film ≈2" (5 cm) above top of shoulder.
• Left arm at side, holding cup with right hand, straw in mouth.

Central Ray

• CR ⊥, to center of film (≈3" (7 cm) distal to jugular notch (T6).

SID: 40–48" (102–122 cm)

Collimation: To area of interest (5–6" [12–15 cm] wide).

Respiration: With thin barium expose while swallowing (after 3 or 4 swallows). With thick barium expose immediately after swallowing, while holding breath.

Technique: kVp (100–115) _____

mrad

S	51	G <0.01 M
ML	19	0.1 F

	cm	kVp	mA	Time	mAs	SID	Film–Screen	Grid	F.S.
Model	15	110			3	44"	Kodak 400	12:1	L
Room									
S									
M									
L									

Bontrager Textbook, 3rd ed., p.437

Upper GI – PA

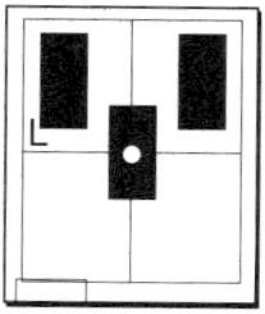

- 11 x 14" L.W. (or C.W.) (30 x 35 cm) or 10 x 12" (24 x 30 cm)
- Grid

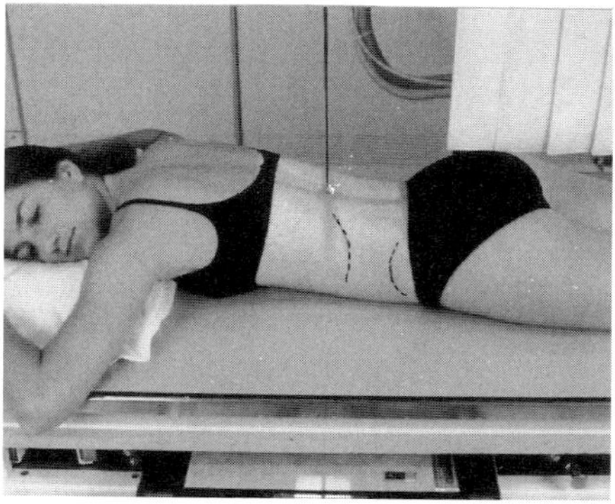

PA upper GI (stomach)

Position

- Prone, arms up beside head.
- Align and center patient and cassette to CR.

Central Ray

- CR ⊥, centered to pylorus and lesser curvature.

Average: Center ≈1" (2.5 cm) above lower rib margin and ≈1" (2.5 cm) to left of vertebral column.

Hypersthenic: Center 1–2" (3–5 cm) higher, film C.W.

Asthenic: Center ≈2" (5 cm) lower and nearer midline.

SID: 40–48" (102–122 cm)

Collimation: To outer margins of cassette.

Respiration: Expose at end of full expiration.

Technique: kVp (110–125) _____(80–95 for double contrast) ___

	cm	kVp	mA	Time	mAs	SID	Film–Screen	Grid	F.S.
Model Room	15	125			4	44"	Kodak 400	12:1	L
S									
M									
L									

Bontrager Textbook, 3rd ed., p. 441

mrad

S 88	G 0.1 M	
ML 30	7 F	

Upper GI – RAO

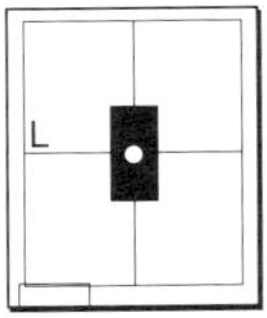

- 11 x 14" L.W. (or C.W.)
  (30 x 35 cm)
  or
  10 x 12" (24 x 30 cm)
- Grid

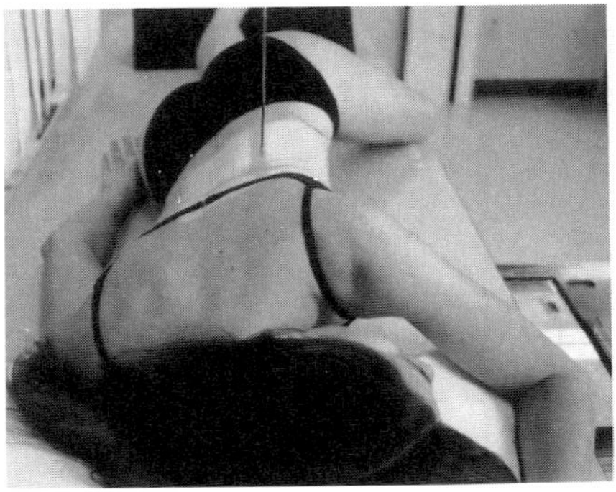

40–70° RAO, upper GI (stomach)

Position
- Semi-prone, rotate 40–70° from prone toward right side.
- Right arm down, left arm up, partially flex left hip and knee.
- Align and center patient to CR.

Central Ray: CR ⊥, to duodenal bulb region.

Average: Center ≈1" (2.5 cm) above lower ribs and midway between vertebrae and left lateral abdominal border, 45–55° oblique from prone.

Hypersthenic: Center 1–2" (3–5 cm) higher, ≈70° oblique.

Asthenic: Center ≈2″ (5 cm) lower, ≈40° oblique.

SID: 40–48" (102–122 cm)

Collimation: To outer margins of cassette.

Respiration: Expose at end of full expiration.

Technique: kVp (110–125) _____ (80–95 for double contrast) ___

	cm	kVp	mA	Time	mAs	SID	Film–Screen	Grid	F.S.
Model Room	17	125			5	44"	Kodak 400	12:1	L
S									
M									
L									

Bontrager Textbook, 3rd ed., p. 440

mrad

S 115	G 0.1 M	
ML 40	9 F	

Upper GI – Lateral

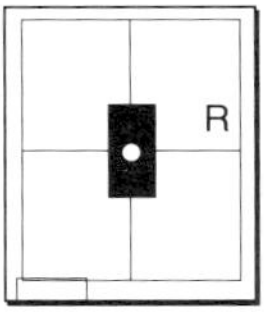

- 11 x 14" L.W. (or C.W.)
  (30 x 35 cm)
  or
  10 x 12" (24 x 30 cm)
- Grid

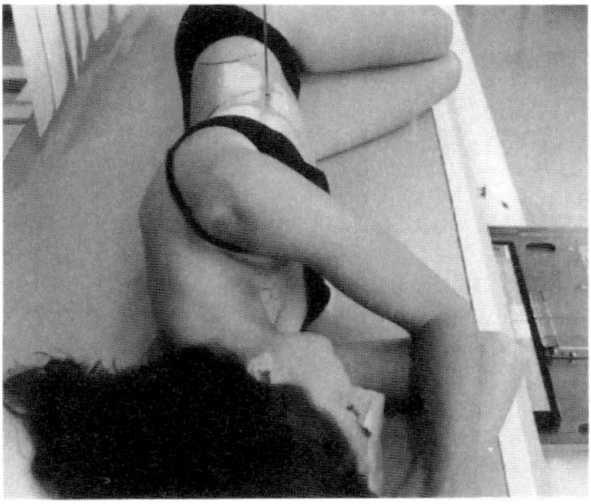

Right lateral upper GI (stomach)

Position

- Patient on right side, arms up, hips and knees partially flexed.
- Align and center patient and cassette to CR.

Central Ray

- CR ⊥, to region of pylorus.
  Average: Center to midway between xiphoid tip and lower ribs, and to anterior 1/3 of abdomen.
  Hypersthenic: Center ≈1" (2.5 cm) higher.
  Asthenic: Center ≈2" (5 cm) lower.

SID: 40–48" (102–122 cm)

Collimation: To outer margins of cassette.

Respiration: Expose at end of full expiration.

Technique: kVp (110–125) ____ (80–95 for double contrast)___

	cm	kVp	mA	Time	mAs	SID	Film–Screen	Grid	F.S.
Model	27	125			7	44"	Kodak 400	12:1	L
Room									
S									
M									
L									

Bontrager Textbook, 3rd ed., p. 442

mrad

S 207	G 0.1 M
ML 37	16 F

Upper GI – AP

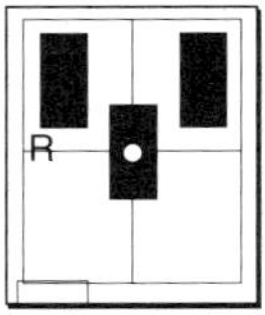

- 11 x 14" L.W. (or C.W.)
  (30 x 35 cm)
  or
  10 x 12" (24 x 30 cm)
- Grid

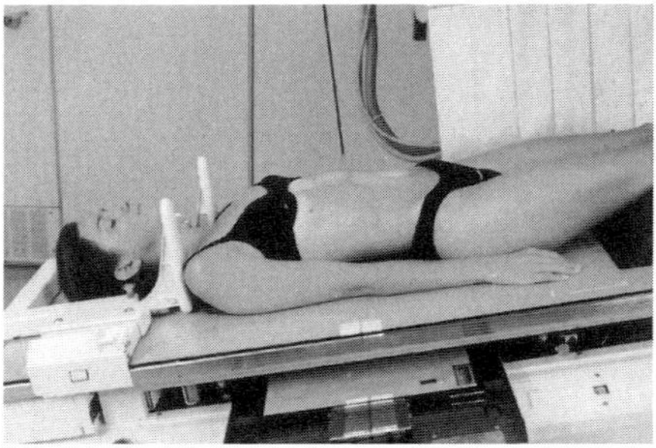

AP supine Trendelenburg, upper GI (stomach) (Trendelenburg position best demonstrates hiatal hernia)

Position

- Supine, arms at side.
- Align and center patient and cassette to CR.

Central Ray

- CR ⊥, centered to 1–2" (2.5 – 5 cm) to left of MSP.

Average: Center to level of L1 (midway between xiphoid tip and level of lower lateral ribs).

Hypersthenic: Center ≈1" (2.5 cm) higher, 11 x 14 C.W.

Asthenic: Center ≈2" (5 cm) lower, 11 x 14 L.W.

SID: 40–48" (102–122 cm)

Collimation: To outer film margins.

Respiration: Expose at end of full expiration.

Technique: kVp (110–125) ____ (80–95 for double contrast) ___

	cm	kVp	mA	Time	mAs	SID	Film–Screen	Grid	F.S.
Model	18	125			5	44"	Kodak 400	12:1	L
Room									
S									
M									
L									

Bontrager Textbook, 3rd ed., p. 444

mrad		
	S 118	G 0.1 M
	ML 38	8 F

Upper GI – LPO

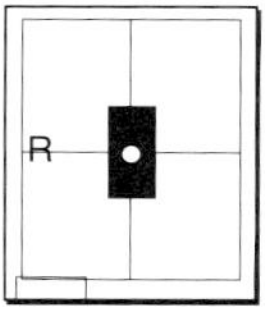

- 11 x 14" L.W. (or C.W.) (30 x 35 cm)
  or
  10 x 12" (24 x 30 cm)
- Grid

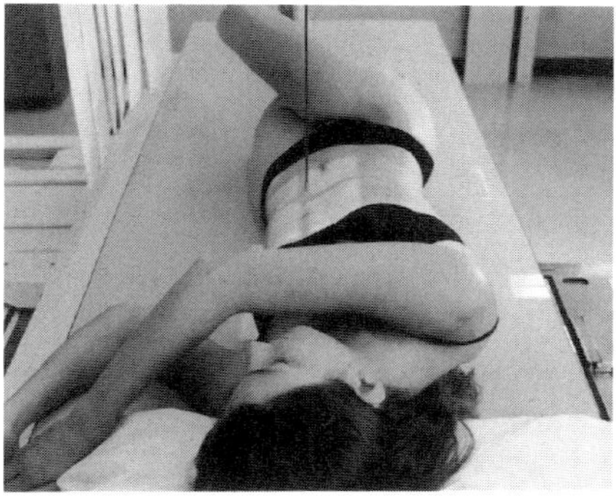

30-60° LPO, upper GI (stomach)

Position

- Semi-supine, 30–60° obli., left side down, partially flex right knee.
- Center patient and cassette to CR.

Central Ray

- CR ⊥, centered to left half of abdomen.

Average: Center to L1 (midway between xiphoid tip and level of lower lateral ribs), 45° oblique.

Hypersthenic: Center 1" (2.5 cm) higher, film C.W., 60° obli.

Asthenic: ≈2" (5 cm) lower and nearer midline, film L.W., 30°.

SID: 40–48" (102–122 cm)

Collimation: To outer film margins.

Respiration: Expose at end of full expiration.

Technique: kVp (110–125) ____ (80–95 for double contrast) ___

	cm	kVp	mA	Time	mAs	SID	Film–Screen	Grid	F.S.
Model Room	19	125			5	44"	Kodak 400	12:1	L
S									
M									
L									

Bontrager Textbook, 3rd ed., p. 443

mrad

S 121	G 0.2 M
ML 37	9 F

Small Bowel Series - PA

A common routine includes films at 15 or 30 minute intervals until barium reaches ileocecal valve.

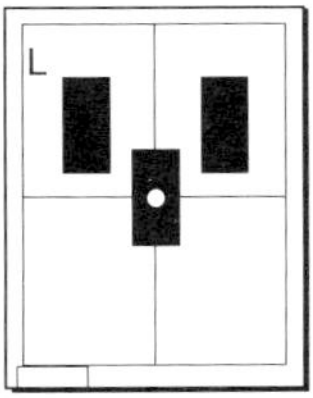

- 14 x 17" L.W. (35 x 43 cm)
- Grid

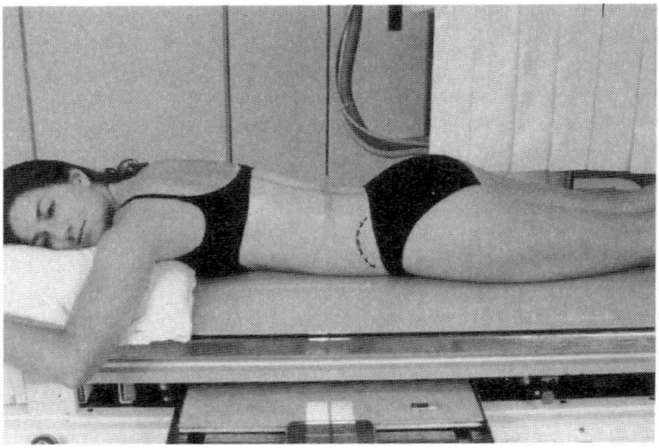

PA small bowel (15 or 30 min.)

Position

- Prone preferred (may be taken AP supine if necessary).
- MSP aligned to centerline, no rotation.
- Center patient and cassette to iliac crest (center higher on early films).

Central Ray: CR ⊥, to center of cassette, ≈**2" (5 cm) above level of iliac crest for early films** (15 or 30 min.), and **at iliac crest for later films**.

SID: 40–48" (102–122 cm)

Collimation: To outer margins of cassette.

Respiration: Expose at end of full expiration.

Technique: kVp (110–125) _____

mrad		
	S 91	G 0.1 M
	ML 26	26 F

	cm	kVp	mA	Time	mAs	SID	Film–Screen	Grid	F.S.
Model Room	16	125			4	44"	Kodak 400	12:1	L
S									
M									
L									

Bontrager Textbook, 3rd ed., p. 470

Barium Enema - PA or AP

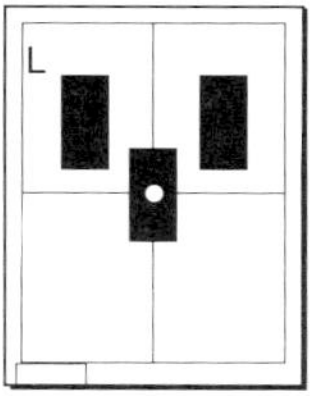

- 14 x 17" L.W. (35 x 43 cm)
- Grid

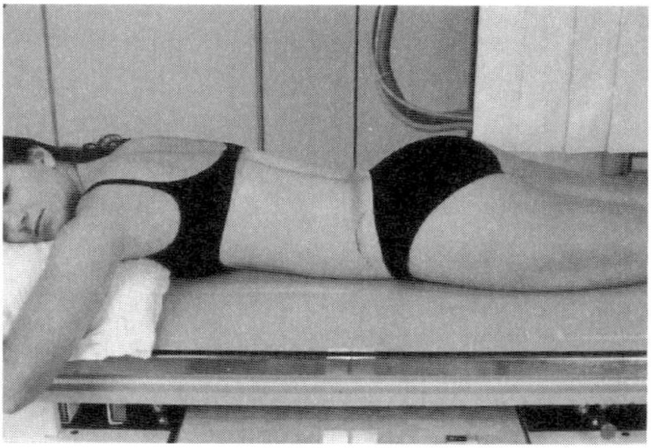

PA barium enema

Position

- Patient prone (PA) or supine (AP); work quickly.
- Patient aligned and centered to centerline, no rotation.
- Center cassette to level of iliac crest (see note).

Central Ray

- CR ⊥, to center of cassette, at level of iliac crest.

Note: For large or hypersthenic patients, the use of two films may be necessary, placed crosswise if the entire colon is to be included (one centered for lower abdomen and one for upper abdomen).

SID: 40–48" (102–122 cm)

Collimation: To outer film borders.

Respiration: Expose at full expiration.

mrad			
S	68	G	16 M
ML	20		20 F

Technique: kVp (110–125) ____ (80–95 for double contrast)___

	cm	kVp	mA	Time	mAs	SID	Film–Screen	Grid	F.S.
Model Room	16	125			3	44"	Kodak 400	12:1	L
S									
M									
L									

Bontrager Textbook, 3rd ed., p. 472

Barium Enema - RAO and LAO
(or RPO and LPO)

Both right and left obliques are commonly taken.

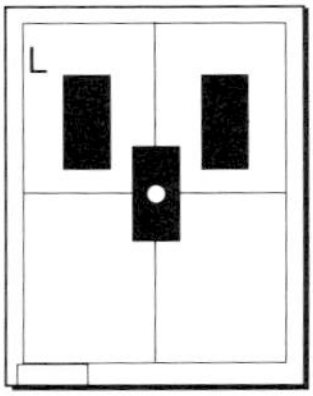

- 14 x 17" L.W. (35 x 43 cm)
- Grid

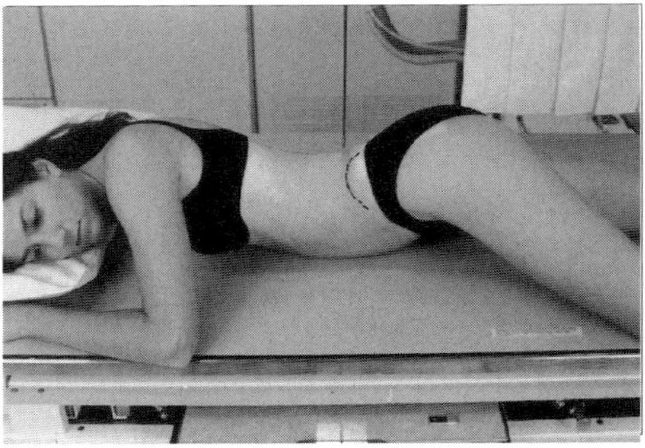

35–45° RAO barium enema

Position

- Semi-prone (PA) or semi-supine (AP), rotated 35–45°.
- Align and center abdomen to centerline.
- Cassette centered to level of iliac crest (include rectal area).

Central Ray: CR ⊥ to center of cassette (at level of iliac crest).

Note: Many patients require a second film centered ≈2" (5 cm) higher if the left colic flexure is to be included – most important on **LAO** or **RPO** (determine departmental routine).

SID: 40–48" (102–122 cm)

Collimation: To outer film borders.

Respiration: Expose at expiration.

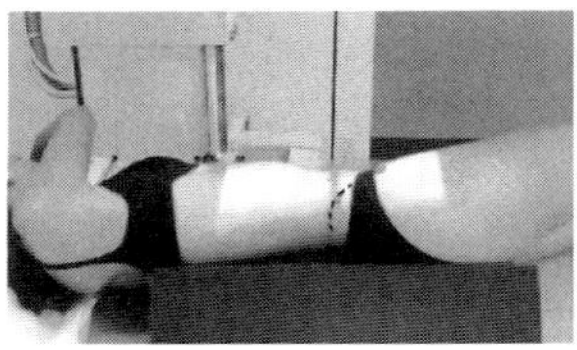

35–45° LPO

Technique: kVp (110–125)____(80–95 for double contrast)____

	cm	kVp	mA	Time	mAs	SID	Film–Screen	Grid	F.S.
Model Room	20	125			4	44"	Kodak 400	12:1	L
S									
M									
L									

Bontrager Textbook, 3rd ed., pp. 476-477

mrad

S	100	G 4 M
ML	22	38 F

Barium Enema – Lateral Rectum

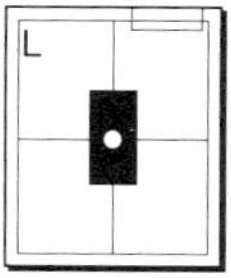

- 10 x 12" L.W. (24 x 30 cm) or 11 x 14" L.W. (30 x 35 cm)
- Grid

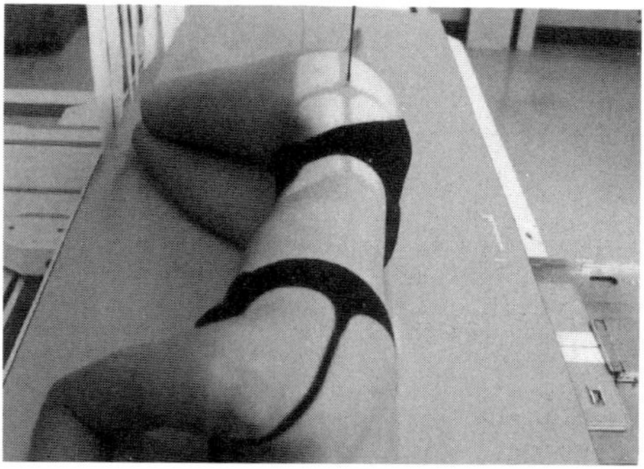

Left lateral for rectum

Position

- Recumbent in true lateral position, work quickly.
- Center midaxillary plane to centerline, knees and hips partially flexed.
- Center patient and cassette to CR.

Central Ray: CR ⊥, to ≈1" (2.5 cm) distal to level of ASIS, centered to midaxillary plane (midway between ASIS and posterior sacrum).

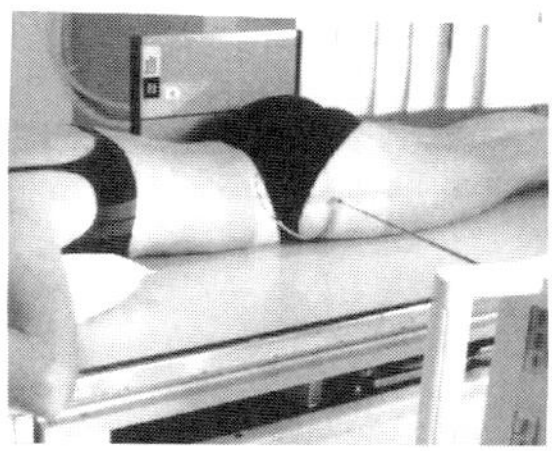

Ventral decub lat. rectum (Alternate projection with double contrast exam)

SID: 40–48" (102–122 cm)

Collimation: To outer film borders.

Respiration: Expose at full expiration.

mrad

S 2054	G 19 M
ML 241	275 F

Technique: kVp (110–125) _____ (single and double contrast)

	cm	kVp	mA	Time	mAs	SID	Film–Screen	Grid	F.S.
Model Room	30	125			64	44"	Kodak 400	12:1	L
S									
M									
L									

Bontrager Textbook, 3rd ed., p.473

Barium Enema – Lateral Decub.

Both right and left lateral decubitus are commonly taken as part of a double-contrast series.

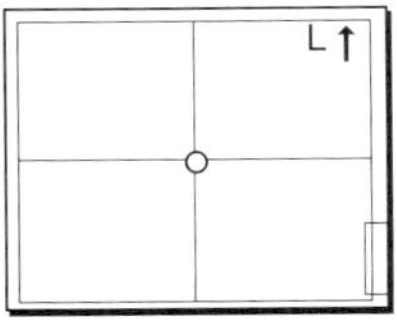

- 14 x 17" L.W. to patient (35 x 43 cm)
- Grid (portable grid or Bucky)

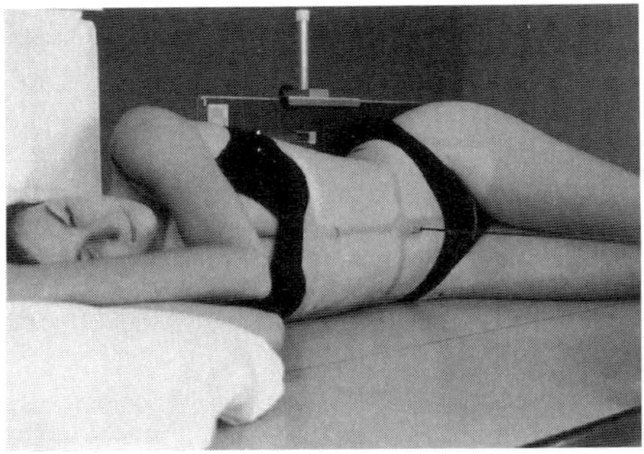

Right lateral decubitus (AP)

Position

- Patient on side, arms up, knees partially flexed, back against grid cassette or table.
- MSP aligned and centered to centerline of cassette (and CR), no rotation. (Lock wheels if stretcher is used.)
- Cassette centered to level of iliac crest.

Central Ray: CR horizontal to center of cassette (to level of iliac crest at mid-sagittal plane).

SID: 40–48" (102–122 cm)

Collimation: To outer film borders.

Respiration: Expose at full expiration.

Technique: kVp (80–100) _____(+20–30 kVp for single contrast)

	cm	kVp	mA	Time	mAs	SID	Film–Screen	Grid	F.S.
Model	17	90			6	44"	Kodak 400	12:1	L
Room									
S									
M									
L									

Bontrager Textbook, 3rd ed., p. 475

mrad

S 59	G	1 M
ML 13		16 F

Barium Enema – AP (PA) Axial (Butterfly position)

*Special views of rectosigmoid: A 30–40° left posterior oblique may result in less superimposition of bowel segments than a straight AP or PA.

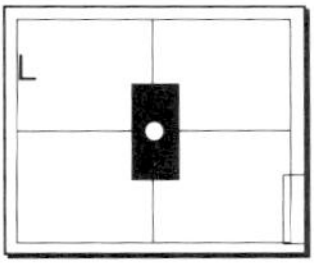

- 11 x 14" C.W. (30 x 35 cm) or 10 x 12" C.W. (24 x 30 cm)
- Grid

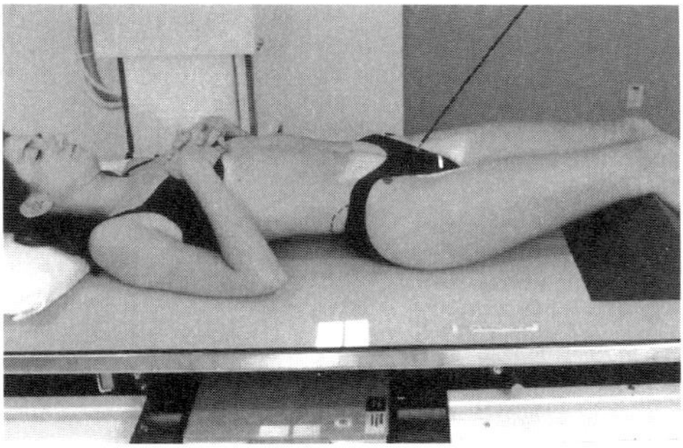

AP, CR 30–45° cephalad

Position

Supine (AP) or **prone (PA)**, patient aligned and centered to centerline.

***Alternate oblique –** LPO or RAO: Oblique patient 30–40°.

Central Ray: CR 30-45° cephalad for AP; 30–45° caudad for PA (30–35° for heavy to average; 40–45° for slender to asthenic).

AP: CR to 2" (5 cm) inferior to ASIS'.

PA: CR to enter at level of ASIS'.

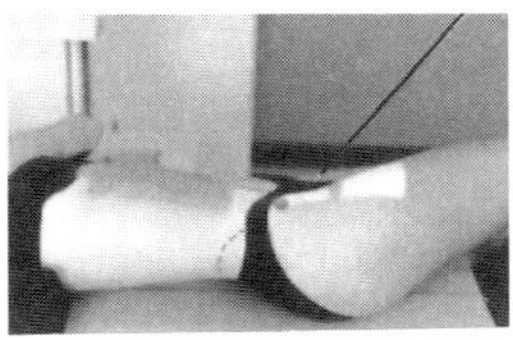

*35° LP0 axial - CR 30–45° cephalad

SID: 40–48" (102–122 cm)

Collimation: To outer film borders.

Respiration: Expose at full expiration.

Technique: kVp (110–125) ____ (90–100 for double contrast)___

	cm	kVp	mA	Time	mAs	SID	Film–Screen	Grid	F.S.
Model Room	16	125			6	44"	Kodak 400	12:1	L
S									
M									
L									

Bontrager Textbook, 3rd ed., p. 479

mrad

S	135	G	5 M
ML	41		51 F

Barium Enema

9

Barium Enema – PA Post-Evac

Take only after sufficient time has been allowed for evacuation

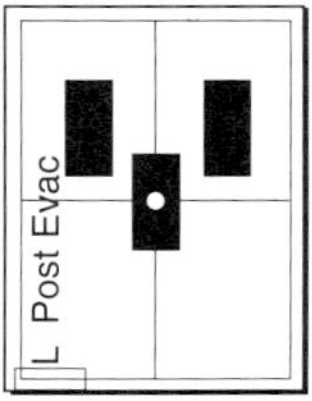

- 14 x 17" L.W. (35 x 43 cm)
- Grid
- Post-evac marker included on film

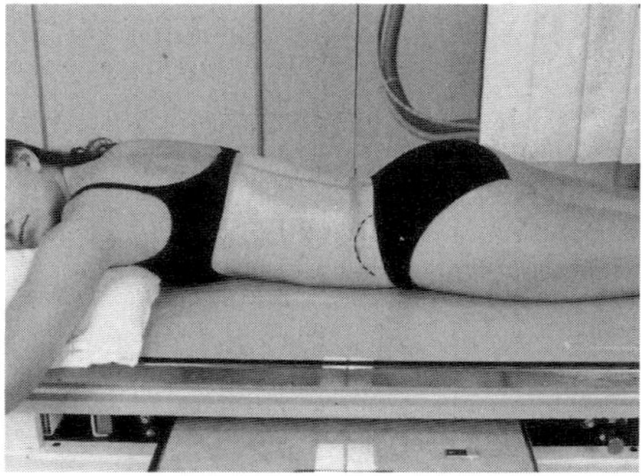

PA post-evac

Position

- Patient prone (PA), may also be taken supine (AP) if necessary
- Patient aligned and centered to centerline, no rotation.
- Cassette centered to level of iliac crest.

Central Ray

- CR ⊥, to center of casette (to level of iliac crest, at MSP).

SID: 40–48" (102–122 cm)

Collimation: To outer film borders.

Respiration: Expose at end of full expiration.

Technique: kVp (90–100) _____

mrad

S	58	G	9 M
ML	15		14 F

	cm	kVp	mA	Time	mAs	SID	Film–Screen	Grid	F.S.
Model Room	16	100			4	44"	Kodak 400	12:1	L
S									
M									
L									

Bontrager Textbook, 3rd ed., p. 478

Gall Bladder – PA Scout

Some routines include a full 14 x 17" KUB for a gall bladder scout.

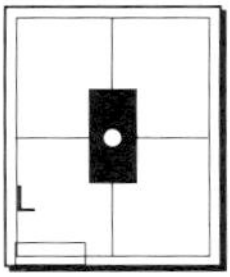

- 10 x 12" L.W. (24 x 30 cm)
- Grid

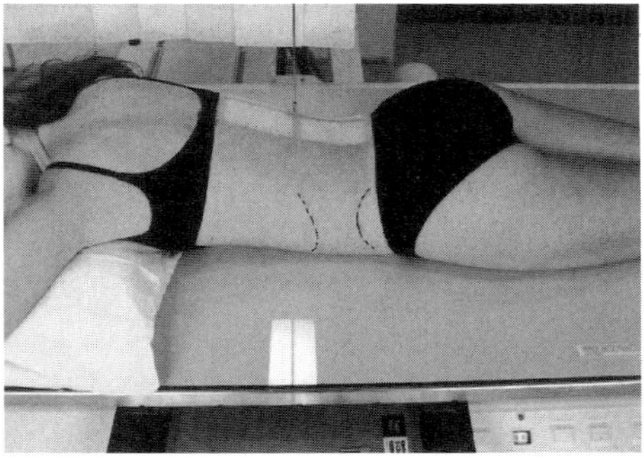

PA scout gall bladder

Position

- Prone, arms up beside head, no rotation.
- For smaller film, align and center right half of patient to CR (for large film, center at iliac crest as for a KUB).
- Center patient and cassette to CR.

Central Ray: CR ⊥ to film.

Average: Center to level of L2 (slightly above level of lowest lateral ribs) to mid right abdomen.

Hypersthenic: Center ≈1" (2.5 cm) higher and more lateral.

Asthenic: Center ≈2-3" (5-7 cm) lower and nearer midline.

Note: Mark location of GB on patient for follow-up films.

SID: 40–48" (102–122 cm)

Collimation: To outer margins of cassette.

Respiration: Expose at end of full expiration.

Technique: kVp (75±5) _____

mrad

S 140	G <0.1 M
ML 37	5 F

	cm	kVp	mA	Time	mAs	SID	Film–Screen	Grid	F.S.
Model Room	16	70			22	44"	Kodak 400	12:1	S
S									
M									
L									

Bontrager Textbook, 3rd ed., p. 498

Gall Bladder – LAO (or RPO)

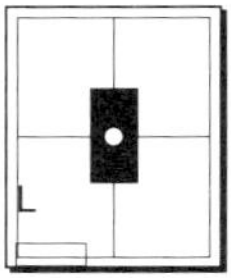

- 10 x 12" L.W. (24 x 30 cm) or 8 x 10" L.W. (20 x 24 cm)
- Grid

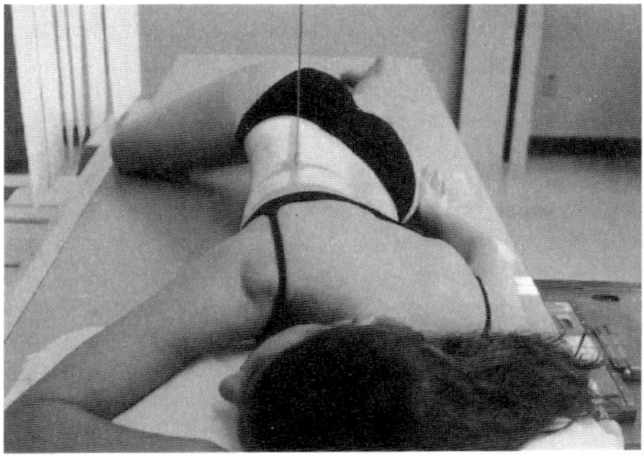

15–40° LAO gall bladder
More obliquity (30-40°) on thin asthenic patient, less (15-20°) on broad hypersthenic type

Position

- Semi-prone, left side down, flex right knee and elbow for support (degrees of obliquity dependent on body habitus).
- Center to gall bladder as determined on scout film (right half or elevated side of abdomen centered to CR and centerline.

Alternate: May also be taken as a 15–40° RPO.

Central Ray: CR ⊥, to gall bladder (location determined from scout).

SID: 40–48" (102–122 cm)

Collimation: To margins of cassette.

Respiration: Expose at expiration.

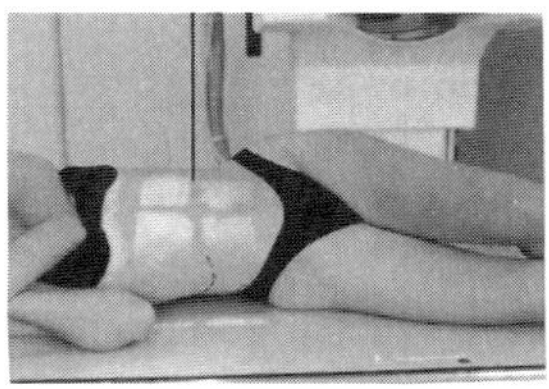

Alternate: 15–40° RPO

Technique: kVp (75±5) _____

mrad

S 205	G <0.1 M
ML 42	7 F

	cm	kVp	mA	Time	mAs	SID	Film–Screen	Grid	F.S.
Model Room	19	70			30	44"	Kodak 400	12:1	S
S									
M									
L									

Bontrager Textbook, 3rd ed., p. 499

Gall Bladder – Right Lat. Decub.

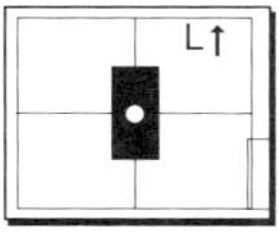

- 10 x 12" L.W. to patient (24 x 30 cm)
- Grid
- Include up-side or decub. marker

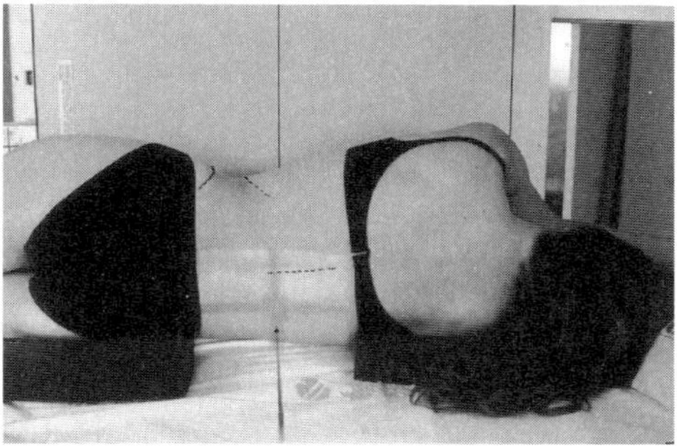

Right lateral decub. (PA) with horizontal CR

Position

- Patient on right side, pads placed under hips and shoulders (allows GB to drop away from vertebrae).
- PA or AP projection (PA preferred, facing film, places GB closer to film).
- Center cassette to CR (to right half of abdomen to GB location per scout film).

Central Ray

- CR horizontal, to gall bladder location per scout film.

SID: 40–48" (102–122 cm)

Collimation: To outer margins of cassette.

Respiration: Expose at end of full expiration.

Technique: kVp (75±5) _____

mrad		
	S 138	G <0.1 M
	ML 35	5 F

	cm	kVp	mA	Time	mAs	SID	Film–Screen	Grid	F.S.
Model Room	17	70			26	44"	Kodak 400	12:1	S
S									
M									
L									

Bontrager Textbook, 3rd ed., p. 500

Gall Bladder – Erect PA (or AP)

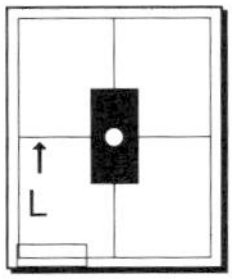

- 10 x 12" L.W. (24 x 30 cm)
- Grid
- Include erect marker

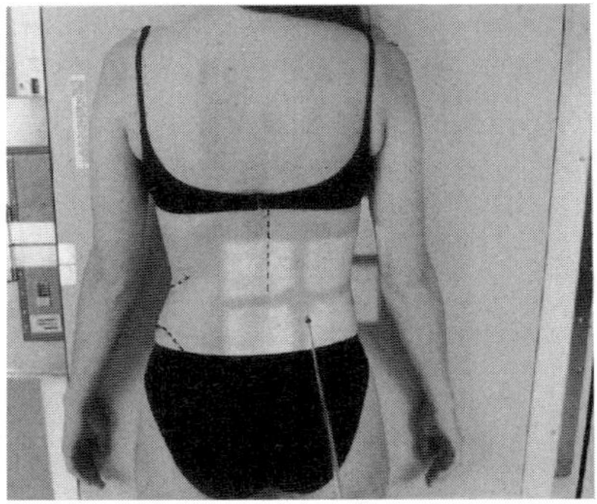

Erect gall bladder, PA

Position
- Erect PA (or AP), right half of abdomen aligned and centered to centerline. (PA preferred due to the more anterior location of GB).
- Cassette centered CR.

Central Ray
- CR horizontal, to gall bladder location determined from scout film, allowing for ≈1-2" (2.5 -5 cm) dropping of GB in erect position.

SID: 40–48" (102–122 cm)

Collimation: To outer margins of cassette.

Respiration: Expose at end of full expiration.

Technique: kVp (75±5) _____

mrad

S 196	G <0.1 M
ML 47	6 F

	cm	kVp	mA	Time	mAs	SID	Film–Screen	Grid	F.S.
Model Room	17	70			30	44"	Kodak 400	12:1	S
S									
M									
L									

Bontrager Textbook, 3rd ed., p. 501

Intravenous Urogram
AP Scout and Series

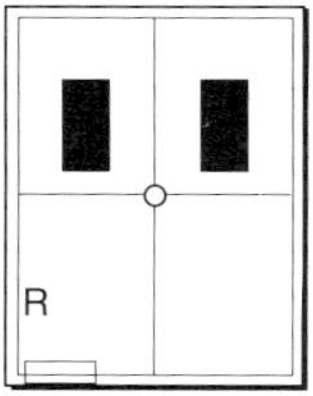

- 14 x 17" L.W. (35 x 43 cm)
- Grid
- Include minute marker

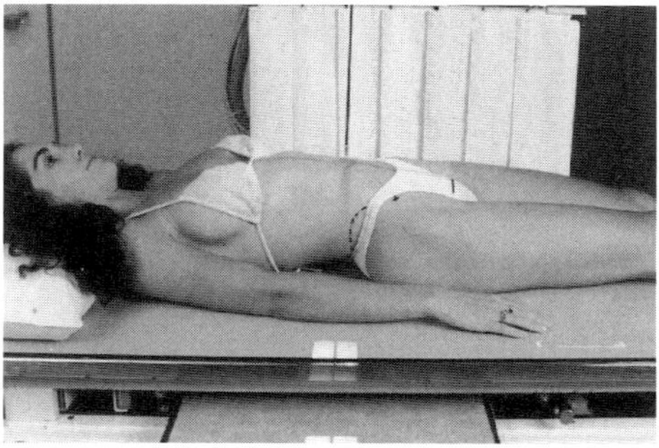

AP IVU

Possible filming sequence (fill in your departmental routine):
20-60 sec. nephro., 5 min. AP, 15 min. AP, 20 min. obli.'s, Post-void

________, ________, ________, ________, ________

(Note that early films may be nephrotomograms.)

Position – shield gonads for males
- Supine, midsagittal plane aligned and centered to centerline, support placed under knees, no rotation.

Central Ray: CR ⊥, to center of cassette, at level of iliac crest, or 1–2" (3–5 cm) above crests on long torso patients with second smaller film cross wise for bladder area, to include symphysis pubis on lower border of film.

SID: 40–48" (102–122 cm)

Collimation: To outer margins of cassette.

Respiration: Expose at end of full expiration.

Technique: kVp (75±5) _____

mrad per projection (without shields)

S 117	G	2 M
ML 28		26 F

	cm	kVp	mA	Time	mAs	SID	Film–Screen	Grid	F.S.
Model Room	19	75			15	44"	Kodak 400	12:1	S
S									
M									
L									

Bontrager Textbook, 3rd ed., p. 523

Intravenous Urogram

RPO and LPO

Both R and L posterior obliques should be part of routine.

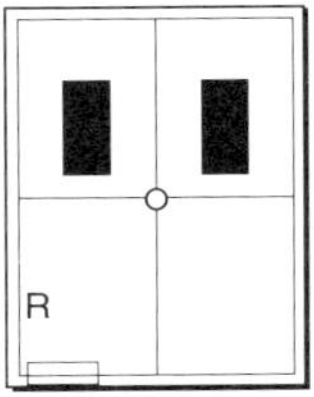

- 14 x 17" L.W. (35 x 43 cm)
- Grid
- Include minute marker

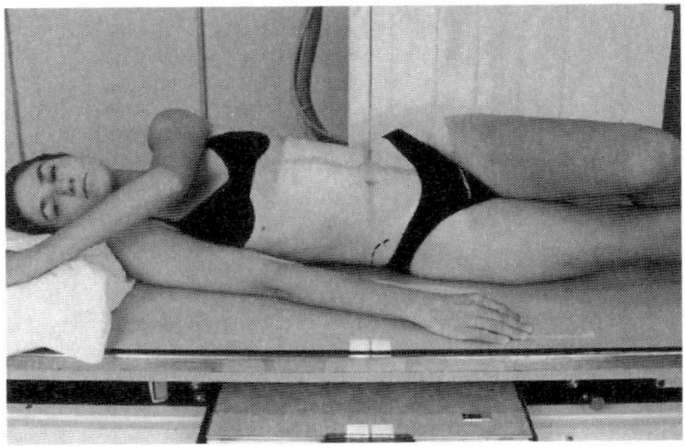

30°, RPO

Position – shield gonads for males

- Semi-supine, obliqued 30° to right (or left), flex elevated knee and elbow as shown for support. (Place angled support under back if needed.)
- Align and center abdomen to centerline.
- Center cassette to level of iliac crest

Central Ray

- CR ⊥, to center of cassette, at level of iliac crest.

SID: 40–48" (102–122 cm)

Collimation: To outer margins of cassette.

Respiration: Expose at end of full expiration.

without shields

mrad		
S 205	G	4 M
ML 41		46 F

Technique: kVp (75±5) _____

	cm	kVp	mA	Time	mAs	SID	Film–Screen	Grid	F.S.
Model Room	19	75			25	44"	Kodak 400	12:1	S
S									
M									
L									

Bontrager Textbook, 3rd ed., p. 525

Intravenous Urogram
AP Erect Post-Void

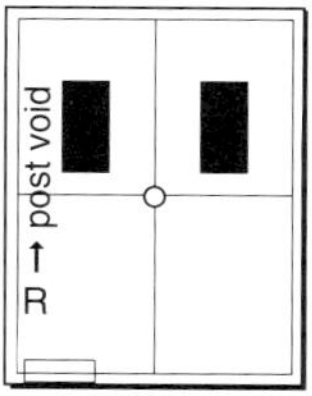

- 14 x 17" L.W. (35 x 43 cm)
- Grid
- Erect and post-void markers

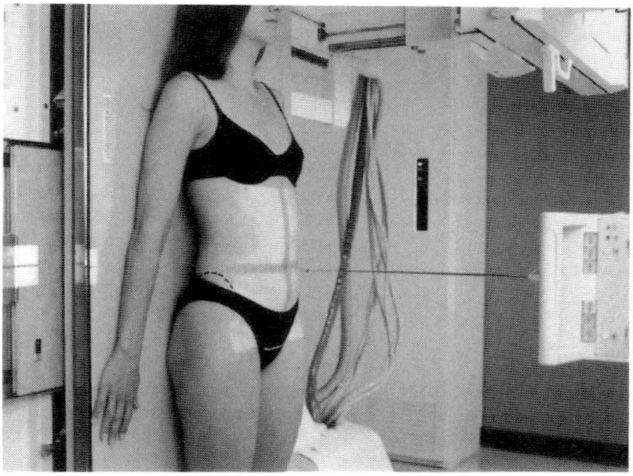

AP erect post-void

Position
- Erect, midsagittal plane aligned and centered to centerline, no rotation.
- Center cassette to iliac crest – ensure that bladder area including the symphysis pubis is included at lower film margin.

Central Ray
- CR ⊥, to center of cassette (at level of iliac crests or ≈1" or 2.5 cm lower than crest to include bladder area).

SID: 40–48" (102–122 cm)

Collimation: To outer margins of cassette.

Respiration: Expose at end of full expiration.

without shields

mrad		
S 176	G	3 M
ML 38		39 F

Technique: kVp (75±5) _____

	cm	kVp	mA	Time	mAs	SID	Film–Screen	Grid	F.S.
Model	18	75			22	44"	Kodak 400	12:1	S
Room									
S									
M									
L									

Bontrager Textbook, 3rd ed., p. 526

Cystogram - AP

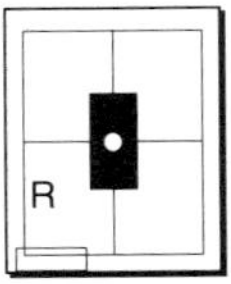

- 10 x 12" L.W. (24 x 30 cm)
- Grid

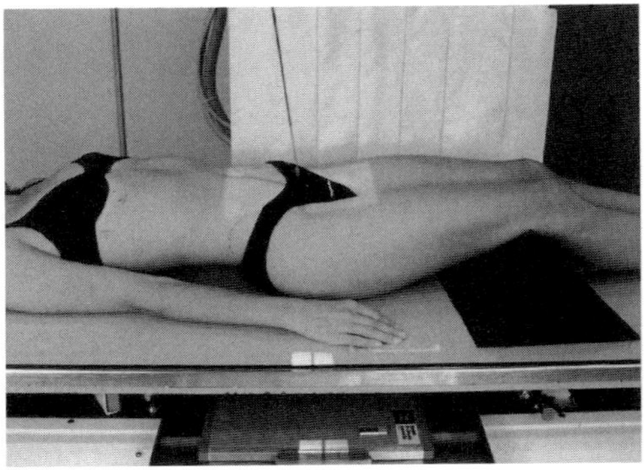

AP, CR 10–15° caudad

Position

- Supine, midsagittal plane aligned and centered to centerline, legs fully extended.
- Center cassette to projected CR.

Central Ray

- CR 10–15° caudad, centered to ≈2" (5 cm) superior to symphysis pubis at MSP (projects anterior pelvis inferiorly to better visualize bladder region).

SID: 40–48" (102–122 cm)

Collimation: To outer margins of cassette.

Respiration: Expose at end of full expiration.

without shields

mrad

S 112	G	44 M
ML 32		21 F

Technique: kVp (75±5) _____

	cm	kVp	mA	Time	mAs	SID	Film–Screen	Grid	F.S.
Model Room	16	75			15	44"	Kodak 400	12:1	S
S									
M									
L									

Bontrager Textbook, 3rd ed., p. 529

Cystogram – Posterior Obliques
(RPO, LPO and Optional Lateral)

Note: Cystogram routine may not include a lateral due to high gonadal dose.

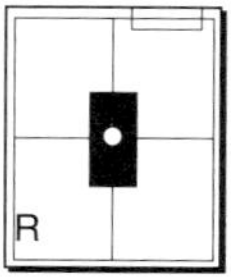

- 10 x 12" L.W. (35 x 43 cm)
- Grid

mrad

S	168
ML	33
G	65 M 32 F

75 kVp
20 mAs

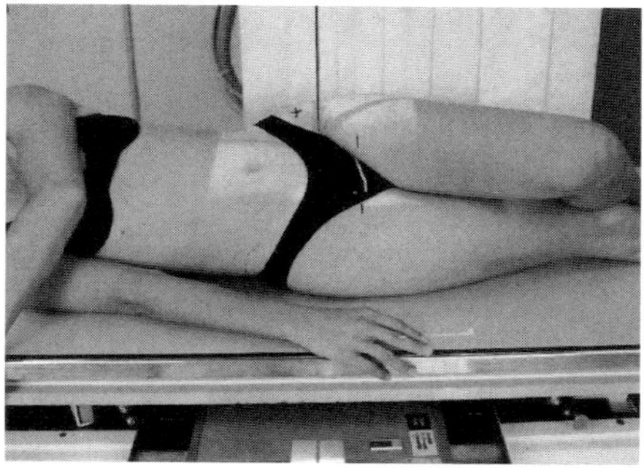

45° RPO

Position

- Semi-supine, obliqued 45–60° (60° oblique best demonstrates posterolateral bladder and UV junction).
- Flex elevated arm and leg to support this position.
- Center patient and cassette to CR.

Central Ray: CR ⊥, to ≈2" (5 cm) superior to symphysis pubis, and 2" (5 cm) medial to elevated ASIS.

SID: 40–48" (102–122 cm)

Collimation: To margins of cassette.

Respiration: Expose at expiration.

mrad

S	815
ML	76
G	76 M 76 F

90 kVp
48 mAs

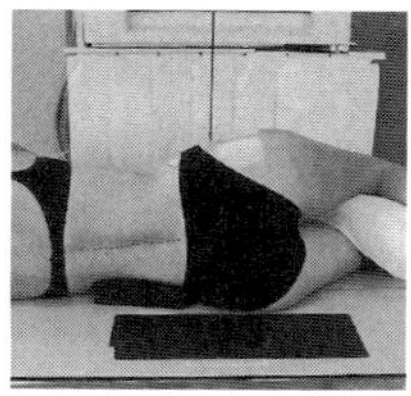

Optional lateral
- CR ⊥, 2" (5 cm) superior & post. to symphysis pubis

Technique: AP - kVp (75±5) _____ **Lat.**- kVp (90±5) _____

	cm	kVp	mA	Time	mAs	SID	Film–Screen	Grid	F.S.
Model Room	Obli. 20	75			20	44"	Kodak 400	12:1	S
S									
M									
L									

Bontrager Textbook, 3rd ed., p. 529

Abdomen and Contrast Media Studies

Position:

Central Ray:

SID:

Collimation:

Respiration:

Technique:

	Room	cm	kVp	mA	Time	mAs	SID	Film–Screen	Grid	F.S.
S										
M										
L										

Chapter 10

Mammography

Contributions and photographs by
Eugene D. Frank, MA, RT(R), FASRT

Breast Tissue and Exposure Factors

Breast tissue types based on relative amounts of glandular-fibrous tissue compared to fatty tissue are important in determining exposure factors. Three broad categories of breast types used in addition to breast thickness in determining exposure factors are as follows:

Breast Types[1]

Suggested kVp range

A. Fibro-glandular breast – greatest density. **(25-28 kVp)**
- Postpubertal adolescent through approximate age 30; also pregnant or lactating breasts. (Plus [+] density compensator may have to be used.)

B. Fibro-fatty breast – average density. **(25 kVp)**
- 30-50 age group (multiple pregnancies accelerate development of this breast type).

C. Fatty breast – least density. **(22-25 kVp)**
- Postmenopausal age (average 50+ years). (Minus [-] density compensator may have to be used.)

Automatic Exposure Controls (AEC)

AEC systems are incorporated in most modern mammography equipment wherein the ionization chamber cells are located in the area where the thickest part of the breast near the chest wall is placed. This AEC system determines the density of the mammogram by controlling the exposure time (and the mAs) as well as the kVp in some equipment.

Kilovoltage (kVp)

Suggested kVp ranges for the different breast types are listed above. Generally however, kVp values are set or predetermined by departmental policy and are only adjusted for certain type A breasts.

The kVp– density rule states that a 15% change in kVp is equivalent to a 100% change in mAs. Therefore even a 1 or 2 kVp change will change the dose and also the contrast on mammograms.

Mammogram – Craniocaudad (CC)

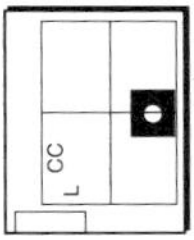

CR and AEC cell

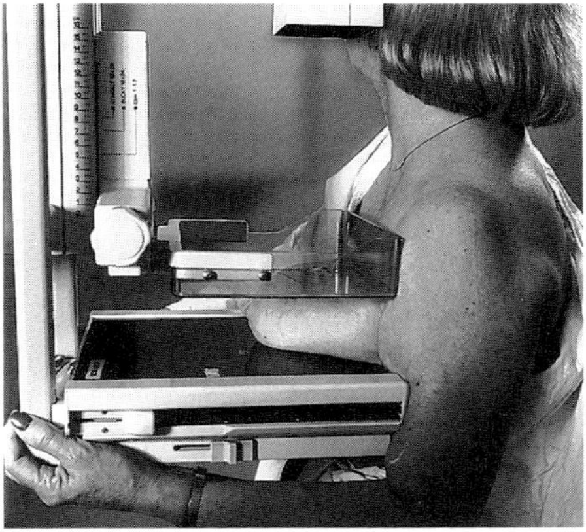

- Match film size to breast size.
- Grid
- Marker placed on axillary side of film.

CC projection

Position

- Erect, standing or seated facing the film, head turned to side, affected side arm down and relaxed shoulder pulled back.
- Film raised to upper limits of inframammary crease.
- Breast fully extended onto film, nipple in profile.
- Firm compression applied (final step before exposure).

Central Ray: CR perpendicular, to center of breast and photo-timer sensor.

Collimation: Match cone size to breast size.

SID: 60 cm (23.6"), may vary with manufacturer.

Respiration: Suspend during exposure.

Technique: kVp range 25–28_____.   mrad | S 867 | MGD 133

	compressed cm	kVp	mA	Time	mAs	SID	Film Size	Screen	Grid	1 Ø / 3 Ø
Model	4	25	80	AEC		60 cm	18x24cm	150	4:1	1 Ø
Average										
Dense (type A)										

Bontrager Textbook, 3rd ed., p. 540

Mammogram – Mediolateral Oblique (MLO)

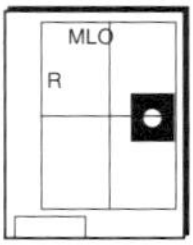

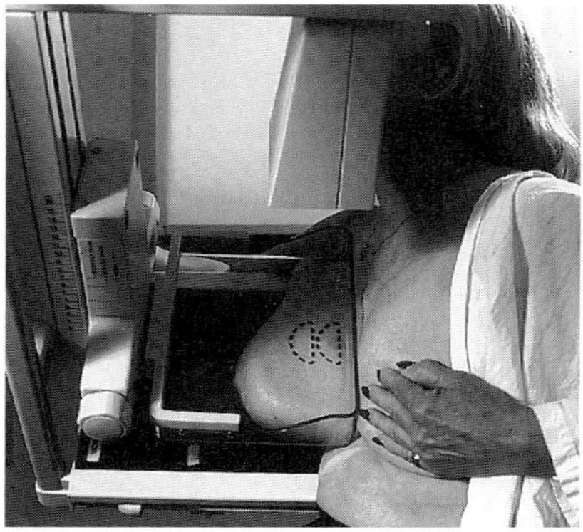

MLO, tube and film angled 45°

- Match film size to breast size.
- Grid
- Marker placed at axillary side of film.

Position

- Tube and film angled 45–70° from vertical, (large breast 40–60°, smaller breast 60–70°).
- Erect, standing or seated facing the film, slightly turned with arm of affected side forward holding on to support.
- Film raised to place upper margin of film at axilla.
- Extend breast and tail of breast over film as far as possible, nipple in profile.
- Firm compression applied (final step before exposure).

Central Ray: CR ⊥ to film, centered to center of breast and AEC cell.

Collimation: Match cone size to breast size.

SID: 60 cm (23.6"), may vary with manufacturer.

Technique: kVp range 25–28_____.   mrad | S 867 | MGD 133

	compressed cm	kVp	mA	Time	mAs	SID	Film Size	Screen	Grid	1 Ø 3 Ø
Model	4	25	80	AEC		60 cm	18x24cm	150	4:1	1 Ø
Average										
Dense (type A)										

Bontrager Textbook, 3rd ed., p. 541

Mammogram – Exaggerated Lateral CC (XLCC)

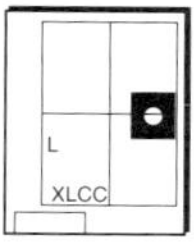

- Match film size to breast size.
- Grid
- Marker placed at axillary side of film.

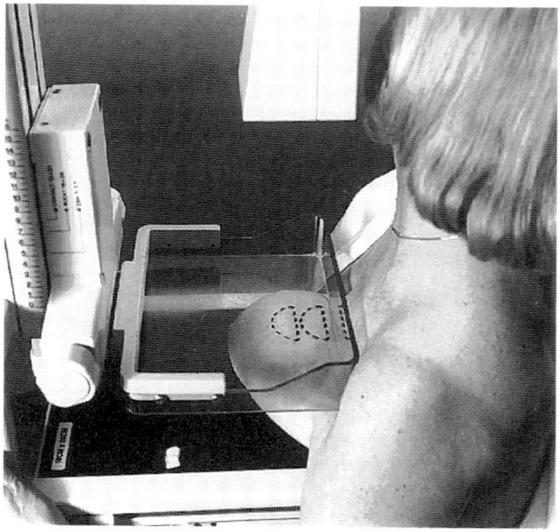

XLCC projection

Position

- Erect, standing or seated, partially turned to include axillary tissue, arm forward holding on to support, head turned to side.
- Breast extended onto film without tissue folds or wrinkles, nipple in profile.

Central Ray: CR ⊥ to center of breast and AEC cell.

Collimation: Match cone size to breast size.

SID: 60 cm (23.6"), may vary with manufacturer.

Respiration: Suspend during exposure.

Technique: kVp range 25–28_____.

mrad	S 867	MGD 133

	compressed cm	kVp	mA	Time	mAs	SID	Film Size	Screen	Grid	1 Ø 3 Ø
Model	4	25	80	AEC		60 cm	18x24cm	150	4:1	1 Ø
Average										
Dense (type A)										

Bontrager Textbook, 3rd ed., p. 542

Mammogram – Eklund Technique[2]

A common routine for mammograms involving implants includes standard CC and MLO projections with the implant image included on the radiograph. In addition a second CC and MLO projection is taken wherein a special technique is used for pushing back or "pinching" the implant to better visualize breast tissue. (There are exceptions wherein the implants become encapsulated in breast tissue and thus cannot be pushed back in this way.)

Ecklund "pinch" technique demonstrated

Step 1
Position as for a standard CC projection, then gently push the implant back with finger tips as shown.

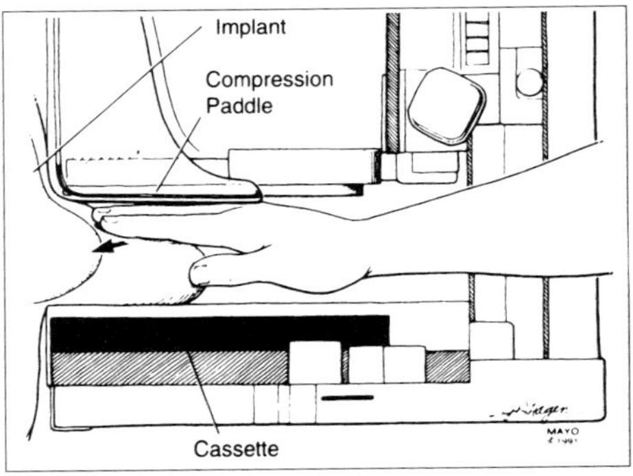

Step 2
Breast and implant are in position with compression applied holding implant back out of exposure field.

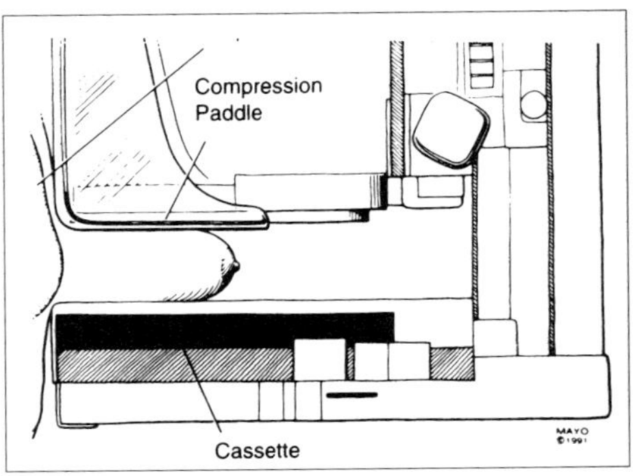

Used by permission, Mayo Clinic

AEC should not be used with implants because the dense implant over the AEC cell will result in overexposed radiographs.

Mammogram

Position

Central Ray:

Collimation:

SID:

Respiration:

Technique:

	compressed cm	kVp	mA	Time	mAs	SID	Film Size	Screen	Grid	1 Ø 3 Ø
Model										
Average										
Dense (type A)										

Mammogram

Position

Central Ray:

Collimation:

SID:

Respiration:

Technique:

	compressed cm	kVp	mA	Time	mAs	SID	Film Size	Screen	Grid	1 Ø 3 Ø
Model										
Average										
Dense (type A)										

Chapter 11

Personal Notes on Portables (Mobile), Surgical Procedures, Tomography and Others

The routines for portables, surgical procedures, tomograms and other special procedures vary greatly among different hospitals and in different regions of the country. Therefore, these outline pages are provided for each person to fill in descriptions and techniques that are being used in their departments for these portables (mobile) procedures.

Portables (bedside)

Body Part:

Patient Position Description:

Central Ray Location and/ or Angle:

Technique:

	Machine or Room	cm	kVp	mA	Time	mAs	SID	Film Size	Screen	Grid	1 Ø 3 Ø
S											
M											
L											

Portables continued

Body Part:

Patient Position Description:

Central Ray Location and/or Angle:

Technique:

	Machine or Room	cm	kVp	mA	Time	mAs	SID	Film Size	Screen	Grid	1 Ø 3 Ø
S											
M											
L											

Body Part:

Patient Position Description:

Central Ray Location and/or Angle:

Technique:

	Machine or Room	cm	kVp	mA	Time	mAs	SID	Film Size	Screen	Grid	1 Ø 3 Ø
S											
M											
L											

Surgical Procedures

Body Part:

Patient Position Description:

Central Ray Location and/or Angle:

Technique:

Machine or Room	cm	kVp	mA	Time	mAs	SID	Film Size	Screen	Grid	1 Ø 3 Ø
S										
M										
L										

Body Part:

Patient Position Description:

Central Ray Location and/or Angle:

Technique:

Machine or Room	cm	kVp	mA	Time	mAs	SID	Film Size	Screen	Grid	1 Ø 3 Ø
S										
M										
L										

Body Part:

Patient Position Description:

Central Ray Location and/or Angle:

Technique:

Machine or Room	cm	kVp	mA	Time	mAs	SID	Film Size	Screen	Grid	1 Ø 3 Ø
S										
M										
L										

Body Part:

Patient Position Description:

Central Ray Location and/or Angle:

Technique:

Machine or Room	cm	kVp	mA	Time	mAs	SID	Film Size	Screen	Grid	1 Ø 3 Ø
S										
M										
L										

Chapter 12

Additional Imaging Procedures

Special radiographic surveys and series, and long bone measurements

Additional Imaging Procedures

(Special surveys and series, and long bone measurements)

Certain diagnostic imaging procedures require a specific series or survey of projections for various purposes. Following are suggested routines for these series and surveys. Check off boxes are provided for marking specific departmental routines and space to write in the projections which differ from those listed. (Suggest that these be written in pencil.)

1. Bone Survey

(Possible metastatic)

	Suggested Routines	Departmental Routines
❒ Chest	PA	
❒ Abdomen	AP, (KUB)	
❒ Pelvis	AP	
❒ Skull	PA, Caldwell & Lat.	
❒ C. spine	AP, Lat & Swimmers	
❒ T. spine	AP & Lat (breathing)	
❒ L. spine	AP & Lat	
❒ Ribs	AP (upper & lower)	
	RPO & LPO	
❒ Upper limbs	Bilateral AP humeri	
	& AP forearms	
❒ Lower limbs	Bilateral AP femora	
	& AP lower legs	
❒		
❒		

2. SNAT Series

(Pediatrics, Suspected NonAccidental Trauma)

	Suggested Routines	Departmental Routines
❒ Ribs	AP	
❒ Abdomen	AP	
❒ Skull	AP & lat	
❒ Upper limbs	AP & lat	
❒ Lower limbs	AP & lat	
❒		
❒		

3. Trauma Series

(Adult or pediatric)

	Suggested Routines	Departmental Routines
❒ Chest	AP	
❒ Abdomen	AP	
❒ Pelvis	AP	
❒ C. spine	AP, lat, open mouth & Swimmers	
❒		

4. Shunt Series (Drainage of ventricles into abdomen)

	Suggested Routines	Departmental Routines
❒ Abdomen (To check for abdominal shunt)	AP	
❒ Skull to include neck	AP & lat	
❒ Chest to include neck	AP	
❒		

5. Bone Age

	Suggested Routines	Departmental Routines
❒ Hand and wrist (If less than one year, include from shoulder to fingers.)	PA (or AP)	
❒		

6. Long Bone Survey

	Suggested Routines	Departmental Routines
❒ Humerus	AP & lat	
❒ Forearm	AP & lat	
❒ Femur	AP & lat	
❒ Lower leg	AP & lat	
❒		

7. Long Bone Measurements

(Scanogram or orthoroentgenogram, with Bell-Thompson ruler)

A. Lower Limb Measurements

Three separate exposures are made on one film with the tube and film moved between exposures. Each exposure requires accurate centering of the CR directly over the **hip, knee** and **ankle joints** (see next page).

The film in the Bucky tray is moved between exposures so the three separate and well collimated exposures are made on one film. A lead numbered measuring device is placed on the table top directly beside the leg ensuring no movement of either the leg or ruler between exposures.

The length of the femur and the tibia-fibula can be calculated from the ruler readings at each of these joints.

Individual Limbs: The most precise measurements are possible when each limb is radiographed separately as shown.

Optional bi-lateral limbs: An alternate method reducing patient exposure but resulting in less precise measurements is exposing both the right and left limb simultaneously with the ruler placed midway between the limbs, or with a ruler under each limb. Three individual exposures are again made on one larger film including both right and left joints. Some bilateral distortion does occur from the divergence of the x-ray beam.

B. Upper Limbs

Measurements of the upper limbs can also be made by taking three separate exposures of the **shoulder, elbow** and **wrist joints** respectively. Each limb is examined separately. The tube and film are again moved for each exposure with the CR centered directly over each individual joint. The metal ruler is also placed on the table top directly under each limb.

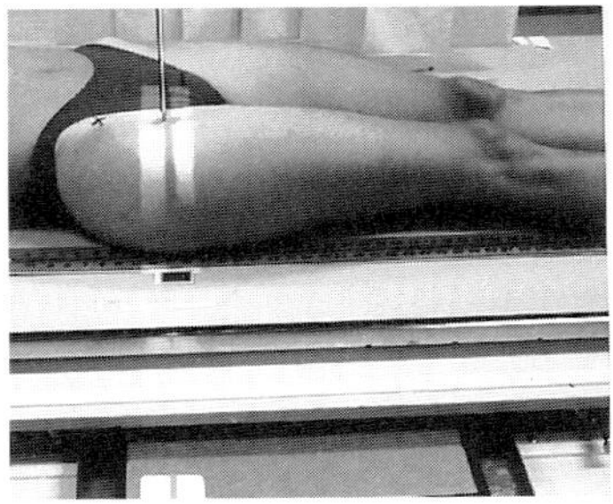

1.**AP** - **hip joint** (include head & neck area)
- CR: 1/2 - 3/4" (1-2 cm) superior to level of symphysis pubis.
- Ruler under and beside leg, do **NOT** move leg or ruler between these three exposures.
- Collimation field to upper film region.

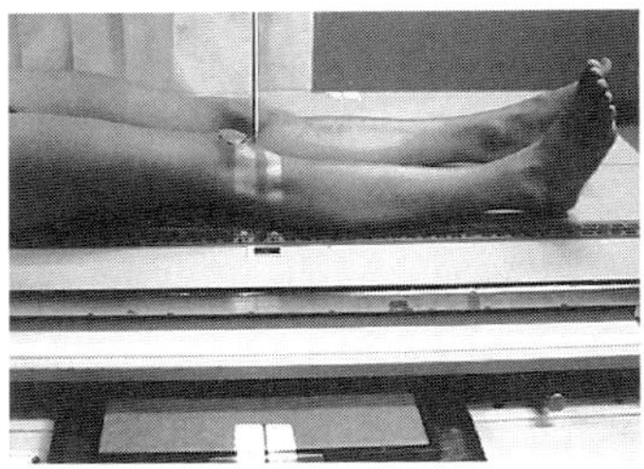

2. AP - knee joint
- CR: ≈ 3/4" (2 cm) distal to apex of patella.
- Narrow collimation to mid film region.

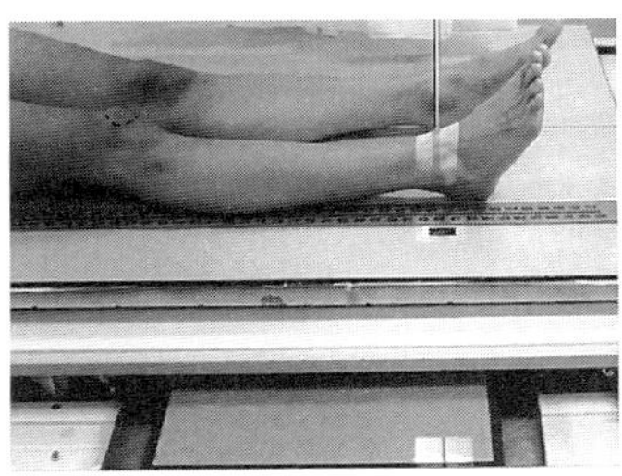

3. **AP - ankle joint**
- CR: midpoint between malleoli.
- Narrow collimation to lower film region.

Chapter 13

Computed Radiography (CR)

General Diagnostic CR and Digital Fluoroscopy (DF)

Contributions and illustrations by
James A. Sanderson, BS, RT(R)

General Diagnostic CR

Digital Fluoroscopy (DF)

Computed Radiography (CR)

Principles

Computed radiography (CR) is an imaging modality used to produce radiographic images in a digital format for output to a computer monitor or x-ray film. General diagnostic CR as described in this section uses standard sized cassettes containing a **reusable imaging plate** instead of intensifying screens and film. Exposures are achieved using **ordinary fixed or portable radiographic equipment.**

A plate reader or processor converts the exposed image to digital form using a laser scanner. During the scanning process, image data is automatically adjusted for contrast, brightness, and detail enhancement. The processed and adjusted digital image can then be viewed on a computer monitor, or may be output to x-ray film.

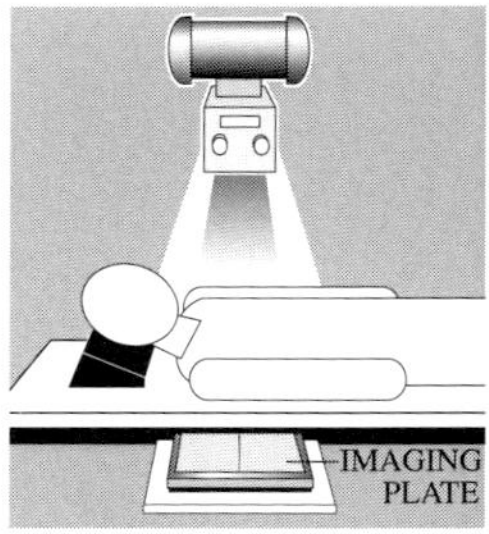

CR uses standard x-ray equipment (except for imaging plate)

Components

Cassettes with IP

A cassette is used to house the **image plate (IP).** Though the CR cassette is similar to the standard radiographic film cassette in external appearance, it has several distinctive features. For example, the IP inside the CR cassette is not sensitive to light. Therefore since the CR cassette does not contain film or intensifying screens, it does not need to be "light tight" and is primarily designed to hold and protect the removable IP.

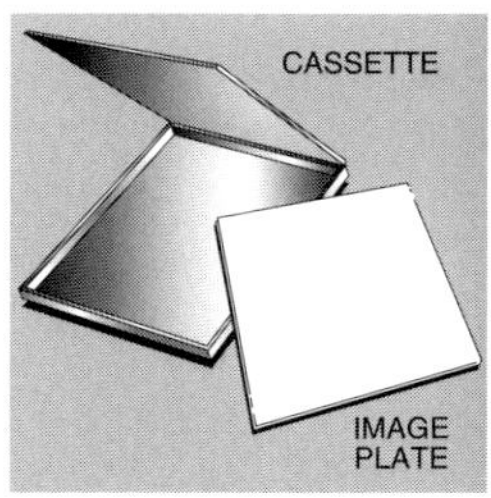

CR cassette holds removable image plate (IP)

Patient information is placed on the CR image using bar codes or other digital technology which eliminates the typical name blocker found on conventional cassettes.

Image Reader (Processor)

After it is exposed to ionizing radiation, the CR cassette is placed into a reading apparatus called the **IP processor.** Inside the processor the IP is removed from the cassette and placed into a reading stand where it is scanned by a red laser. As the laser scans line by line, the IP phosphors release electrons which emit light equal to their stored energy.

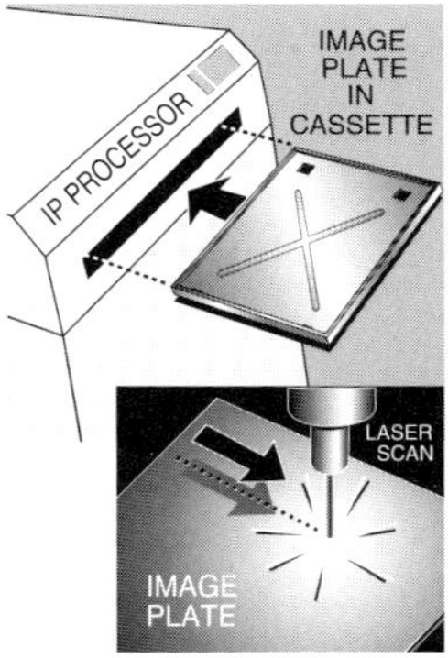

IP processor removes image plate for laser scanning and image processing. Erased IP is returned to cassette.

A detector mechanism senses the light intensity and converts the detected light signal into a digital format capable of manipulation, enhancement, viewing and printing from a computer workstation. Equipment used to display, print, transmit, and store images is configured much the same as a common personal computer system.

Image Display and Recording

The **display monitor** is used to view and manipulate images. Various monitor sizes and resolution are available depending on the application. Large, high resolution monitors are required for reading and interpretation whereas small, medium resolution monitors are used for viewing and manipulation of the image prior to film output.

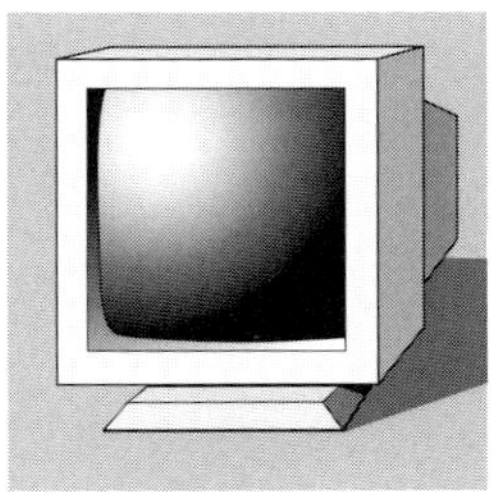

Display monitor

Computer Workstation

Image manipulation is achieved by using a standard computer **keyboard** with a **mouse** or **trackball** to select desired contrast, brightness, and edge enhancement tools. Menus and controls are displayed in a user friendly windows format for ease of use.

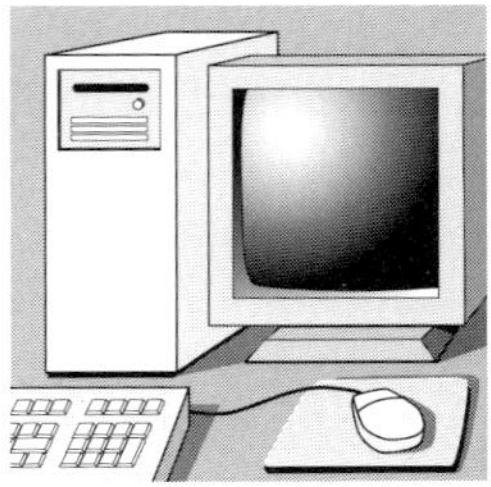

Workstation with keyboard and mouse

The **computer workstation** provides the option of printing the final displayed image to x-ray film using a **laser printer**. During printing, a laser beam imprints line by line onto a single emulsion film sensitive to laser light.

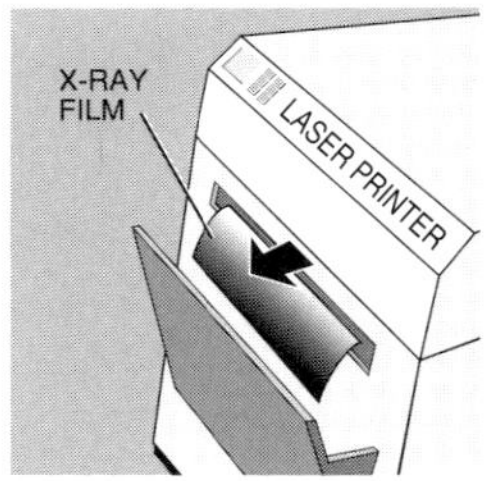

X-ray film generated by laser printer

Image Transmission

The computer workstation also allows the option of **electronic transmission** of image data to a remote computer or viewing monitor and console. Connection to local or national networks is possible when digital image data is converted to an industry standard protocol recognized by different computer equipment manufacturers. This can be done over telephone lines or through fiberoptics or satellite transmission.

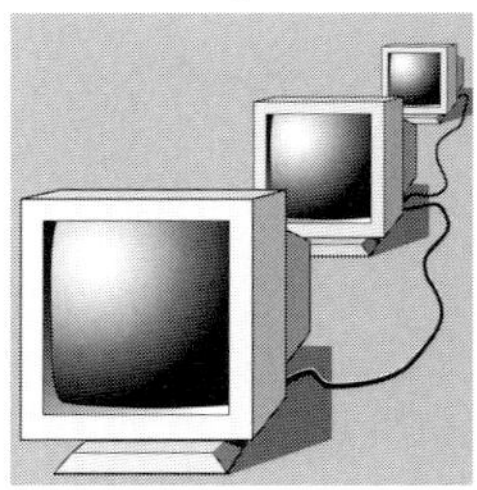

Electronic transmission

Image Storage

Hard disk drives, optical disks or other high capacity storage devices permanently archive (store) the image data in a digital form. Film storage is not necessary with this system.

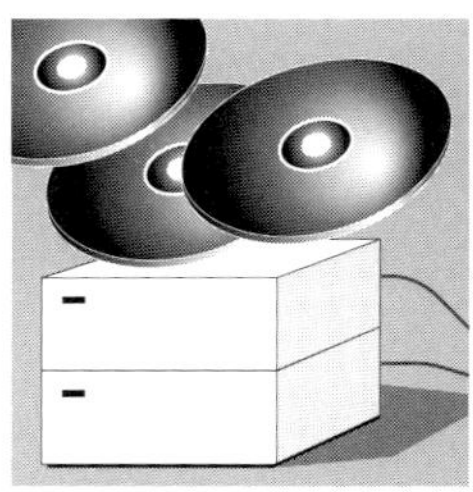

Image storage on hard drive or optical disk

Determining Exposure Factors

When selecting a technique (exposure factors) using CR the radiographer must consider the following:

- During image manipulation, CR uses digital processing algorithms also known as Exposure Data Recognition (EDR) to compensate for exposure as needed.
- EDR can compensate for approximately **500% over exposure** and **85% underexposure**.[1]

Exposure Index

The exposure index is a representation of the number of x-rays reaching the image plate forming the latent image. The radiographer uses this index number as an indicator of whether the best exposure was used to produce **the highest quality radiograph with the least possible exposure to the patient.**

In CR the final density and image quality is **not** primarily dependent on technique (exposure factors) because of image adjustments which occur during processing. Therefore the appearance of the radiograph cannot be used to judge correct technique. **The exposure index is the only indicator used to provide feedback as to whether the exposure factors or techniques were correct or best for that image**.

Fuji™ CR System and "S" Numbers

Each image is assigned a specific exposure index number. With the Fuji system this is referred to as an "S" number (for "sensitivity") representing an approximation of the screen-film speed required for a given exposure. Therefore as demonstrated on the next page, with the Fuji system a **higher "S" number** represents a faster speed system, indicating **less exposure** was used. A **lower "S" number** indicates a **greater exposure** was used. The optimal range of "S" numbers should be determined by each facility or institution.

Normal Exposure

When proper exposure settings, positioning, collimation, and image processing factors are employed, generally the index number on the radiographic image will reflect a number in the desired exposure range. For example when a portable AP chest using Fuji CR is exposed correctly at the x-ray tube, and the assigned exposure index is 400, then the "S" number on the radiograph will be near 400.

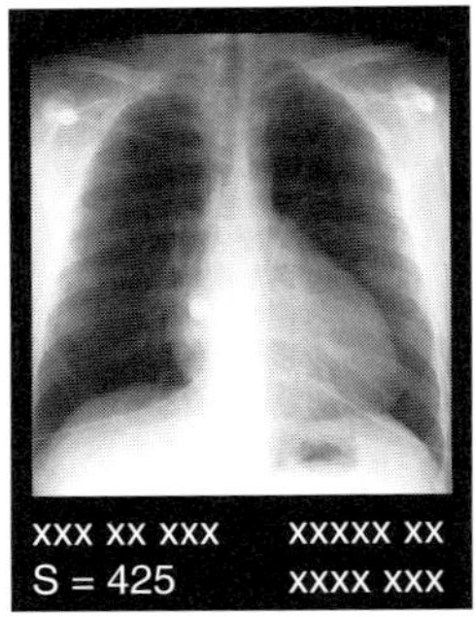

Normal exposure with a desirable Fuji "S" number

Underexposure

When the IP is underexposed within the 85% margin of error, the image will be compensated to appear normally exposed. For example if the exposure index for a portable AP chest was set at 400 using Fuji CR, and the film was underexposed by 6-8 kVp, the "S" number appearing on the radiograph would be higher, or near 600 indicating some underexposure. EDR however compensates for under exposures within 85%, so the image still appears sharp and normally exposed.

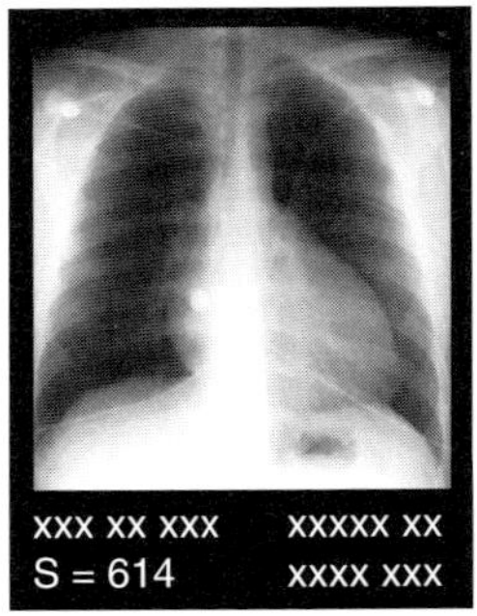

Slightly underexposed, compensated correctly (slightly higher "S" number)

However as underexposures begin to exceed the ability of EDR to compensate, the image may appear near normal in overall density, but becomes "grainy" in appearance with image noise known as **quantum mottle.** The Fuji "S" number would be much higher on such a radiograph.

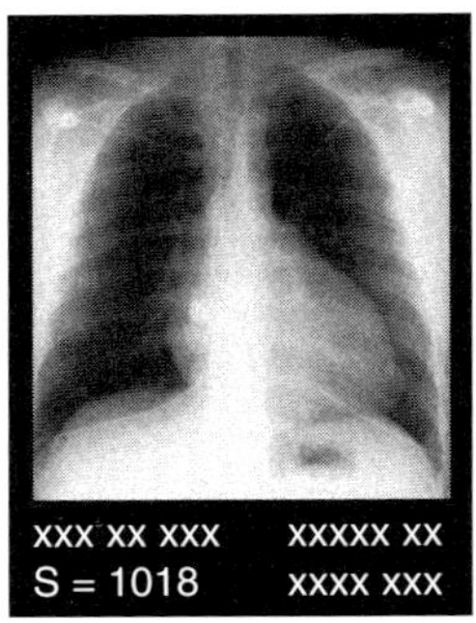

Unacceptable underexposure results in grainy image (high "S" number)

Greatly underexposed: Images with very high Fuji "S" numbers often appear both overexposed (dark) and grainy. A dark grainy image with a very high Fuji "S" number occurs when the EDR over compensates for too little image data on the IP resulting from too much of an underexposure.

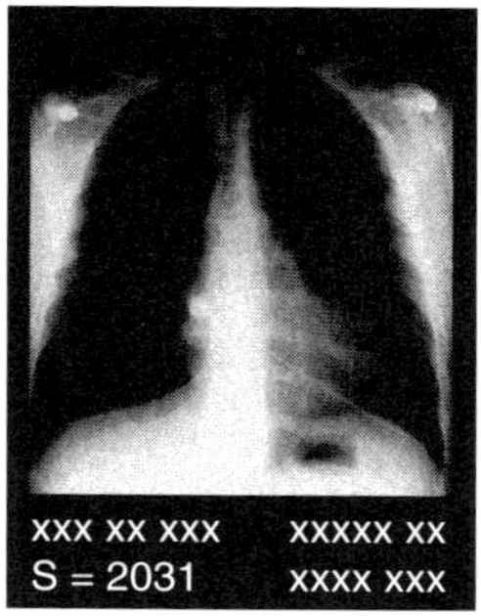

Greatly underexposed could not compensate correctly (very high "S"

Overexposure

A compensation range of 500% over exposure provides a wide latitude for EDR adjustment. A significantly over exposed IP will still result in a radiograph appearing nearly correctly exposed. For example if the exposure index is correctly set at 400 using the Fuji system for an AP chest, but the film is overexposed by 6-8 kVp, the "S" number would be low, nearer 100 indicating some overexposure. EDR compensates for overexposures within 500%, so the image still appears sharp and normally exposed.

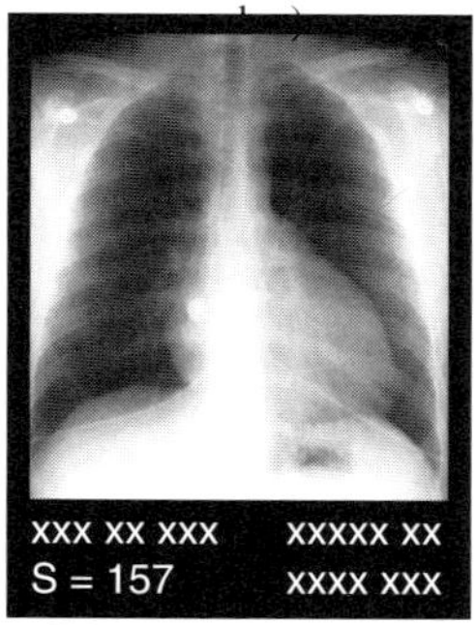

Slightly overexposed, compensated correctly (lower "S" number)

However when overexposures exceed the ability of EDR to compensate, the image will appear underexposed (light). An underexposed (light) appearing radiograph with a very low Fuji "S" number generally indicates an extreme overexposure.

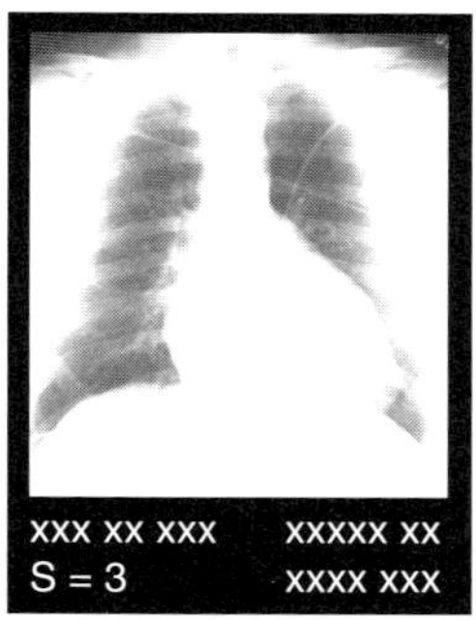

Greatly overexposed, could not compensate correctly (very low "S" number)

NOTE: Although EDR is very forgiving with overexposures, radiographers must always strive for the **lowest possible exposure dose to the patient**.

Image Enhancement

Digital image processing offers the user image enhancement capabilities for examinations requiring additional visualization techniques. One form of image enhancement is referred to as **edge enhancement** (non-linear unsharp masking). This is used to define or enhance edge sharpness and is useful in visualizing lines or catheters in chests and abdomens. Fracture lines of bony anatomy can also be enhanced for better visualization.

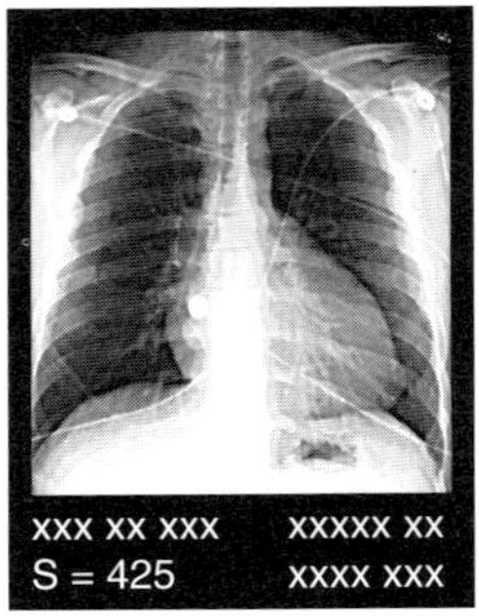

Enhanced image
(edge enhancement)

Kodak™ CR System

Other CR systems utilizing an image plate may use a different exposure indexing system. For example the Kodak system also uses an exposure index based on screen-film speed but in a different way in that the index numbers change in the same direction as the exposure changes. Therefore **overexposures** result in **higher index numbers** on the radiograph, and **underexposures** result in **lower index numbers**. This is the opposite of the Fuji system already described and illustrated.

Kodak CR Imaging Index Comparisons

CR Index	Screen-film speed
1400	400 (high)
1700	200
2000	100 (medium)
2300	50 (detail)

As seen on the right, with the Kodak system a higher index number corresponds to a slower speed screen-film indicating a higher technique was used. Doubling the exposure increases the exposure index by 300.

Kodak CR
Example: Chest Exposures

Chest Radiograph	Index Numbers
Greatly underexposed	500-1000
Slightly underexposed (-6-8 kVp)	1300-1400
Correctly exposed	**1500-1600**
Slightly overexposed (+6-8 kVp)	1700-1800
Greatly overexposed	3000-4000

Critical Considerations of CR

Since CR differs from conventional film technology, the radiographer must thoroughly understand the characteristics of the specific computed radiography equipment being utilized. In general, CR is very sensitive to **centering**, **collimation**, and **image processing parameter selection**.

Centering

CR exposure compensation uses a center sampling technique which is often compared to a phototimer or AEC pick-up cell where **accurate centering of anatomy over the detector area is critical** to attain a proper appearing exposure.

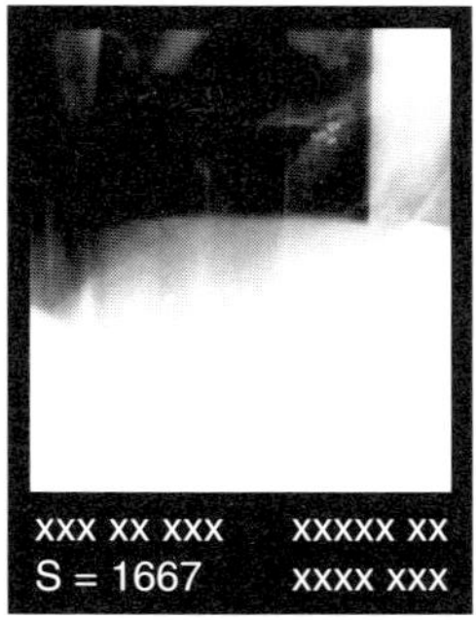

Centering error-odontoid view. Compensation failure due to off centering.(EDR could not compensate correctly.)

Collimation

IP processors are programmed to locate the collimated edges of an exposure and concentrate processing within the collimated borders. This reduces any unnecessary information outside of the collimated area from being heavily averaged into the processing of the desired image. Therefore **careful collimation to the required anatomy is essential** to improve image quality by reducing the averaging of unwanted information during image processing.

Use of Correct Image Processing Parameters (algorithms)

Image processing parameters (algorithms) of optimal contrast and density are preprogrammed into the IP processor for each radiographic projection. For example, a cassette exposed with an AP chest is placed into the IP processor with "AP Chest" selected on the IP processor display panel. A lateral chest would require a specific "lateral chest" selection. Therefore it is essential that **the radiographer must somehow identify and remember which cassette is used for which specific projection**. Tape or "stick-on" notes placed on each cassette can be used for this purpose. **Selection of an incorrect image processing parameter (algorithm) may produce undesirable image quality.**

Digital Fluoroscopy (DF)

Principles and Spot Filming

Digital fluoro (DF) as described in this chapter, is a type of computed radiography used in fluoroscopy and cine wherein a digital image receptor and processor are incorporated into a fluoroscopy tower. As in conventional fluoroscopy systems, the x-ray tube is located under the table and the image receiving mechanism (fluoroscopy tower) is above the patient. Images are captured in digital form with an image intensifier and a high resolution video camera which transmits image information to a computer for storage. Images can then be displayed on a high resolution video monitor for manipulation and output to film.

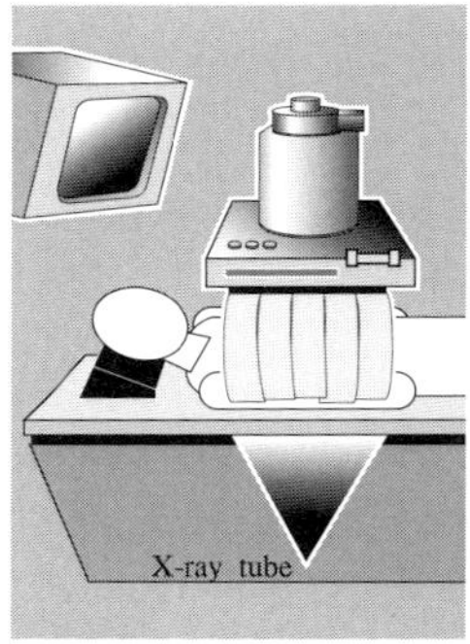

Digital fluoro system

Features and Capabilities of DF

No Cassette Required

DF image acquisition is similar to exposing a "spot film" during conventional fluoroscopy except no cassette is required. Image data is stored in computer memory for later printout on x-ray film. Image plates as used in general diagnostic CR are **not** used with DF systems.

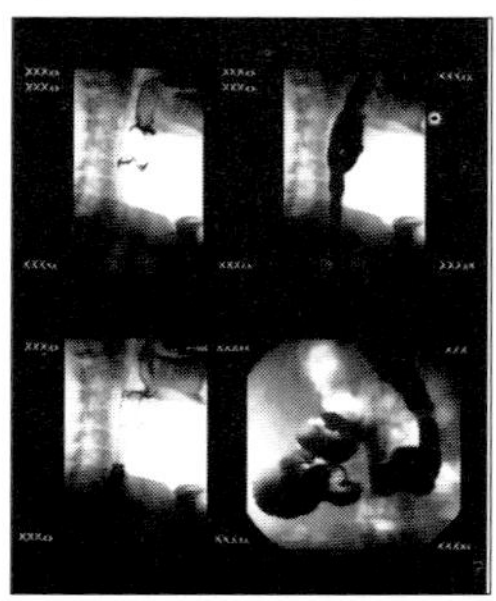
4:1 format (four digital images on 14 x 17" film)

Multiple Frame Formatting

Multiple images can be formatted on one film. These can be 4:1, 6:1, 9:1 or 12:1 depending on the size of the image.

Cine Loop Capability

Digital images can be exposed in rapid succession without the delay of changing cassettes. Therefore cine images (e.g. 4 image/sec) can be easily obtained eliminating the use of a 105mm film device. Moving image sequences can be played back immediately on the display monitor.

Image Enhancement

DF images can be manipulated in much the same way as with general CR images (i.e. edge enhancement, zoom, brightness and contrast). Additional digital image enhancement features for specific use by DF may include:

- Adjustable shutters or electronic coning.
- Equalization filter to bring out detail in under or over-exposed areas of an image.
- Mask and subtract filters for road-mapping and digital subtraction studies.

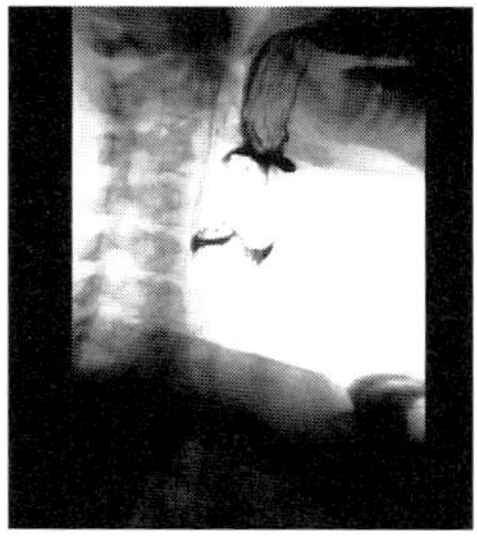
Without equalization filter

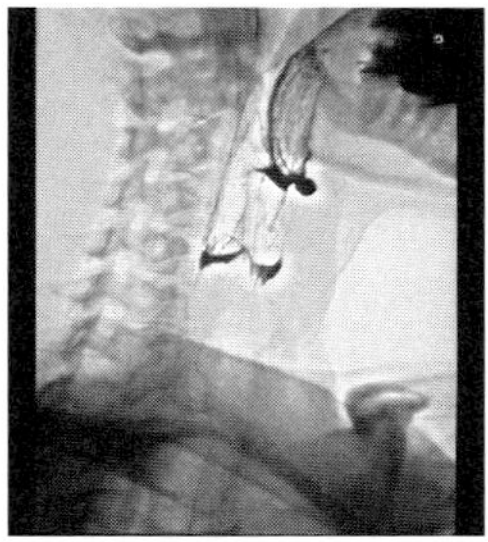
With equalization filter

Hand-held Remote Control

A convenient hand-held remote control (cordless) provides instant access to review stored images or cine studies during fluoroscopic procedures without interrupting the examination.

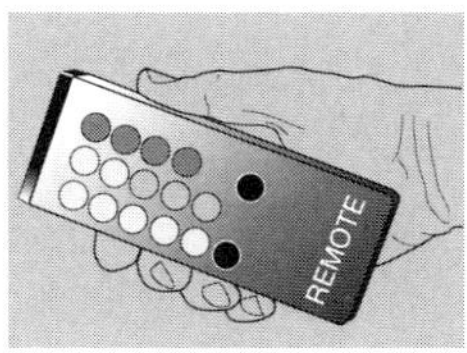

Hand-held remote

Remote Console and Networking

An optional remote console can be utilized to perform DF image post-processing and filming functions. DF images can also be transmitted through local and/or national networks in a manner similar to general CR.

Multiple "Original" Films

Every film printed from the digital is an "original". Therefore with both general CR and DF new films can be generated at any time if a film gets lost or another copy is needed.

Reduced Exposure

Both general CR and DF imaging can reduce patient exposure 30–50%[3,4] due to increased sensitivity of image receptors as compared to conventional fluoroscopy. This is especially valuable for DF imaging in pediatric applications.[5]

Personal Notes:

Appendix A: mAs Chart

Time In seconds		mA 50	75	100	150	200	250	300	400	500	600	800
1/500	.002	.1	.15	.2	.3	.4	.5	.6	.8	1	1.2	1.6
1/200	.005	.25	.38	.5	.75	1.0	1.25	1.5	2	2.5	3	4
1/120	.008	.4	.6	.8	1.2	1.6	2	2.4	3.2	4	4.8	6.4
1/100	.01	.5	.75	1	1.5	2	2.5	3	4	5	6	8
≈1/80	.013	.65	.98	1.3	1.95	2.6	3.25	3.9	5.2	6.5	7.8	10.4
≈1/60	.016	.8	1.2	1.6	2.4	3.2	4	4.8	6.4	8	9.6	12.8
≈1/50	.019	.95	1.43	1.9	2.85	3.8	4.75	5.7	7.6	9.5	11.4	15.2
1/40	.025	1.25	1.88	2.5	3.75	5	6.25	7.5	10	12.5	15	20
1/30	.033	1.65	2.48	3.3	4.95	6.6	8.25	9.9	13.2	16.5	19.8	26.4
≈1/24	.041	2.05	3.08	4.1	6.15	8.2	10.25	12.3	16.4	20.5	24.6	32.8
1/20	.05	2.5	3.75	5	7.5	10	12.5	15	20	25	30	40
≈1/15	.064	3.2	4.8	6.4	9.6	12.8	16	19.2	25.6	32	38.4	51.2
1/12	.08	4	6	8	12	16	20	24	32	40	48	64
1/10	.1	5	7.5	10	15	20	25	30	40	50	60	80
1/8	.125	6.25	9.38	12.5	18.8	25	31.25	37.5	50	62.5	75	100
1/6	.16	8	12	16	24	32	40	48	64	80	96	128
1/5	.2	10	15	20	30	40	50	60	80	100	120	160
3/10	.3	15	22.5	30	45	60	75	90	120	150	180	240
2/5	.4	20	30	40	60	80	100	120	160	200	240	320
1/2	.5	25	37.5	50	75	100	125	150	200	250	300	400
3/5	.6	30	45	60	90	120	150	180	240	300	360	480
4/5	.8	40	60	80	120	160	200	240	320	400	480	640

Warning: Check tube rating chart for maximum T & mA combinations

Appendix B: Exposure–Distance Conversion Chart

This conversion chart contains multiplication factors which are used for determining new exposure factors when the SID is to be changed. (Factors are rounded off to the nearest tenth, and can be used with either mA, Time or mAs.)

New SID	**Original SID**								
	36" (91 cm)	40" (102 cm)	42" (107 cm)	44" (112 cm)	48" (122 cm)	60" (152 cm)	72" (183 cm)	100" (254 cm)	120" (305 cm)
30" (76 cm)	.7	6	5	.5	.4	.3	.2	.1	.1
36" (91 cm)	1	.8	.7	.7	.6	.4	.3	.1	.1
40" (102 cm)	1.2	1	.9	.8	.7	.4	.3	.2	.1
42" (107 cm)	1.4	1.1	1	.9	.8	.5	.3	.2	.1
44" (112 cm)	1.5	**1.2**	1.1	1	.8	.5	.4	.2	.1
46" (117 cm)	1.6	1.3	1.2	1.1	.9	.6	.4	.2	.2
48" (122 cm)	1.8	1.4	1.3	1.2	1	.6	.4	.2	.2
50" (127 cm)	1.9	1.6	1.4	1.3	1.1	.7	.5	.3	.2
55" (140 cm)	2.3	1.9	1.7	1.6	1.3	.8	.6	.3	.2
60" (152 cm)	2.8	2.3	2	1.9	1.6	1	**.7**	.4	.3
72" (183 cm)	4	3.2	3	2.7	2.3	1.4	1	.5	.4
100" (254 cm)	7.7	6.3	5.7	5.2	4.3	2.8	2	.1	.7
120" (305 cm)	11.1	9	8.2	7.4	6.3	4	2.8	1.4	1

Example 1: Determine mAs with SID changed from 40 to 44". (Look down the 40" column to the 44" box and locate **1.2** as the conversion factor.) Original mAs = 8.
Answer: 8 x 1.2 = 9.6 or **10 mAs**

Example 2: A chest technique @ 72" is 6 mAs @ 90 kVp. If the SID needs to be decreased to 60", what mAs should be used if other factors remain unchanged?
Answer: Conversion factor is **.7**. 6 mAs x .7 = **4.2 mAs**

Appendix C: Screen–Speed Conversion Chart

New Screen Speed	Original Screen–Speed											
	25	50	80	100 (PAR)	200	250	300	350	400	500	800	1200
25	.1	2	3.2	4	8	10	12	14	16	20	32	48
50	.5	1	1.6	2	4	5	6	7	8	10	16	24
80	.31	.63	1	1.25	2.5	3.13	3.75	4.38	5	6.25	10	15
100 (PAR)	.25	.5	.8	1	2	2.5	3	3.5	**4**	5	8	12
200	.125	.25	.4	.5	1	1.25	1.5	1.75	2	2.5	4	6
250	.1	.2	.32	.4	.8	1	1.2	1.4	1.6	2	3.2	4.8
300	.08	.17	.27	.33	.67	.83	1	1.12	1.33	1.67	2.67	4
350	.07	.14	.23	.29	.57	.71	.85	1	1.14	1.4	2.29	3.4
400	.06	**.13**	.2	**.25**	.5	.63	.75	.88	1	1.25	2	3
500	.05	.1	.16	.2	.4	.5	.6	.7	.8	1	1.6	2.4
800	.03	.06	.1	.13	.25	.31	.38	.44	.5	.63	1	1.5
1200	.02	.04	.07	.08	.17	.21	.25	.29	.33	.42	.67	1

This conversion chart allows for a quick conversion of exposure factors when changing from one speed screen to another.

Example: If the exposure factors for an AP knee with high speed (400) screen is 4 mAs @ 70 kVp, and a 100 speed detail screen is to be used, how much of an increase in mAs is required? *Answer:* Find the conversion factor by looking down the 400 speed column to the 100 speed box row and locate the conversion factor of **4.** 4 mAs x 4 = **16 mAs.**

To check your answer, convert back from the 100 to the 400 screen technique by looking down the 100 column to the 400 box, for a conversion factor of **.25.**
16 mAs x .25 = **4 mAs** (original mAs).

Appendix D:
Grid Ratio Conversion Chart

New Grid Ratio		Original Grid Ratio (Original Exposure Factors): Non Grid	InSight Grid	5:1 or 6:1	8:1	12:1	16:1
	Recommended kVp Range	<60–70	60–90	60–75	70–90	70–125 (95-125)	70–125 (95-125)
Non Grid	<60–70	1	.5	.33	.25	.2 (.17)	.17 (.14)
InSight Grid (4 or 5:1 equivalent)	60–90	2	1	.67	.5	.4	.33
5:1 or 6:1	60–75	3	1.5	1	.75	**.6**	.5
8:1	70–90	4	2	1.33	1	.8	.67
12:1	70–125 (95–125)	5 (6)	2.5	**1.67**	1.25	1	.83
16:1	70–125 (95–125)	6 (7)	3	2	1.5	1.2	1

This conversion chart can be used for general grid conversions based on mid recommended kVp ranges of each grid type. See page 26 of Chapter 1 for more specific grid conversion considerations.

To use this chart, determine the correct conversion factor (multiplication number) by looking down the chart to the new grid being used and multiply by this factor.

Example: If 7 mAs @ 70 kVp is the technique for a shoulder using a 12:1 grid, what mAs should be used with a 5:1 portable grid? *Answer*: The conversion factor for converting from 12:1 to 5:1 is **.6.** 7 mAs x .6 = **4.2 mAs** at 70 kVp.

To check your answer, convert the other way from a 5:1 to a 12:1 grid. An increase in technique would be needed and the conversion factor is **1.67**. (4.2 mAs x 1.67 = **7 mAs,** the original technique for the 12:1 grid.)

Appendix E: Patient Doses

Calculations by Richard A. Geise, Ph.D., Certified Radiological Physicist

All doses as calculated for this handbook are for a three phase generator with a half-value layer of 3 mm aluminum at 80 kVp and an output at one meter at 80 kVp of 6 mR/mAs. The skin entrance dose (S) was determined by using certain adjustment factors considering the source-skin distance and adjusting for back-scatter. Midline (ML) dosages approximate specific organ doses within mid body regions.

Each of these doses were determined for the part thickness and the kVp and mAs indicated in the technique boxes. The female models as shown in this handbook are smaller than many adult patients meaning the technique factors and the resultant patient doses would also be greater for larger patients than the values listed.

Gonadal Doses: The gonadal doses (G) as listed for both male and female assume no gonadal shields were used unless so indicated. For example the hip projection photos in Chapter 6 demonstrate ovarian shields in place, which **if correctly placed would reduce these ovarian doses to only about 10% of those listed without contact shields.** The male testes doses when in the primary beam would also be only approximately 10% of the listed male gonadal doses if lead contact shields were correctly placed over the testes area. This demonstrates the importance of using gonadal shields whenever possible, especially on patients of childbearing age when the gonads are in or adjacent to the primary x-ray beam.

These gonadal doses should remind the radiographer of the significant doses received by these radiosensitive organs on projections involving the pelvis and lower abdomen region, and the importance of using correctly placed gonadal shields. In general **organs within about 3 cm (1.25 inch) of the edge of the x-ray field will receive a dose of about 10% of that received in the field. A distance of 10 cm (4 inches) from the edge of the exposure field reduces the dose to only about 1%.** This demonstrates the importance of careful collimation to the area of interest only.

Effect of kVp: The patient dose for a 90 kVp technique can be compared to 80 kVp for the bilateral hips on page 140. This demonstrates the advantage of using higher kVp and lower mAs whenever possible, especially for the pelvic areas within close proximity to the ovaries and testes.

Departmental Policy: Each radiographer should determine departmental policy concerning the use of higher kVp and the use of ovarian shields for female patients of reproductive age for lower abdominal and pelvic areas. For example ovarian shields for females generally would not be used for any abdomen or GI study films including the mid and lower abdomen. This is also true for the lower spine or the pelvis regions involving the entire pelvic girdle unless so indicated by a radiologist because they would obscure essential anatomy. However ovarian shields **can** be used for exams of the hips and proximal femurs if placed correctly as demonstrated in this handbook. Also shielding of the testes on all males of reproductive age is important for exams of the hips and pelvis because **they can be shielded** without obscuring essential anatomy.

NDC: The initials "**NDC**" stand for "**No Detectable Contribution"** and are used in radiation dose handbooks for certain body regions implying that a calculation was done and the contribution to the dose was insignificant. These initials are used for both male and female gonadal doses for the upper and lower limb exams, and for exams of the head and upper body areas.

Mammography Doses: The mammographic doses as shown are for the kVp indicated with exposures controlled by AEC with a 50/50 breast phantom using Kodak Min-R screens and extended processing. The "**MGD**" is the "**Mean Glandular Dose**" rather than the midline dose.

Note: Organ doses were calculated based on tables in the *CRC Handbook of Radiation Doses in Nuclear Medicine and Diagnostic X-ray* by James Keriakes and Marvin Rosenstein (CRC Press, Boca Raton, 1980). These doses were adjusted considering the approximate collimation field size as indicated in the film box drawing beside each positioning photo.

References

Chapter 1

1. Carroll, QB *Fuchs's Principles of Radiographic Exposure, Processing and Quality Control*, 4th ed. Springfield, IL: Charles C. Thomas, 1990, p70
2. Carlton, RR, Adler, AM *Principles of Radiographic Imaging*. Albany: Delmar, 1992, p188
3. Tortorici, M *Medical Radiographic Imaging*, Philadelphia: WB Saunders, 1992, p89
4. Kebart, RC, Jame, CC Benefits of Increasing Focal Film Distance. *Radiologic Technology* 62-6, 1991, p434
5. Carlton, p373
6. Bontrager, KL *Textbook of Radiographic Positioning and Related Anatomy*. 3rd ed. St. Louis: Mosby-Year Book, Inc., 1993, p109
7. Bushong, SC *Radiologic Science for Technologists.* 5th ed. St. Louis: CV Mosby, 1993, p303
8. Carlton, p368
9. Bushong, p303
10. Carroll, p168
11. Bushong, p227-230
12. Carlton, p333
13. Kodak InSight portable imaging system, Eastman Kodak, Rochester
14. Ibid
15. Ibid
16. Ibid
17. Ibid
18. Carlton, p261
19. Bontrager, p109
20. Carroll, p154
21. Kodak
22. Ibid
23. Bushong, p263
24. Characteristics and Application of X-ray Grids, Liebel-Flarsheim, Cincinnati: 1989
25. Carlton, p267
26. Gratale, P, et al, Using the Anode Heel Effect for Extremity Radiography, *Radiologic Technology* 61-3, 1990, p195

27. Hendee, WR, Ritenour, R *Medical Imaging Physics,* 3rd ed. St. Louis: Mosby-Year Book, 1992, p130
28. Carlton, p502
29. Carroll, p284
30. Carroll, p286
31. Hagler, MJ, *The Pocket Rad Tech*. Philadelphia: WB Saunders, 1993, p502
32. Bontrager, p14

Chapter 2 Chest and Bony Thorax

1. Bontrager, p63
2. Bontrager, p64
3. Long, GW, Rafert, JA *Orthopaedic Radiography*. Philadelphia: WB Saunders Co.,1995, p212

Chapter 3 Upper Limb

1. Bontrager, p125
2. Long/Rafert, p94
3. Coyle, GF *Radiographing Immobile Trauma Patients* Unit 7, Special Angled Views of Joints - Elbow, knee, Ankle. Denver: Multi-Media Publisning, Inc., 1980

Chapter 4 Shoulder Girdle

1. Long/Rafert, p192
2. Ballinger, PW *Merrill's Atlas of Radiographic Positions and Radiologic Procedures*. 8th ed. St. Louis: Mosby-Year Book, Inc., 1995, Vol 1, p 146
3. Garth, WP et al, Roentgenographic Demonstration of Instability of the Shoulder: The Apical Oblique Projection. *Bone Joint Surgery* 66-A, 1453, 1984
4. Sloth, C, Lundgren, JS The Apical Oblique Radiograph in Examination of Acute Shoulder Trauma. *Europ J. Radiology* 9:147, 1989
5. Bontrager, p164
6. Cullinan, AM, *Optimizing Radiographic Positioning*. Philadelphia: J B Lippincott, 1992, p79

Chapter 5 Lower Limb

1. Bontrager, p41
2. Bontrager, p191
3. Bontrager, p192
4. Ballinger, p1-200
5. Ballinger, p1-206
6. Swallow, RA, Naylor, E *Clark's Positioning in Radiography*. 11th ed. Rockville: Aspen Publications, 1986, p95
7. Long and Rafert, p384
8. Frank, ED, et al, Mayo Clinic Radiography of the Ankle Mortise. *Radiologic Technology* 62-5, 354, 1991
9. Martensen, KM Alternate AP Knee Method Assures Open Joint Space. *Radiologic Technology* 64:1, 19, 1992
10. Manaster, BJ *Handbooks in Radiology, Skeletal Radiology*. Chicago: Year Book, 1989, p249
11. Bontrager, p206
12. Ibid
13. Ballinger, p1-243
14. Ballinger, p1-257
15. Bontrager, p206
16. Merchant, AC, et al, Roentgenographic Analysis of Patellofemoral Congruence, *J Bone and Surgery* 56-A:1391, 1974
17. Ibid

Chapter 6 Proximal Femora and Pelvis

1. Bontrager, p227
2. Bontrager, p231
3. Ballinger, p1-288

Chapter 7 Vertebral Column

1. Bontrager, p253, 281
2. Bontrager, p279
3. Ballinger, P1-328, 330
4. Long/Raefert, p252
5. Bontrager, p250

Chapter 8 Skull

1. Bontrager, p314, 316
2. Ballinger, p2-217
3. Swallow (Clark's) p243

Chapter 9 Abdomen and Common Contrast Media Procedures

1. Bontrager, p80
2. Ballinger, p1-40
3. Bontrager, p420-422
4. Ballinger, p1-41
5. Bontrager, p558
6. Bontrager, p559

Chapter 10 Mammography

1. Bontrager, p535
2. Eklund, GW, et al, Improved Imaging of the Augmented Breast. *American Journal of Radiology,* 151:469, 1988

Chapter 13 Computed Radiography

1. Fugi CR imaging literature
2. Kodak CR imaging literature
3. Hendee/Ritenour, p388
4. Fugi and Kodak CR imaging literature
5. G.E. Medical Systems, *Advantx DRS* (Digital Radiology System) Milwaukee, 1993

Bibliography

Ballinger, PW *Merrill's Atlas of Radiographic Positions and Radiologic Procedures.* 8th ed. St. Louis: Mosby-Year Book, Inc., 1995

Bontrager, KL *Textbook of Radiographic Positioning and Related Anatomy.* 3rd ed. St. Louis: Mosby-Year Book, Inc., 1993

Bushong, SC *Radiologic Science for Technologists.* 5th ed. St. Louis: CV Mosby, 1993

Carlton, RR, Adler, AM *Principles of Radiographic Imaging.* Albany: Delmar, 1992

Carroll, QB *Fuchs's Principles of Radiographic Exposure Processing and Quality Control.* 4th ed. Springfield: C C Thomas, 1990

Coyle, GF *Radiographing Immobile Trauma Patients* Unit 7. Denver: Multi-Media Publishing, Inc., 1980

Cullinan, AM *Optimizing Radiographic Positioning.* New York: JB Lippincott, 1992

Frank, ED, et al, Mayo Clinic Radiography of the Ankle Mortise. *Radiologic Technology* 62-5, 354, 1991

Godderidge, C *Pediatric Imaging*. Philadelphia:W B Saunders, 1995

Gratale, P, et al, Using the Anode Heel Effect for Extremity Radiography. *Radiologic Technology* 61-3, 195, 1990

Hagler, MJ *The Pocket Rad Tech.* Philadelphia: WB Saunders, 1993

Hendee, WR, Ritenour, R *Medical Imaging Physics.* 3rd ed. St. Louis: Mosby-Year Book, 1992

Kath, K *Pocket Reference to Radiographic Exposure Techniques.* St. Louis: CV Mosby, 1993

Kebart, RC, Jame, CC Benefits of Increasing Focal Film Distance. *Radiologic Technology* 62-6, 1991 p434

Long, BW, Rafert, JA *Orthopaedic Radiography.* Philadelphia: WB Saunders, 1995

Manaster, BJ *Handbooks in Radiology, Skeletal Radiology.* Chicago: Year Book, 1989

Martensen, KM Alternate AP Knee Method Assures Open Joint Space. *Radiologic Technology* 64:1, 19, 1992

Swallow, RA, Naylor, E *Clark's Positioning in Radiography.* 11th ed. Rockville, MD: Aspen, 1986

Tortorici, M *Medical Radiographic Imaging.* Philadelphia: WB Saunders, 1992

Watkins, GL, Moore, TF *Atypical Orthopedic Radiographic Procedures.* St. Louis: Mosby-Year Book, Inc., 1993